Medical Care for the Roman Army on the Rhine, Danube and British Frontiers in the First, Second and Early Third Centuries AD

Medical Care for the Roman Army on the Rhine, Danube and British Frontiers in the First, Second and Early Third Centuries AD

Patricia Anne Baker

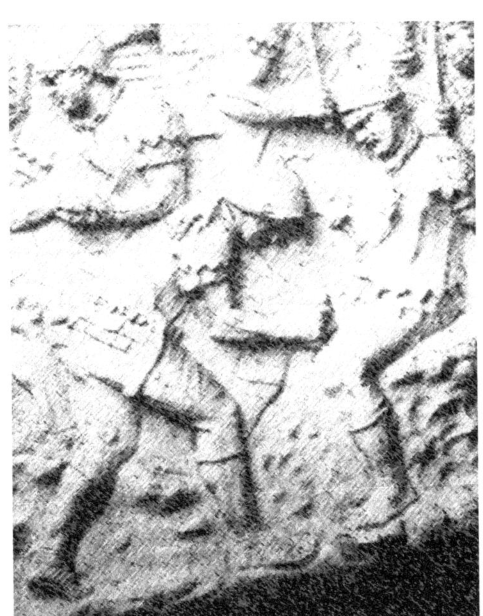

BAR International Series 1286
2004

Published in 2016 by
BAR Publishing, Oxford

BAR International Series 1286

Medical Care for the Roman Army on the Rhine, Danube and British Frontiers in the First, Second and Early Third Centuries AD

ISBN 978 1 84171 378 6

Volume Editor: John W. Hedges

BAR Publishing is the trading name of British Archaeological Reports (Oxford) Ltd. British Archaeological Reports was first incorporated in 1974 to publish the BAR Series, International and British. In 1992 Hadrian Books Ltd became part of the BAR group. This volume was originally published by John and Erica Hedges Ltd. in conjunction with British Archaeological Reports (Oxford) Ltd / Hadrian Books Ltd, the Series principal publisher, in 2004. This present volume is published by BAR Publishing, 2016.

Printed in England

BAR
PUBLISHING

BAR titles are available from:

BAR Publishing
122 Banbury Rd, Oxford, OX2 7BP, UK
EMAIL info@barpublishing.com
PHONE +44 (0)1865 310431
FAX +44 (0)1865 316916
www.barpublishing.com

For Josh

TABLE OF CONTENTS

List of Figures

Appendix Three

List of Tables within the Text and Appendices

ACKNOWLEDGEMENTS

This study began as my PhD thesis, which was undertaken at the University of Newcastle upon Tyne, England. I was fortunate to have received a number of awards to complete this project: The Wellcome Trust, the British Federation of Women Graduates, the Sir Richard Stapley Educational Trust, the NB Print and Design Company Award, the Excavation and Fieldwork Committee of Newcastle and Durham Universities and the Catherine Cookson Trust.

I travelled to a number of museums for my research and am grateful for the help I received. Therefore I would like to thank a number of people for their help providing me with useful information. In Britain I would like to thank S. Fox (Legionary Museum, Caerleon), G. Plowright (Corbridge and Chesters Museum), B. Trett (Newport Museum), staff at the Tulley House Museum, Carlisle, D. Robinson (Grosvenor Museum, Chester), J. McElvey (Wallsend Site), E. Hartley (Yorkshire Museum), R. Jackson (British Museum) and L. Allason-Jones (Museum of Antiquities, Newcastle). In Germany: H. E. Joachim and U. Heimberg (Rheinisches Landesmuseum, Bonn), I. Jensen (Reiss-Museum, Mannheim), F. J. Hassel and E. Künzl (Römisch-Germanisches Zentralmuseum Forschungsinstitut für Vor- und Frühgeschichte, Mainz), F. Naumann-Steckner (Römisch-Germanisches Museum, Cologne), G. Weber (Römische Sammlung Cambodunum, Kempten im Allgäu), A. Boos (Stadt Regensburg Museen, Regensburg) and H. Kronenwelt (Stadtmuseum, Baden Baden). In Switzerland: R. Hänggi and J. Fuchs (Kantonsarchaeologie, Vindonissa Museum, Brugg) and B. Meier (Historisches Museum, Baden). In Austria: H. Uble (Museum Lauriacum, Enns). In the Netherlands: M. Brouwer (Rijks Museum van Oudheden, Leiden), H. F. J. Horstmannshoff and S. Braadbaart (the Rijks Universiteit, Leiden). In Hungary: P. Zsidi and M. Németh (Aquincum Museum, Budapest).

I owe my heartfelt gratitude to my PhD supervisor, Professor Philip J. van der Eijk who offered continuous encouragement, critical discussions and comments on my work. I would also like to thank Dr. K. Greene (University of Newcastle) for comments on the early stages of the work, Dr. M. Gillings (University of Leicester), J. Longrigg (Department of Classics, Newcastle), Charles Young and John Harris (University of Kent), K. Gostenčnik (Magdalensburg Archaeological Unit, Austria) and Dr. C. van Driel-Murray (Universiteit van Amsterdam). Ralph Jackson (British Museum), Kathryn Lomas (UCL) and John Lazenby (Newcastle) provided very useful comments on the text. I am also grateful for the support of Diana Meijne, Antje Streuber, and Nathalie Verplaetse, my parents Peter and Agnes, my brother and sister Philip and Paula who encouraged me along the way. Finally I would like to thank Joshua Pollard for his never-ending support and encouragement throughout the time of the entire process and for our many stimulating and critical discussions on archaeological interpretation.

Chapter One

Introduction

Standardisation is both expected and accepted by many scholars who study the Roman army as a factor of military organisation. Discussions made about the rank, daily and social life of the soldiers, the design of the frontiers and the construction of fortifications almost universally apply this concept of homogeneity. The units of soldiers in the Roman army are even described as if they comprised an homogeneous group of people, with little to no consideration of their cultural or ethnic background. (e.g. Johnson 1983: 19-20; Watson 1969: 24). Since the army occupied a vast area that covered the outer edges of the empire as well as having stations within the provinces and cities, expectations would be that a uniform system of operation would have been a necessity in order to control such a large group. In some instances this is the case: military rank, the structure of the legions, auxiliary and cavalry units and the uses of Latin and Greek as official languages for documentation were just some ways to manage a widely dispersed army. Yet, more recent academic work is demonstrating that the idea of 'a Roman army' is becoming less easy to demonstrate in the historical and archaeological record. Although being part of a larger system, evidence coming to light is pointing to an army where different units were, in many ways, adopting or keeping to a lifestyle that provided them with a separate identity from other units (James 2002: 38-9, 44). In some cases a number of separate cultural identities were even maintained and recorded within a single unit (Haynes 1999). Further evidence for variations is supported by the archaeological remains, as each military instillation had its own layout. Although most fortifications have a central headquarters building and barrack blocks located near the fortress walls, the remaining internal buildings are generally not built on the same plan, nor are they placed in the same position, disparities rather than similarities in structure and plan are the norm.

Since there are suggestions that the Roman army was more varied than previously believed, it is important to scrutinise specific components of the military to see if there is further evidence to support this recent argument. Medical practice in the army is one of the elements that is believed to have been managed uniformly by all units throughout the empire. However, anthropological studies of medicine have established that beliefs about illness and its treatment are culturally defined and constructed. Ideas about the formation and etiology of diseases, their care and cure, the anatomy and physiology of the body are all based on specific cultural viewpoints, which manifest themselves in a very varied range of medical practices even within superficially homogeneous cultural systems.

In relation to classical medicine, scholars of many specialisms such as classical philology, philosophy, history and archaeology have, by examining various aspects of Greek and Roman medicine, contributed much to our understandings of the subject. From the philological and philosophical studies we know that there was not one school of thought on the subject, but that there were many different philosophical ideas about how diseases were believed to have originated and to have been treated. Archaeologists have added to the subject by identifying, in conjunction with literary sources, artefactual evidence of many surgical instruments and their functions. The descriptions of the intended use of the instruments also show evidence of a possible understanding of anatomy by those who might have used or described their function (Jackson 2002: 92). The literary and archaeological evidence hint, and in some cases the literature makes it clear, that there was much concern about how the body should be treated when sick, how the body functioned and how it was to be cared for on a daily basis. With this in mind, it is necessary to re-evaluate the system of medical care to see if there remains enough evidence to support the idea of uniformity in medical practice and ultimately in the running of the army.

1.1 Aims of the Study

It is the central aim of this work to examine military medical practice on the Roman frontiers of the Rhine, upper and middle Danube and Britain in the 1st, 2nd and early 3rd centuries AD. This will challenge the above mentioned supposition that there was a universal system of health care provided to the legionary and auxiliary units in the Roman army (i.e. Davies 1969a & b; 1970; 1972; Jackson 1988: 133-4; Nutton 1969; Penn 1964; Richmond 1952; Salazar 2000: 76-81; Wilmanns 1995a & b). Other issues to be considered are whether the available information can illustrate differences in care provided to the legionary and auxiliary units; if the data suggests any treatment having been offered by military doctors to civilians who lived in the area of the fortifications, or vice versa; and if the location of the soldiers' treatment can be determined. To try and answer these questions, one must look at what the remaining material evidence (including literary sources) can tell us, and consider how medical care might have been influenced by other factors such as military events, provincial policy and the cultural background of the soldiers. An attempt will be made to understand the perceptions of illnesses and how this might have affected possible variations in medical practice between the different military units and between the civilians and the army. By looking at the questions raised from a more critical and anthropological angle, the complex cultural matrix of the Roman army will be brought to the fore-ground.

Anthropological work on medical practice is an important consideration for any study of medical history because it teaches us to be critical of our understandings and assumptions of medicine in past societies. Medical anthropology also informs us that there are invariably complicated underlying beliefs and perceptions about health care and the body. Although, from an archaeological perspective, we may never be able to gain a precise understanding of these complexities, we are at least made aware that they would have existed. Obviously one cannot use an anthropological example as a direct analogy to past events, but the understanding provides a critical awareness of the idea that people in both the present and the past do not understand the world in the same way. The same can be said for understandings of the body and medicine. The reason this issue has not been raised in the majority of scholarship on Roman military medicine can be found in the nature of Roman military studies (James 2002).

It has only been recently that consideration of the interaction between the Romans and other societies has gazed beyond concepts of Romanisation, which is generally a one-sided approach concerned with the influence of Rome on the indigenous population who lived in the provinces and on or around the frontiers (e.g. Creighton and Wilson 1999; Cunliffe 1988: 126-7; Millett 1990; Wilmanns 1995b: 133-4). Romanisation is commonly described in terms of progress and civilisation passed from the sophisticated Romans to the backward 'barbarian' (Hingley 1999: 139). The validity of a one-sided approach to understanding the Roman provinces has only recently been questioned. Concentration on the reversal of cultural influences – the native groups onto Rome – is rare, but Barrett (1989) and Okun (1989) discuss the importance of considering such. Clarke, for example, looks at the architecture of indigenous peoples living around the Roman fort at Newstead in Scotland where there seems to be little Roman influence, and argues that this could have resulted from the deliberate strategies on the part of the native population to maintain their identity (1999: 36-45). Post-colonial theory - a study part of which examines how incoming societies of settlers have influenced the native population of the land they colonised and vice versa - has also been used to interpret interaction and attitudes of the conqueror and the conquered (e.g. Gosden 1999; 197-203; Webster 1994). One might expect that such theories would be used in Roman military studies, but in a recent examination of cultural interaction with the Roman army and Germanic societies (Creighton and Wilson 1999) the contributors to this volume continue to examine Roman structures and artefacts, but say very little about those of the Germanic societies unless they show Roman influences (e.g. Krausse 1999: 54-70; Sommer 1999: 160-98; Wigg 1999: 99-124). Thus there is still a bias towards the Roman world in some areas of scholarship and this has affected the way in which data has been interpreted and collected.

There is a need to examine the methodology used by those who study the frontiers, as this area has also remained fairly traditional, with scholarly opinion frequently incorporating the concept of Romanisation as a tool for interpretation. With the exception of a recent trend to define the term frontier (e.g. Whittaker 1994; Elton 1996), it is clear from one of the most recent volumes of papers from the 1995 *Limes Congress* (Groenman-van Waateringe *et al.* 1997) that critical interpretative stances are not being employed very frequently. Much of the scholarship presented in this volume of the *Limes Congress* is very similar to the first conference held in 1949 (Birley 1952). Many of the papers concentrate on descriptions of sites (e.g. Manning 1997: 33-40; Ottaway 1997: 135-42), developments, dating and phasing of the frontiers and fortifications (e.g. Stather 1997: 159), supply of the frontiers (e.g. Birley 1997: 273-80; Bounegru 1997: 311-16) and recent excavations of military sites (e.g. Szirmai 1997: 527-30; Wilmott 1997: 581). No one can deny the importance of these studies, as they are useful sources of information to draw upon when making interpretations. However, when looking through these volumes, one is struck by the paucity of discussions on topics relating to soldiers' lives, identity and even religion, which could be made when using the information brought forward in the more traditional examinations. Those studies that do address these issues tend to simplify situations by describing the military as an homogeneous unit, or in discussions of Roman and native contact, emphasis is placed on the superiority of the Romans over the natives (e.g. Allason-Jones and Dungworth 1997: 318, 319; Wilson 1997: 589). The main challenge is to ask more questions from the wealth of information available to provide new interpretations in this area of classical archaeology and frontier studies.

To break from this traditional means of interpretation this study is approached with the methodology of historical archaeology. A general definition of historical archaeology, as defined by Deetz, is "the study of cultural remains of literate societies that were capable of recording their own histories" (1977: 5). Since the Romans did write their own histories, along with leaving records through inscriptions, papyrus fragments and military diplomas, to name a few, there is no reason why the archaeology for that time should not be broached from an interpretative standpoint common in much post-medieval archaeology and even in prehistory. When one is interested in making interpretations about the lifestyles of those who lived in the past using both literary and artefactual remains, an understanding of such methodologies makes for more critical evaluations of the evidence. Although the common approaches to classical archaeology are helpful when it comes to dating and understanding specific styles of artefacts, the descriptive approach does not allow for much interpretation beyond the identification, date, possible function and stylistic relations of objects, or structures.

Classical archaeology has come under much critical observation recently by anthropologically-trained archaeologists, not because of the typological approach used, although it is an issue, but mainly because other means of interpretation are not being considered (e.g. Barrett 1989: 236; Jones 1997; Johnson 1999: 154; Shanks 1996, 1999; Small 1999: 122-3). Such criticism of the subject should not be perceived as a means of discrediting the study, but rather as an exciting way of creating new understandings of the classical world and expanding on topics that have been frequently covered. On a more general level, it might also be asked why there is such reluctance in classical archaeology to use new methods of interpretation associated with material culture studies and anthropology? Shanks observes that the subject began with an idea that the Greek and Roman worlds were considered the zenith of western civilisation, and this attitude remains deeply ingrained in the basis of classical archaeology (1996: 96-7). Moreover, he supports this with a statement from the former editor of the *American Journal of Archaeology* who stated that 'the achievement of classical archaeology was to recover and reconstruct as much as possible the betterment of mankind; this is Hellenism'. He further observes that "classical archaeologists have not, like anthropological archaeologists, been examining the ideological and theoretical basis of the discipline, but have subconsciously accepted the late 19th century founding ideology of their discipline, while dropping the most imaginative components" (Shanks 1996: 97-8). This expresses a prejudicial nature to the subject, because there is an assumption that classical societies were somehow superior to other groups of people who lived and interacted with them. Attitudes like this allow scholars to be dismissive of the fact that Greek and Roman societies were heterogeneous and influenced by other cultures with which they came into contact.

There has been an attempt to rectify this with the emergence of the Theoretical Roman Archaeology Conference that began in 1991. Many areas of Roman archaeology have been re-assessed, or considered for the first time in these conferences such as new approaches to funerary ritual, colonisation and the role of architecture in the social construction of space (e.g. Baker *et al.* 1999; Carr *et al.* 2003; Cottam *et al.* 1994; Forcey *et al.* 1998; Medows *et al.* 1996). Another area that is gaining greater awareness is the study of attitudes towards ethnicity in the classical world. Greek identity in Rome or Italy is being considered (e.g. Cornell and Lomas 1997), but it was not only the Greeks who lived in Italy and it is important to make note of this. There was no single Roman society, but one that was influenced by a variety of cultures (Woolf 1998: 6). To show that there were mixed cultures within the classical world a recent study by Isaac (2004) argues that racist views were common.

Since it is clear that the Roman empire was heterogeneous there is difficulty in defining the term Roman. One can ultimately become embroiled in a semantic discussion of its meaning, yet for this examination it is used simply to define groups from Italy and Rome itself, as opposed to others who lived within different parts of the empire: the empire consisted of many different societies of people with varied cultural practices, languages and no doubt different understandings about their bodies and its care. One must always use care in attempting to not create a dualistic categorisation of Roman versus Other, as even those living in Italy or Rome itself were not a 'pure' unmixed group of people. Nonetheless, with the lack of a better word, the term Roman is used simply to define a group from a particular area, with the understanding that even in these places there were many different cultures and medical practices.

1.2 Variations in Medical Care

The cultural background of the soldiers must be considered to understand how the organisation of the army and ultimately its medical care worked. Batavian auxiliary soldiers retained their own traditions in burial practice and treated their dead comrades differently to other units, showing a distinct selection of their Iron Age values over the Roman ones (Woolf 1998: 245). Material culture also shows that soldiers were not always adopting a Roman lifestyle. The pottery remains from Saalburg and Zugmantel, for example, are stylistically similar to that of, if not actually made by, people living on the borders of Germania Superior (Wells 1999: 136). Much of the pottery at Roman military sites in Germany is indigenous rather than imported from Italy (Wells 1999: 142-3). Thus, if soldiers were continuing to use their own pottery, or that of a local group, it is possible that they continued to maintain the use of other aspects of their background, or adopted cultural practices that were not particularly Roman, but those of the local population.

Medical texts even point to the fact that there were no standard medical practices, as there were many different medical philosophies and beliefs. Celsus (*proem.* 30-1) stated that medical treatments were not the same in all areas of the empire. According to him the methods of practice were subject to the nature of localities, and he exemplifies that one method was required in Rome, another in Egypt and another in Gaul. He felt that if the causes of disease were understood by all cultures to be the same, then the different groups should employ the same remedies. Despite this, he was aware that even if different groups had the same understandings of a specific cause for a disease, for example, ophthalmia, or wounds, different treatments were still employed:

> *"Differre quoque pro natura locorum genera medicinae, et aliud opus esse Romae, aliud in Aegypto, aliud in Gallia. Quod si morbos haec [causae] facerent, quae ubique eadem essent, eadem remedia quoque ubique esse debuisse. Saepe etiam causas apparere, ut puta lippitudinis, vulneris neque ex his patere medicinam"* (proem. 30-1).

Soranus mentioned the different ways Germans, Scythians and even some Hellenes treated their new-born infants in comparison to Roman practices, by plunging the infants into cold water to test their ability to survive (*gyn* II. 12), suggesting either that there was some knowledge of cultural differences in medical treatment throughout the classical world, or that there were at least perceived understandings of variation. It could be argued that these views of different medical practices were simply devices of propaganda. Hygiene and medical practices are often used in a derogatory manner by one society to differentiate themselves from another or even denigrate another group of people.

The variations of medical practice discussed by both writers did not, however, simply differ between groups within the empire, but within practical Roman medicine itself. There were different philosophical viewpoints on ways to treat the body, and no universal means of training or testing doctors (Nutton 1995a: 44-6). In conjunction with this, there were many folk remedies and religious ideas about treatments in existence (e.g. Pliny *NH*) that contradicted the medical writings, indicating that a doctor's care in the Roman world would differ according to the way in which the individual was taught medicine. Wilmanns' (1995b: 133-4) argues that the military units in the 2nd and 3rd centuries would have adopted Roman medical practice without question, this being based on evidence that there were more inscriptions from the frontiers mentioning *medici* dating from this period. Moreover, she believes that the Roman army would have been a good means for the spread of Roman medicine to other groups of people who had contact with the military (1995a: 121). It is possible that ideas about classical medical practices were transferred through the army to auxiliary units, or groups of indigenous people living in the provinces. Yet, knowing there were differences in medical teaching in the Roman world and most likely cultural differences in practice, one would need to question the type of medical knowledge that was being transferred. On a basic level, the culture within which a patient is living influences their experience and understanding of the disease and the healing process (Lupton 1994: 13). At the same time the doctors' knowledge and perceptions of treatment are also influenced by local knowledge (Commelles 1997: 43-4). Kleinman argued in 1980 that he wished to advance the notion that cultural categories are intrinsic to all cultures and that their analysis and cross-cultural comparisons are essential for understanding medical systems (1980: xii). With these variations in mind, it is questionable why, so frequently, studies made of medical care in the Roman army describe the organisation of medical care as if it were a uniform system throughout the entire empire (e.g. Callies 1968; Davies 1969b; 1972; 1989; Jackson 1988: 133-4; Nutton 1969; Salazar 2000: 74-81; Scarborough 1968; Wilmanns 1995a & b). Although there are different views about how the system was organised (e.g. compare Davies 1989 with Wilmanns 1995a & b or Scarborough 1968 with Nutton 1969) it is most frequently referred to as a medical service, implying homogeneity.

Ancient medicine was not approached and learned by the doctors of the classical era in a purely scientific, or 'rational' manner, as one would understand it from a modern western point of view. A recent issue in the fields of anthropology, sociology and certain areas of archaeology is an examination of the way that Cartesian thought has structured modern writers' scientific practice into defining the world around a series of binary oppositions, such as male:female, nature:culture, wild:civilised and sacred:profane (e.g. Lévi-Strauss 1963; 1969). There is a growing recognition that such dualistic reasoning does not have a universal validity (e.g. Johnson 1999: 101-8; Moore 1999a: 19; 1999b). The reason for bringing this issue to the fore is that in some cases classical archaeologists tend to look at the classical world as being structured in such a way that religion and daily life, or the sacred and the profane, are treated as opposites. From what is understood about perceptions of religion in the classical world, the sacred was incorporated into most everything; rivers and streams for example, were thought not only to have had an associated deity, but in some respect these bodies of water were actually thought to be the deity (e.g. Burkert 1979; Morford and Lenardon 1985: 12-15). Sometime there is an attempt to make divisions between what was written from a 'rational' point of view, that is without religious overtones, folk remedies or magic, as opposed to medical practices that included these elements (e.g. Longrigg 1993; 1998). Many medical texts from the classical era seem to be written without the influences of folk treatments, causing scholars to make this division between the so-called rational and irrational; yet, even if the medical writers did not refer to divine aspects, their world was still surrounded and imbedded within the sacred (e.g. Gladigow 1995; Gordon 1995; Lloyd 1983).

It is clear in the epigraphic and archaeological evidence that some Roman doctors were practicing 'practical' medicine, a term used in this study to mean the basic technical areas of medicine such as bandaging or surgery, alongside practices with more explicit religious overtones, as some altars were dedicated by doctors asking for the help of healing deities (Appendix 2, numbers 7, 8, 10, 24, 25, 29, 31, 34, 36, 37, 38). Certain religious sanctuaries were also dedicated to healing, such as Epidauros on the Peloponnese. Amulets, charms and anatomical votive offerings also occur in the archaeological record, indicating an embedded belief that medicine and religion were intertwined. Recently a set of surgical instruments from Stanway near Colchester was found with a possible set of divining rods (Crummy 2002; Jackson 1997). These rods may imply that even the most practical surgical procedures had embedded magical practices, that might have been seen as purely 'rational' from the doctor and patient's perspective, and necessary for the treatment to be effective. Medical anthropology has demonstrated that people's perception of the healing process is embedded in their beliefs: therefore, if they believe that some form of magic or ritual was intrinsic to healing then the action becomes a necessary part of the procedure (Kleinman 1980; Landy 1977: 472-3; Morley 1978: 6; Morsy 1993: 83-4). To understand medicine in the classical world, one must attempt to erase the structural world with which we are so familiar and understand that even the 'rational', or perhaps 'practical', aspects of medicine were thought about and used by a society whose belief system embodied the sacred and the profane on the same level (Baker 2002a; Lloyd 1983). Even though this study concentrates on the 'practical' elements, such as the surgical instruments that have been identified in the archaeological record, there is the potential that it is only presenting half of the picture, as only the instruments commonly recognised as having a 'practical' function tend to be discussed in the archaeological literature on medicine. However, the possible divining rods from Colchester indicate that perhaps the full range of instruments employed in the medical practice could include objects such as amulets, divination rods, curse tablets or charms.

When units of non-Roman soldiers, with medical backgrounds and understandings divergent to those of the Romans, were approached with different ideas of illnesses and their treatment a reaction either for or against its acceptance would most likely have occurred. An example of peoples' reactions to new medical practice is demonstrated in a study of medical treatment made in Grenada and Trinidad in the 1950s. The study showed people were more willing to approach a local doctor rather than one trained in western medicine, unless the healer realised that western medicine would be more beneficial to the patient's treatment (Landy 1977: 472-3). Kleinman discusses the combination of western and traditional medicine in his study on the doctor and patient relationship in Taiwanese medical practices. He describes how infants often suffered from a culturally defined disorder called 'fright', which could be one of a number of problems such as colic or measles. The traditional treatment usually involves a healing ceremony and wearing charms to ward off the disease, and this is usually performed on children who might have been inoculated by western medical practitioners only a few hours earlier (1980: 12-13). Here it is seen that western medicine was basically rejected until there was no other hope for a cure by traditionally accepted means, or in some cases the traditional practices were performed in conjunction with foreign ones.

More specifically, medical practice is bound up in behaviour that is significant to a culture, and affects beliefs about how treatments are to be executed. The people of Fatiha in rural Egypt use bodily ornamentation as medicine, such as tattooing the forehead veins to relieve the pressure from the frequent hauling of loads of goods. They also use ear piercing as a means of curing a fever, which has to be done by the females of the society with pointed earrings instead of a tool specifically designed for the purpose, allowing for the fever to escape through the hole in the ear (Morsy 1993: 83-4). These anthropological observations encourage one to question understandings of past societies, because in areas where western medicine has been thought to have influenced traditional medicines in reality it is seen to have been adapted in different ways. With Roman medicine would one not expect to find similar reactions between provincial natives, soldiers from different backgrounds and the Romans who brought medical practices from Italy?

More directly related to classical medicine is Nijhuis' philological examination of Roman reactions to Greek doctors. In it she argues how cultural constructions of illness caused problems with the two societies interacting, because Roman doctors would have prescribed chants and Greek doctors had other ideas about curing (1995: 57-60). She borrows her methodology from Kleinman (1980: 259-310), demonstrating that anthropological methods can be used in philological studies of medicine. With this she discusses the reactions, sometimes hostile, that occurred because of the misunderstandings of foreign practice (1995: 60). Nijhuis' paper is a demonstration that an interpretative anthropological approach can lead scholars to distinguish aspects of a problem or question that might not have been visible to them by using less interpretative approaches. Moreover, it is an indication that there were cultural conflicts about medicine in the classical world, and one should not expect that soldiers with different medical traditions would have openly accepted Roman ones.

1.3 Data Analysis

Before moving on to a consideration of Roman military medical practice, some concepts on the nature of the evidence are necessary. The manner in which data is collected and analysed in Roman military archaeology must also be reconsidered because there is a limited interpretative focus in relation to material culture. Artefacts are normally described and organised according to typological group, such as pottery, bronze finds and iron finds. Rarely is full contextual information provided with details of material associations for individual artefacts, making it very difficult to understand the full character of particular assemblages (Hingley 1999: 141; Jones 1997: 131). Shanks and Tilley argue that in earlier studies of archaeology, artefacts were sorted in a manner equivalent to biological classifications. Finds were expected to fit a tight category according to date and classification. This practice divorces the object from its context, rarefying it, and limiting the potential of sound interpretation (1987: 79-80). According to Deetz classifying artefacts in this manner can mislead scholars (1977: 13). The conventional typology does not allow one to take into account all the variables that humans consider, consciously or unconsciously, when they use, make or own an object; nor is it possible for an archaeologist to use the information to see if there are any unusual patterns in the way artefacts were deposited (Shanks 1996: 39-41). As Small argues in a discussion on the deficiency of material cultural studies in Roman archaeology, the failure to question more about the artefacts "can miss underlying structures and clues to the social strategies of past societies, which are contained in different community contexts" (1999: 123). In the same discussion, Small notes that classical archaeologists tend to view the material remains as a subordinate means to support the literature and history. However, the artefacts can often demonstrate an opposing point of view from that mentioned in the literature, and in some cases can demonstrate subtle features neglected in the textual sources. Matthews (1994), for example, discusses how one might possibly find evidence for a gay male sub-culture in Roman society. He notes that there are some Roman writers who mention effeminate men in a derogatory manner, but he is curious to see if it was only the writers who expressed such feelings, or if homosexual men were able to openly display their sexuality. Matthews suggests one way to identify this is to examine the material remains found with sexed skeletons. He realises that there are difficulties in determining gender specific artefacts, for example men today wear earrings as they did in the Elizabethan era, but we often associate them with females. Yet, by comparing finds in biologically sexed male burials with those in female burials he points to two possible burials that have 'female' jewellery, possibly suggesting an open demonstration of gay sexuality that may imply a different attitude from that mentioned in the classical literature. Some men may have openly displayed their sexuality in spite of the attitudes we are aware of through the written record of the time (1994: 125-8).

Another example denoting contradictions between the literature and material culture is mentioned by Deetz, who uses lists of livestock in Colonial

America to show how misinterpretations can occur in what has been written and what was actually transpiring. In one instance he observed that farm animals in Colonial America were listed in documentary records, and many archaeologists used these records as a means of determining the types and numbers of animals that were owned by specific farmers, assuming that the animals listed were the only ones owned by the farmers. However, Deetz argues that only those animals listed on documentary records were intended to be used for food because the archaeological remains of animal bones showed that the specific farmers owned other animals. The bones of the animal types not mentioned on the lists did not show signs of butchering, whilst the types listed did (1977: 12); thus, warning archaeologists and historians that literary sources of any type must not be taken as the exact truth to a situation.

An additional problem with classifying artefacts in strict groups is that certain objects tend to be given higher status over others. Painted Greek pots, for example, are referred to as vases and are often discussed individually as objects of art, whilst the unpainted and coarse wares are generally perceived as anonymous works, hence of lower culture and status (Shanks 1996: 31-9). It is the archaeologist and the art historian who are responsible for assigning the significance and importance to the objects, as we understand them to be today. This modern identification of pottery as objects of art can create abstract ideas about how they were understood by those who used and made them, and it is likely that the designations say more about the scholars' perception of the artefact than past value systems.

Of particular importance in respect to this examination is the fact that Roman medical instruments do not escape such categorisation either. Riha (1986) and Künzl (1983), for instance, use a classification for medical artefacts: strictly surgical, strictly toilet and those instruments that could have been used for both purposes. In general, the categorisation is useful as a means of defining the possible intended function of an instrument in conjunction with the description of their use by classical writers of medical treatment. However, it soon becomes clear that the majority of instruments could be used for a variety of purposes: medical, pharmaceutical and even non-medically related functions. The most common types of instruments are classed as surgical/toilet instruments, which can be used for a variety of purposes. Yet, a certain hierarchy seems to have been ascribed to strictly surgical instruments because they do not have the perceived intended dual functions as the surgical/toilet instruments and are not as common in the archaeological record. It is possible that the strictly surgical instruments had a dual function as well. As a consequence, the dual-purpose instruments tend to be 'played down' in their importance. For example, more articles are written on individual types of surgical instruments such as specula (Longfield-Jones 1986), uvula forceps (Jackson 1994a) and syringes (Bliquez 1985; Bliquez and Olesen 1994) than are on the more common instruments such as spatula and spoon probes. It is interesting that the uncommon instruments are discussed more than the surgical/toilet instruments. Yet, multi-functional instruments could have been used for surgical purposes just as often, if not more so, than the less common strictly surgical instruments.

An analogy to this is that the same pattern appears in the collection of art and antiques. Value is equated with rarity, though modern values might be a distortion, or an inversion of past ideals. By looking at 17th century London delftware, some of the most valuable pieces on the market today are plain white wares, though these pieces were the ones that were produced in more abundance, and as a consequence these were the ones that were looked after with less care and were used and discarded with greater frequency. On the other hand, the blue and white delftware was more expensive in the 17th century, so these were looked after with greater care, causing them to be more abundant and, therefore, less expensive in today's antique's market (Britton 1987: 116-19). The prevalence of surgical/toilet instruments may be able to tell us much more about how people viewed health care and the body. Since they could have been used more for personal use perhaps this says something about individual hygiene practices, and from this more can be drawn out about attitudes towards bodily treatment (Hill 1995; Hill and Jundi 1998). Although, at the moment, the assigned category and the commonality of an instrument helps to define how it is regarded in typological discussions, more interpretation needs to be developed about the social meanings of the instruments (see Baker 2002a: 23-6; 2004 for a discussion on this).

1.4 Deposition of Finds

Understanding the deposition of finds is an important interpretative aspect to material cultural studies and one that should be employed more in Roman military studies. Deposition is a complex process that can range from accidental to deliberate disposal regimes and even votive offerings. What recent work on the anthropology and archaeology of deposition suggests is that all modes of deposition (excluding accidental loss) were worked through culturally specific understandings of the world. How artefacts were discarded can say much about the people one is observing. Deetz demonstrates that in early 18th century America the colonists threw their trash outside their houses, and often just outside the door. This practice appears to change in both rural and urban areas in the mid-18th century with garbage being thrown and buried in pits, which Deetz argues to be the result of a change in mind set to more 'Georganised' practices - concurrent with new architectural and culinary orders. Deetz notes that some archaeologists argued that the reason for the change was purely functional, relating to an increase in population penetrating urban spaces and, therefore, the need to clear rubbish away from the streets. However, Deetz notes that even before this period the more highly populated areas practised discarding trash in the streets (1977: 125-6), which seems unhygenic in modern western thought, but rational thought, or 'common sense', is also culturally defined (Deetz 1977: 23; Geertz 1984).

In Roman military studies deposition, when it is discussed, tends to be described in very functional terms, if consideration is given to it at all. For example, articles and reports on ceramics and metalwork tend to describe objects alone with little or no discussion of their associated finds. Recycling of metals is frequently used as an argument for a lower number of metal finds than one might expect, and overall this offers a sound interpretation. Nonetheless, not every bit of metalwork was recycled and it is the status of those objects that were not recycled which needs to be questioned. In the context of this study, given that medical instruments are intrinsically associated with the body, disease and wounds, it is entirely feasible that they may have been discarded in different manners depending upon the beliefs of the people using the instruments.

1.5 Limitations of the Study

With any historical research there are always limits to the answers to the questions that are raised because of a dependence upon the sources available. The material examined here was mainly gathered by visiting museums that housed unpublished medical finds and by looking through site reports and finds catalogues. Given the nature of the questions asked in this study the more traditional typological and descriptive analysis was not undertaken. The only descriptive elements recorded were instrument type, size and material, and a written description was provided for the more unusual tools, though this was rare, as the majority were easily recognised. Thus it was not the recording of specific typological detail of the instruments that was of utmost importance to the study, but rather gaining information about the context of the artefacts that was needed for the nature of the questions being raised. It became a noticeable problem, on account of poor archaeological recording, that the contextual information was not as readily available as had been hoped. At the same time, there was still enough information gathered to begin to answer the questions that have not been considered in previous scholarship. Despite these limitations, the material has been employed in this study in a way that generates the possibility of broadening the scope of Roman military medicine.

1.6 Order of the Book

The chapters of this study are arranged in a successive manner so that the reader will first gain a basic understanding of the history of the scholarship related to the field of study, and the methodology used in the examination, before the evidence is looked at to consider the main concerns. Before looking at the evidence for medical care a general background of the history of classical medicine, classical medical literature and the scholarship related to Roman military medical care will be provided (Chapter 2). In Chapter 3 an historical review will be given for the area of study: the Roman frontiers on the Rhine, Britain and the upper and middle Danube. Theories of what constitutes a frontier will be described, followed by a discussion on how anthropological approaches might be used to enhance our understanding of the frontiers and the interaction that occurred between various groups of people. The chapter will conclude with a general survey of the main military events that occurred in each of the relevant frontier provinces. It is crucial for this background to be presented to appreciate how the development of the frontiers and interaction between the Roman army and the native communities may have influenced the health care provided for each frontier and unit type.

In Chapter 4 the main question will begin to be addressed. It is here that the classical philological sources, including literature, papyri and epigraphic remains will be reviewed to provide an account of what is most probably known about health care for the soldier from recruitment to retirement. The expectations of health regulations for military recruitment, the question of what the Romans thought to be a fit and healthy body and how this relates to interaction and variation will be addressed. A comparison of the epigraphic evidence relating to the type of doctors will be made as a means to determine whether certain provinces and/or types of units were receiving different standards or types of health care.

Taking further the examination of the organisation and standardisation of medical care offered to the soldiers, a consideration of the archaeological remains of surgical instruments will be the focus of Chapter 5. It will be questioned whether a certain type of implement was common in all areas, only specific regions, or in fortifications with units from the same areas, and the possibility will be explored that medical procedures were regionally and/or culturally distinct. There will also be a consideration of whether different tools appear in legionary fortresses and/or auxiliary forts. Such a juxtaposition might help to demonstrate whether certain units or areas were receiving more, or rather, different types of care than others, or whether procedures were fairly consistent throughout the frontiers. The deposition of the instruments will also be noted and examined as a means of determining whether there were differences in attitudes towards medical treatment and the body that might be reflected in the disposal of tools. Finally, the instruments might provide some insight into whether certain doctors might have cared for civilians, as is suggested by a single inscription from Dacia (Appendix 2, Table A.2.8, number 41). At the moment the only means to test this consideration is to study the artefactual remains of gynaecological instruments. Since one of the main functions of these instruments, if related to the literary sources, was to be used on females, they can be used to try and designate whether there was medical treatment for people other than soldiers.

The topic of *valetudinaria* is the main issue of Chapter 6. The structures will be examined to see if there are signs of architectural variation among military units. Secondly, the question of the identification of *valetudinaria* will be raised. The identification of Roman military hospital buildings (*valetudinaria*) was made at the beginning of the 20th century (Koenan 1904) and has only recently been challenged in spite of many new archaeological interpretations and methodologies (Baker 2002b). Questions have not been asked about the context of material remains in many of the structures identified as *valetudinaria*, or if it is possible to identify a structure on the basis of a ground plan alone, which has been the main means in previous scholarship to determine the function of many of the buildings within fortifications. An important issue that has yet to be raised with much critical discussion about hospitals is how the Romans perceived a *valetudinarium* to be. Hyginus (Gromat. *Lim.* 4), the only extant source providing information about military *valetudinaria*, mentions that they were to be placed in quiet areas inside the fortifications, but he does not describe their architectural plan. In spite of having no other written evidence about the structures, Roman *valetudinaria* are often described as if they were modern hospitals, having operating theatres, residential areas for the doctors, kitchens, baths, latrines and wards. As no more descriptions are presented of permanent *valetudinaria* in any other extant classical literary source, archaeological evidence is the key to understanding these structures. By re-examining the archaeological material questions will be brought forth to see if these buildings have been properly identified as *valetudinaria*. The provenance of the surgical instruments has been recorded, when available, to see if the majority are appearing in so-called *valetudinaria*, or in another area that might imply a different building for a *valetudinarium* or place of treatment. Artefacts from buildings that have been identified as *valetudinaria* will be discussed, when known, to see if they provide any information about the identity of the structure.

Chapter Two

The Historical Background: A Review of the Classical Medical Literature and Modern Scholarship on Roman Medicine

2.1 Introduction

It can probably be said, perhaps with great certainty, that there was a suspicion of doctors and medical treatment in the Roman era. One reason for this wariness might have been that there was no formalised training for doctors or means of inspection set into place for ensuring a certain standard of medical practice. This allowed for anyone who wished, in spite of education, to set him or herself up as a healer. This could mean that remedies and treatments ranged from the ineffectual and dangerous to care that was fairly safe and effective. Another cause for fear might have been the knowledge of surgery being painful, as there were no truly effective anaesthetics. Since there was no proper understanding of the cause of infections far more deaths were common due to higher risks of infection after surgery, signifying that care offered by surgeons carried a discernible risk to the patient. Some of these anxieties are brought to our attention by Roman satirists. Martial, for example, frequently voiced his opinions of doctors, which were anything but positive. In one instance he remarked that doctors were even incapable of curing a common fever:

> "*Nequius a Caro nihil umquam, Maxime, factum est quam quod febre perit: fecit et illa nefas. Saeva nocens febris saltem quartana fuisses. Servari medico debuit ille suo*".

> "Nothing naughtier, Maximus, was ever done by Carus than his dying of a fever. The fever too did a very bad thing. Cruel noxious fever you might at least have been a quartan. He ought to have been kept alive by his doctor" (Mart. 10. 77, Trans. Bailey)

Martial mentions other worries towards medicine by complaining about doctors' practices and habits for butchering people. Twice he mentions Diaulus, a doctor who had changed his profession to an undertaker. Diaulus is described as having done the same thing as a doctor as he does as an undertaker: "*Chirurgus fuerat, nunc est vispillo Diaulus. Coepit quo poterat clinicus esse modo*" (Mart. 1. 30). "*Nuper erat medicus, nunc est vispillo Diaulus: quod vispillo facit, fecerat et medicus*" (Mart. 1. 47). Pliny explains that there was sometimes a distrust of foreign doctors when he wrote about the first foreign physician to come to Rome, Archagathus, son of Lysanias, a wound specialist nicknamed the 'executioner', and the profession along with those who practised it was seen with much loathing: "*..mox a saevitiae secandi urendique transisse nomen in carnificem et in taedium artem omnesque medicos*" (*HN* 29. 6. 12). A quote in Lucian can probably best be used to show a mixed attitude towards doctors. He says that doctors should not all be trusted, because,

> "*Οῦκ εἰδὼς ὅτι καὶ οἱ ἀμαθέστατοι τῶν ἰατρῶν τὸ αὐτὸ σοὶ ποιοῦσιν, ἐλεφαντίνους νάρθηκας καὶ σικύας ἀργυρᾶς ποιοῦμενοι καὶ σμίλας χρυσοκολλήτους· ὁπόταν δὲ καὶ χρήσασθαι τούτοις δέῃ, οἱ μὲν οὐδὲ ὅπως χρὴ μεταχειρίσασθαι αὐτὰ ἴσασιν· παρελθὼν δέ τις τὸ μέσον τῶν μεμαθηκότων φλεβότομον εὖ μάλα ἠκονμένον ἔχων ἰοῦ τἄλλα μεστὸν ἀπήλλαξε τῆς ὀδύνης τὸν νοσοῦντα*"

> "Unaware that you are doing the same as the most ignorant physicians, who get themselves ivory pill-boxes, and silver cupping vessels and gold inlayed scalpels when the time comes to use them, however, they do not know how to handle them, but someone who has studied his profession comes upon the scene with a knife that is thoroughly sharp, though covered with rust, and frees the patient from his pain" (*Ignorant book collector*. 29. Harmon trans):

In spite of the more disagreeable comments others convey the opposite point of view. Augustus gave preferential treatment to doctors because his personal physician, Antonius Musa, saved his life. To honour Musa, Augustus had a statue constructed of him: "*Medico Antonio Musae, cuius opera ex ancipiti morbo convaluerat, statuam aere conlato iuxta signum Aesculapi statuerunt*" (Suet. *Aug*. 59). According to Dio, Musa, along with the entire population of doctors were granted exemption from taxes: "*...τήν τε ἀτέλειαν καὶ ἑαυτῷ καὶ τοῖς ὁμοτέχνοις, οὐχ ὅτι τοῖς τότε οὖσιν ἀλλα καὶ τοῖς ἔπειτα ἐσομένος, ἔλαβεν.*" (Dio Cassius 53, 30). This exemption is mentioned in the *Theodosian Code*. It states "the reasons of equity demand that the privileges granted to you by former emperors shall be confirmed spend the rest of your lives secure from molestation of all compulsory public services" (13. 3. 4 Trans. Pharr). Further on the code mentions that there was an exemption of taxes for spouses and children of physicians and teachers (13. 3. 10). Other laws state that not only were the children of doctors exempt from taxes, but that they were also excused from public service (13. 3. 3, 8, 10). If one were only to look at the story of Musa and these laws it would seem as if the position of doctors was highly respected and trusted. However, the attitudes of the satirists and other Roman writers make evident that there were mixed feelings in the empire about medicine, and an accurate assessment of how the majority of people felt about doctors is difficult to make. If such opposition existed in Rome itself, than it is likely that there would have been disagreement about classical medical practices in provincial and military areas of the empire, where there was probably an even greater distinction between various groups of people. The point is, however, that people moving to the city of Rome might have wanted to take on more of a Roman life-style, or would at least have been more open to it, whilst those who experienced medicine in the occupied provinces would have probably put up more resistance to a new life-style. In spite of possible opinions of resistance and distrust, doctors still treated patients, treatises were written about many areas of medicine and debates continued between different schools of thought, indicating that there was more to ancient medicine than Martial and Pliny would have us believe.

2.2 Modern Scholarship on Roman Military Medicine

There has been much interest generated in the subject of Roman military medicine over the last 250 years or so. J. Y. Simpson (1856) conducted one of the earliest studies on the subject. He wrote a response to an English translation of an anonymous 18th century French writer's views on the subject (1750: 287, in Simpson 1856: 5). The anonymous writer believed the Roman army was not equipped with doctors, or any form of medical aid (1750: 287, in Simpson 1856: 5). Simpson redirected this course of thinking by questioning the French writer's premise, pointing to both literary and epigraphic sources that proved the army was prepared to handle medical treatment. One of the most convincing quotations Simpson used to support his thesis is from the *Scriptores Historiae Augustae*, (Aurelian 7. 8) that advocates "each soldier should be able to be cured for free by physicians": "*a medicis gratis curentur*", implying that a medical service, or at least doctors, were made available to Roman soldiers. Furthermore, Simpson found confirmation in the *Corpus Iuris Civilis* of Justinian that states that the doctors from the legions were exempt from civil duties when they were absent in the public service:

> "*cum te medicum legionis secundae adiutricis esse dicas, munera civilia quandiu rei publicae causa abfueris, suspicere non cogeris. Cum autem abesse desieris post finitam eo iure vacationem, si in eorum numero es, qui ad beneficia medicis concessa pertinent, ea immunitate uteris*" (10 Tit 52 p. 855, as quoted in Simpson 1856: 7 note 3).

In the case of legionary units, this law proves that doctors did exist (Simpson 1856: 6-7). An inscription from Housesteads of a *medicus ordinarius* (Appendix 2, number 39) was used as evidence to bolster his argument that treatment was also made available to auxiliary soldiers (Simpson 1857: 17-8). These two sources, along with other primary historical literature and inscriptions, helped Simpson to confirm his thesis that there was some form of medical assistance provided to soldiers in the Roman army.

Subsequent studies were made in the earlier decades of the 20th century that expanded upon Simpson's work. Some of the studies mentioned medical care for the army amongst general reviews of Roman medicine, whilst others concentrated specifically on medicine as a particular aspect of the military. In an overview of how soldiers were ranked, Domaszewski included inscriptions of doctors in his study to determine their position in the army and came to the conclusion that all legionary units were equipped with a *medicus* (1908: 45-7, 50-1). Haberling believed there were differences between the care offered to the soldiers living during the republican period to those living in the imperial period. He argued medical organisation was arranged more systematically in the imperial period, and that more doctors were employed to help the soldiers (1910: 4-12). In a broader study of Roman medicine, Meyer-Steineg started his discussion with a history of early Roman medical practice and treatment, which, he maintained, was based on folk remedies, before the introduction of Greek medicine to Rome (1921: 99-103). Following the historical introduction, he continued to discuss Roman medical writers and places for the treatment of the sick (1921: 114-4). Writing specifically on doctors, Gummerus (1932) collected information on all the medical inscriptions available at the time, both military and civilian, to show the prevalence of doctors in the Roman empire.

Although archaeological studies have added information to military medicine, one must apply discretion, as with the literature, when using some of the earlier archaeological examinations because many of the archaeologists who wrote about certain aspects, especially the hospitals, served as soldiers in the two World Wars. They offered their experiences in the military to explain how the daily lives of Roman soldiers functioned. Although it is helpful to make analogies, these are anachronistic, because soldiers fighting in the 20th century would have had an entirely different experience to those who served in the Roman army. During times of war in the modern western tradition a well-organised system of medical care is provided to the soldiers. In comparison, some Roman soldiers might not have participated in much, if any, military action during their 25 years of service, which could have affected the way treatment was provided to them. Since modern soldiers had experienced a uniform system of medical treatment, they would have easily assumed that it was only rational that the systems should be the same, and what may have seemed rational to the archaeologists might not have been to the Romans. Far too often these anachronistic ideas are accepted without question and they have seriously affected the critical study of medical history.

Such acceptance of these anachronistic studies can be seen in the scholarship of the 1950s and early 1960s. During this time some general works were written about the subject, but again they did not offer much in the way of new interpretation (Penn 1964: 253-8; Richmond 1952: 2-6). Richmond discussed how he believed the doctors might have been ranked and organised. According to him, Roman inscriptions provide information about two kinds of doctors: *medici ordinarii,* who he thought were ranked orderlies, and *capsarii*, who were basically people who wrapped wounds. Richmond says both types were exempt from daily fatigue duties (1952: 2); yet he does not present any information about how he came to this conclusion. Penn, on the other hand, looked at the literary evidence to certify the existence of military health care and to see how it may have been organised. He argued that each legion had a doctor, but was concerned with their rank in juxtaposition to the military in the 1960s (1964: 255). His paper makes many assumptions about the system and his uncritical reading of the evidence led him to determine that there was a "highly efficient medical service that was greatly in advance of anything that succeeding civilisations produced until quite modern times" (1964: 257).

In the late 1960s greater interest developed in the topic, and an argument grew between Scarborough (1968; 1976) and Nutton (1969) about the organisation of medical care in the army. The arguments presented by both were more specific than the assumptions previously made by scholars. Scarborough asserted that only the upper ranks of soldiers received treatment, similar to that which is understood for soldiers in the Hellenistic period, whilst the majority of those in the lower ranks were forced to depend upon help from their fellow soldiers. He also maintained that when medical care was provided it was given so the soldiers could heal quickly and return to battle in a very short period of time (1968: 255; 1976: 67). Nutton disagreed with Scarborough for three reasons. Whilst Scarborough (1968: 257) argues that medical care was only provided to the upper ranks, Nutton argued that the doctors were arranged in corps of medical surgeons who were distributed throughout the army, believing that there was the same organised system made available to all the soldiers (1969: 261-2). Secondly he criticises the evidence used by Scarborough for the republican period, feeling it is too scattered and there is not enough to make any firm statements about whether or not the Hellenistic system discussed by Scarborough had been adopted (1969: 261, 267). Finally, the lack of detailed discussion over the epigraphic evidence is noted as a problem (1969: 270). In the end, both agree that there was a system of care in the army, though Nutton points to the fact that doctors were available to the lower ranking soldiers in both legionary and auxiliary units, and he suggests ways to advance the knowledge of military medical care by looking at the evidence of inscriptions in closer detail. There was a study by Callies (1968), written before Nutton's suggestion, that looked at the names of the doctors found on inscriptions to attempt to understand their ethnic identity, but the paper was not focused on the rank of military doctors.

Davies further contributed to the subject by examining more specific elements of military medicine and daily life. His works on medicine are generally in agreement with Nutton in that he believed there was some form of standard health care system set in place for all the ranks. He used the primary literary and epigraphic evidence to expand upon the area to determine details about the rank and order of military medical staff (1969b; 1972; 1974; 1989). Concentrating on the principate, he too expressed the opinion that the system of medical treatment was not organised properly until Augustus was emperor and had sent a large number of troops on campaign (Davies 1969a: 83). In relation to health care, Davies also examined the sanitation, diet, recruitment, *valetudinaria* and some information about surgical instruments to discern more about the topic. Although Davies' papers on the medical service are extensive, he does not look closely at the archaeological evidence, particularly that of the instruments, to determine the calibre of the doctors' skill and the care they were able to provide.

Davies' work is often discussed by scholars who have looked at Roman medicine from a broader perspective (e.g. Conrad *et al.* 1995; Dolmans 1992; Jackson 1988), yet it was not until the mid-1990s that scholarship on military medicine moved on from his work (Wilmanns 1995a & b). In *Der Sanitätsdienst im Römischen Reich,* Wilmanns closely examined the organisation of medical treatment in the army through epigraphic material relating to medical personnel. Like Davies, she used the inscriptions to assess the rank of the doctors and made comparisons between auxiliary and legionary units. However, to help with this comparison she also examined the size of buildings identified as hospitals to see if there was a need for the same arrangement of medical care between the unit types. She concluded that there were more medical and administrative personnel in the legions, whilst the auxiliary units were most likely provided with a single doctor, or minor health care workers, such as *capsarii* and *marsi* (1995b: 116). Unlike previous scholars, Wilmanns also considered the idea of Romanisation; however, she only examines interaction from the Roman perspective, basically how Roman ideas were spread from one place to another. Although she admits that folk remedies would be present, she argues that Roman medicine would have become the main means of treatment in the Roman army in the 2nd and 3rd centuries. Furthermore, she states that the legions were better equipped for the provision of health care than the auxiliary units.

Overall studies of the Roman army tend to agree that the legionary units were provided with a well-organised medical service, whilst the auxiliary units had medical care that was not on the same scale as that of the legions (e.g. Bidwell 1997: 71; Johnson 1983: 159; Webster 1981: 248-54; Wilmanns 1995a & b). In spite of scholars being aware of the provision of doctors for the soldiers, it was the studies of Davies (1969; 1970; 1972), Nutton (1969) and Scarborough (1968) that seem to have initiated the idea that the organisation of medical care was done on a similar, if not the same manner, for every unit throughout the frontiers. Such ideas are continued and reinforced by Wilmanns; although she points out that there would have been varying degrees in the size of the medical staff in accordance with the size of the unit. On a general level there would have been some uniformity throughout the units, such as the arrangement of the soldiers' ranks and the unit types (e.g. the cavalry and infantry) being homogenised. This said, certain aspects of each unit might have been organised and functioned differently, which is evident in the fact that many auxiliaries were allowed to retain their own ways of fighting (Saddington 1997: 493). With other aspects of the army, such as medical care, rigidly institutionalised organisation is expected by scholars, but this underlying supposition is open to question.

2.3 Roman Medicine Juxtaposed to Greek Medicine

It is understood here that there was not a single school of thought in the classical world about how medicine should be approached. Had there been one then it would be easy to say that Roman medicine evolved from that which came before it (i.e. Greek). General introductions to Roman medicine often present it as somehow evolving from the Greek (e.g. Majno 1975: 341-2). All too often, as mentioned in Chapter 1, Roman culture is seen as a homogeneous entity, but such an idea is far from realistic because Roman culture developed from contact and interaction with various groups of people (Woolf 1998: 6). Interactions with different societies would have enabled the Romans to come into contact with various philosophies on the body and its treatment, some of which might have influenced their medical skills, and others of which might have been rejected.

When discussing the history and development of Roman medicine it is commonplace for many scholars to begin their discussions with the Egyptians, because their practices might have had an influence on early Greek medical thought (e.g. Jackson 1988: 14-16; Longrigg 1993; 1998; Majno 1975: 140). Although Egyptian medicine might have had an influence on Greek medicine, it is difficult to say how much of an influence it had on Roman medicine. When Egypt was part of the Roman empire the Romans might have had more medical information from the Hellenistic tradition in comparison to an Egyptian tradition. As it is Roman medicine that is the major concern only a brief account of the possible Greek and Etruscan influences is presented.

One cannot deny the fact that some Roman doctors' techniques and ideas about the body were influenced by certain Greek philosophical and medical texts. Two examples of the various ideas about the body come from the pre-Socratic philosophical texts by Empedocles and Diogenes of Apollonia. Empedocles believed that all things in the universe consisted of four elements: earth, air, fire and water, and these corresponded to dry, cold, hot and wet. When these were not in balance in the body then illness would develop. Galen, a medical writer of the 2nd century AD, appears to have borrowed some of his ideas of Empedocles through the works of Aristotle. As a demonstration of how beliefs differed amongst the pre-Socratics, Diogenes of Apollonia developed the concept of pneuma, something related to or equivalent to air that he felt was the source of all things (Jackson 1988: 17-18). These variations demonstrate, as Edelstein points out "Greek and Roman doctors were not 'scientists' who applied theoretical knowledge to the case at hand on the level of common (modern) medical practice, as biological and physiological inquiries were neither presupposed, nor were they actually made" (1952: 301); indicating that there were entirely different approachs to understanding the body than we have today and that different philosophers, such as Diogenes and Empedocles, would create diverse theories about how the body worked.

Another Greek medical treatise that Roman doctors were influenced by was the *Hippocratic Corpus*. This *Corpus* was not written by a single person named Hippocrates, who is thought to have lived and written at the end of the 5th century BC. The different books within it contain a number of contributions on a variety of topics that were written in different styles, and have contradictory statements about philosophy and the approaches to medicine (Jackson 1988: 20-1). How much of an impact the corpus had on all doctors who did not write about medicine or even read in Roman times is not clear.

One debate that was significant in both Greek and Roman medical texts was the issue of human and animal dissection and vivisection. When dissection and vivisection were first practised on humans cannot be said, but it is certain, however, that both were being carried out in Alexandria in the 2nd and 3rd centuries BC. The two most notable anatomists from that time were Herophilus and Erasistratus. Herophilus is best known for his dissections and vivisections (Longrigg 1998: 93; for a translation of Herophilus see von Staden 1989), while Erasistratus came very close to discovering the circulation of blood and made important advances in understanding the nervous system (Jackson 1988: 27-8; Longrigg 1998: 93). There is a reversal of beliefs in the Roman period and anatomical studies were prohibited, again making it evident that not all aspects of Greek medicine were openly practised by the Romans. However, arguments did continue for the importance of dissection and, in some cases, vivisection. Celsus argued that there was not a need for vivisection, believing it to be cruel; yet, he did believe that there was an educational value in dissecting corpses:

> "*Incidere autem vivorum corpora et crudele et supervacuum est, mortuorum discentibus necessarium: nam positum et ordinem nosse debent, quae cadaver melius quam vivus et vulneratus homo repraesentat. Sed et cetera, quae modo in vivis cognosci possunt, in ipsis curationibus vulneratorum paulo tardius sed aliquanto mitius usus ipse monstrabit.*" (Cels. Proem 74-75).

> "But to lay open the bodies of men whilst still alive is as cruel as it is needless; that of the dead is a necessity for learners, who should know positions and relations, which the dead body exhibits better than does a living and wounded man. As for the remainder, which can only be learnt from the living, actual practice will demonstrate it in the course of treating the wounded in a somewhat slower yet much milder way." (Trans. Spencer)

The most specific demonstration of the ambiguous relationship the Romans had with Greek medical practice was made in 295 BC when a plague struck the people of Rome. Their medicine was not effective so they employed the help of Greek medics. It was not, however, the Greek physicians, or their practices that the Romans trusted, rather they adopted the worship of Aesculapius. More faith was obviously placed in the Aesculapius' capability by the Romans because they built a temple to him on an island in the Tiber (Jackson 1988: 10-12). It is noted from this adoption that some of the Greek physicians were using religion in their medical practices, thus demonstrating Greek medical practice was not as 'rational' as the philosophical texts seem to present. Contact made with the Greek physicians may have influenced some aspects of practical Roman medicine, but it is apparent from Cato that Greek medicine was not trusted by him and possibly many others. As Pliny states, Cato was suspicious of Greek doctors and believed that their introduction to Rome was a conspiracy to kill all Romans, and even worse they would treat people for a fee:

> "*Vincam nequissimum et indocile genus illorum, et hoc puta vatem dixisse: quandoque ista gens suas litteras dabit, omnia conrumpet, tum etiam magis, si medicos suos hoc mittet. Iurant inter se barbaros necare omnes medicina, sed hoc ipsum mercede faciunt, ut fides is sit et facile disperdant*" (Pliny *HN* 29, 7, 14).

Cato insisted on worshipping ancient fertility and agricultural deities as well as using folk remedies instead of trusting the Greek approach to medicine. This situation and attitude towards medical practices of other cultures were quite varied. Later, Julius Caesar confered citizenship to physicians who practised medicine in Rome along with other professions to make Rome a more desirable place to live:

"*Omnisque medicinam Romae professos et liberalium artium doctores, quo libentius et ipsi urbem incolerent et ceteri adpeterent, civitate donavit*" (Suet. *Caes*. 42).

Caesar does not specify where these physicians were to come from, implying that it was possibly not only Greek doctors with whom the Romans came into contact.

Although practical works on medicine were written in the 1st and 2nd centuries AD, along with this people were still practising folk medicine, something that is evident from Pliny's *Natural History*. For example, it has descriptions of treatments that were used to prevent and ward off diseases. Although some treatments were more practical in nature, others involved the use of what we would call superstition, such as spitting to scare away evil spirits: "*despuimus comitiales morbos, hoc est contagia regerimus*" (Pliny *HN* 28, 7, 35; Jackson 1988: 1). Despite the more 'rational' Greek medical texts, it is clear that not all Roman medicine was entirely influenced by it, or evolved directly from it, nor was all Greek medicine 'rational', in our modern, western understanding of the term.

2.4 Cultural Influences as Opposed to Evolution

As seen in the previous section there was some Greek influence on Roman medicine; however, it seems more likely that Roman medicine in the 1st and 2nd centuries AD developed from earlier Roman and Italian practices along with influences from a number of different societies. Since the Greek influence has been mentioned, the discussion shall turn to the Etruscans. The Etruscans were a separate cultural group from the Romans, who had their own language, religion, burial practices and most likely medical care and understandings of the body (Barker and Rasmussen 1998; Bonfante 1986). The Etruscans and Romans are known to have fought, so some aspects of Etruscan society might have appeared antithetical to their own by the Romans. In the context of medicine, however, the Romans may have adapted some Etruscan practices. The archaeological evidence points to the possibility that Etruscan medicine was ritualistic. They may have used the practice of augury and divination as a way of foreseeing an outbreak of disease and possibly aiding treatment (Jackson 1988: 11). The Etruscans had contact with the Greeks, but how much of their medicine was influenced by the Greeks is uncertain.

Remains of false teeth from Etruria demonstrate that the Etruscans did practise dentistry, and it is often assumed that this form of dentistry is 'rational' or practical, unlike traditionally assumed Etruscan medical practices, so it is therefore considered to have been a Greek influence on Etruscan medicine (Jackson 1988: 11). However, a recent study by Becker has noted that the majority of the Etruscan false teeth appear to have been made for females, most are made of gold and they are usually only for the replacement of the incisors. Incisors generally do not decay until later in life, usually when someone reaches their seventies, and the tombs from which these gold teeth were found suggest their use on younger women (Becker: 1999, 2002). This evidence suggests that the gold incisors were intended for some form of bodily adornment, rather than purely medical purposes. Moreover they fade from the archaeological record at a similar point in time as the Etruscan language (Becker 1999: 110). Becker also notes that a similar practice was undertaken on Phoenician men (1999: 103), and they had contact with the Etruscans as well. It can, therefore, be questioned whether such treatment was a Greek influence, a Phoenician influence, or if it was an Etruscan innovation. Thus the practical dentistry it would have taken to make the teeth and extract the incisors need not have evolved from Greek practices, or if it had the practice was adapted to fit Etruscan beliefs. Becker points out that there are no archaeological examples of these in the Roman record, yet there are descriptions of them in the Roman medical literature. A possible reason for this is that such practices might not have been borrowed by Roman women because it might have identified them as Etruscans. This study also shows the use of dental prosthetics varies according to different understandings (Becker 2002). How much of an influence the Etruscans had on Roman medicine is difficult to say; however, one thing that is indicated by the negative archaeological evidence is that the Romans were probably rejecting some Etruscan practices of which they were most likely aware.

Iron Age societies in northern and western Europe might also be examined for medical influences on the Roman world. Künzl asks this question when looking at the early Roman conquest of the Rhine, by examining the name of plants that were thought to have medicinal properties. For the medicinal herbs, he notes that an ointment marker found at Haltern might be an indication that there was contact between the Frisians and the Romans for medicinal remedies because the name of the product was Frisian instead of Latin (1991: 187). The names of some plants used for medicinal purposes that appear in Roman records had Gallic names (Künzl 1991: 189). The names of these herbs might be an indication of contact, but whether both sets of people used them for the same purpose is not known.

To look at this aspect more closely medical tools were examined from the early Roman military sites in Germany (Künzl 1991: 189-96). No clear typologies of instruments exist for the classical world until the 1st through 3rd centuries AD. Before this time there is not much documentation of instrument types, and the archaeological record is slim. By looking at the tools from the sites of Augsburg (although, a fortress has never been found), Haltern and Dangstetten, Künzl notes that the instruments are different from those that are known to date before the military occupation, and he argues that the military instruments were either reshaped on existing designs, or that they were new designs (1991: 196). It is possible the military units were the cause of these changes in design because they do not resemble local Iron Age instruments found in the area. The military at this time would have included many more Italian units, so they could have been bringing Roman styles of tools with them, whilst local instruments could have been of different designs.

Iron Age instruments, although extremely rare, have been found in Germany and Hungary. The instruments that are recorded from these places are not similar to Roman designs. For example, Navarro (1955) mentions two graves of the Middle La Tène period (2nd century BC) that contained medical tools. Both graves are fairly typical of the time since they are found with military items, the only exception is that they were also found with medical tools. One was a cremation grave found in Munich-Obermenzing. Along with the three instruments were a knife, which might be medical, a razor, arm ring, shield-boss, spearhead and a sword with a scabbard (Navarro 1955: 231-40). The three medical instruments are all made of iron, which is unlike the copper-alloys used by the Romans. One instrument has been identified as a cautery and probe, but it has not survived in the best of conditions. The other two survive in much better condition. One is recognised as a double instrument. It has on one of its ends a flat surface with a small hook, identified as a wound retractor. The opposite end is unlike any classical instrument, having a loop made of double wire that runs through two collars. The wire could be tightened and is thought to have been used to snare bodily growths to aid in their removal. The third instrument is identified as a trepanning saw, but it is not circular like the classical varieties (Navarro 1955: 243).

The second set of La Tène finds comes from Baranya in Hungary. This, like the grave from Munich, was found with a spearhead. There are eight instruments in the set, but they are different in their design from those in Munich. They are also unlike classical instruments because they have hooks and loops on their ends. Navarro points out that it is argued in the earlier literature relating to these finds that they were imported from the Greek world, but there are no parallels used to demonstrate this assumption. It is known that these Iron Age cultures did have contact with the Greeks (Navarro 1955: 244); however, there is no evidence to say that the instruments are Greek. One thing that might be indicated is that these two Iron Age groups might have had different surgical practices, implied by the variation in instrument design. Perhaps the doctors or healers who used these tools had different specialities. It is possible that these instruments indicate different cultural medical practices, and hence that there was not just one tradition of medicine in the Iron Age. Furthermore, such practices could have been passed down and used by these people during the Roman period and could have been practised by different groups of soldiers.

The only set of instruments from the Roman imperial period with a possible Iron Age design is from Colchester, Essex already mentioned (Crummy 2002; Jackson 1997; 2002: 92). The instruments, with the exception of one Roman style spoon probe, have different designs from the typical Roman sets of instruments. Like the instruments from Germany and Hungary seven of the Stanway instruments are made of iron, whilst the others are similar to Roman instruments, as two are a composite iron and copper alloy and four are made of bronze (Crummy 2002: 51; Jackson 1997: 1471; 2002: 92). These instruments are not entirely similar to those Iron Age types discussed above. The archaeological evidence for cultural differences in Iron Age medicine may well be more plausible by the variation seen between the Hungarian, Bavarian and Colchester instruments. It is difficult to say with certainty from where the influence for the instruments derived; they might be seen as an amalgam of different Iron Age, Greek and Roman traditions. When the army came into contact with different groups of people, and Roman settlements were established in new areas, then it is quite possible that both groups would have introduced new ideas to one another. The spoon probe from Colchester indicates some Roman influence, but whether the instrument was used for the same purpose as some Roman doctors might have used it is impossible to say.

Thus far, it has been demonstrated that Roman medicine was far more than an evolutionary development from Greek medicine. First of all, there could have been influencing practices on the

Romans from groups who lived in Italy before the Romans. There would also have been contact with different groups other than the Greeks whose traditional remedies were likely to have influenced Roman doctors, who could have drawn upon various understandings and practices of medicine.

2.5 Conclusion

From the preceding discussion, although only intended to be basic, it is evident that certain expectations about medical care in the Roman imperial period are open to question. The topics of the distinction between the sacred and the profane and the evolutionary idea of Roman medicine demonstrate that there were, at that time, many ways that medicine could have been influenced by different cultural values and ideas. Since there were various means by which doctors could have learned their skills, this could have affected the way that practices were applied in the army. However, because scholars assume that the Roman army was a homogeneous group of people, and that soldiers would have experienced the same treatment, regardless of whether they were legionary, or auxiliary soldiers in any unit throughout the empire. This assumption is the foundation on which most of the previous scholarship about military medical care is based.

CHAPTER THREE

DEFINING THE FRONTIERS: AN HISTORICAL OVERVIEW OF THE WESTERN FRONTIERS AND THEORETICAL DISCUSSION OF THE TERM

3.1 WHY THE WESTERN FRONTIERS?

Ideally an examination into Roman military medical care would benefit most from a study of all of the Roman fortifications located throughout the empire that have artefactual remains relating to medicine, but such an undertaking would be impossible given the scale of the empire. Therefore, the most pragmatic approach is to analyse a selection of fortifications from a specific area to make a comparison of medical care between the different types of military units and the areas in which the soldiers occupied. The frontiers selected for the study were in the provinces of Germania Inferior and Superior, Raetia, Noricum, Pannonia Superior and Inferior and Britannia, modern-day Netherlands, Germany, Switzerland, Austria, Hungary and Britain. They were chosen because they appear to have more similarities in military organisation than the provinces of Africa, Egypt, Asia Minor and the lower Danube. The arrangement of their frontiers in the provinces chosen for study are more alike in the construction of their military buildings, arrangement of the frontiers and in the organisation of supply system (Drummond and Nelson 1994: 43). For example, the arrangement of the frontiers in the north-western provinces has a continuous line of auxiliary forts interspersed with watchtowers, unlike the African frontier which has large gaps of a couple hundred kilometres between sections of fortifications (Daniels 2002: 233-65; Whittaker 1994: 78-81). The lower Danube was not examined because of difficulty in gaining access to some of the sites. The frontier of Dacia Porolissensus is also dissimilar to those on the upper Danube and Rhine, consisting of a row of watchtowers with very few fortifications (Maxfield 2002: 184).

One might assume that units stationed in areas sharing a greater likeness in their arrangement of structures had military systems functioning in the same manner, such as medical care and supply of food. Yet, even in these areas each province has obvious differences in the way its frontier was demarcated. For example, the northern frontier in Britain constructed during the reign of Hadrian was a solid wall with fortifications attached to it, whilst parts of Germania Superior had its frontier marked with ditches and wooden palisades. Since there are obvious differences in the construction of each frontier, it begs one to consider the possibility that if certain aspects of similar frontiers were not exactly the same then perhaps this variability spreads to other sectors of the military as well.

The main reason why Egypt, Africa and Asia Minor were not chosen for this study is because differences in military organisation are noted and expected more frequently than in the north-western provinces. For example, the gaps in the African frontier are argued to have been made to allow transhumant groups of people to continue with their traditional lifestyle of herding animals over the land that became the Roman frontiers (Raven 1993: 13, 77). This could be contrasted with Hadrian's Wall, which did not have large breaks to allow for people to cross between Roman and non-Roman territory with as much ease as in Africa. Rather gates within mile-castles were constructed that allowed for even more controlled movement of traffic over the borders. Since the Roman soldiers would have been coming into contact with societies with different ways of living the relationships between the Roman army and the native populations, such as those in Asia Minor, north west Europe and Africa for example, would have been different between the various frontier regions of the empire, which could also have affected the way the frontiers were constructed.

Climatic variations could also be a reason for the organisation of the army to be modified in specific areas. Again using Africa as an example in comparison to the north-west, one sees that its arid climate makes it necessary for people to live a nomadic lifestyle because of the sparse areas for grazing. It is possible that the military food supply was partially dependent upon the native inhabitants and therefore soldiers would have had to allow for them to continue with their means of subsistence. The variations in climate can also be seen in medical care. There were medical specialists called *marsi* who cared for snakebites and scorpion stings and are only known to have been recorded on inscriptions from Africa (CIL VIII 2618 + 18096; CIL VIII 2564 + 18052 = ILS 470; AE 1917/8, 29) most likely because afflictions related to scorpion stings and most snakebites are not expected in the north-western provinces (with the exception of some snakes, these creatures do not generally survive in colder climates). Such a medical specialist would not have been needed in the north-western provinces, making the organisation of medical care different from that in Africa.

Hostilities between the Roman army and the people living on or beyond the frontiers in the different provinces were also reasons for the heterogeneity in their construction. Generally troubles in Africa and Asia Minor rarely had direct effects on the arrangement of the frontiers in the north-west; although sometimes troops were removed to help with wars in the East, but physically the structural development of the north-western frontier was rarely, if ever, affected. On the other hand, military events that took place in one province of the north-western frontier often had repercussions on a neighbouring province, which can be seen in the arrangement of continuous lines of auxiliary forts along the Rhine and Danube.

The location of the fortifications was also an important consideration in choosing the area of study. Only fortifications located on the front lines of the frontiers are to be discussed. The frontier fortifications were selected because they would have been used for similar purposes, such as guarding the borders of the empire, or being active in defence. In contrast to this, military sites located in the interior of the provinces, such as Siscia in Pannonia Superior, would have been used to police the interior of the province. Supplies and the provision of services, including medical treatment, might have been made available in a different manner in comparison to the fortifications on the outer edge of the frontier. The only place where interior legionary fortresses were considered was in Britannia because the fortress of York was the closest to Hadrian's Wall, and Chester and Caerleon were built near auxiliary forts in what is now Wales. Though the fortresses in Britannia seem to be interior fortifications they are still fairly similar to those on the Rhine, which were originally placed on the main line of the frontier, but were not moved forward when the soldiers advanced eastwards, thus the legions were ultimately stationed behind the front line in Germania Superior.

3.2 Problems Defining the Word Frontier

So far I have used the term frontier rather loosely. It is used in this study to designate the fortifications on the fringes of the Roman empire. In spite of this simple explanation of the location of the frontiers, there is a considerable amount of debate about the actual meaning of the term. The definition of what constitutes 'a frontier' is not the main concern of this study, yet, it does require some discussion since it can reveal ways the Romans might have viewed the frontiers, which would have dictated their interaction with people living near, on, or beyond the lines of fortification. The view of what a frontier was might also have varied between different units for a couple of reasons. First of all, different frontiers saw more military action or volatile societies than others, so units on the Rhine and Danube, for example, could have considered the frontier a definite barrier between Roman and indigenous territories. In contrast soldiers stationed in other areas such as Germania Inferior or Africa, which saw less warfare, could have simply seen the frontiers as a more fluid border crossing. The second reason is that soldiers in each auxiliary unit tended to come from similar cultural backgrounds (though there would have been changes through time) and their cultural understandings of boundaries could have played a role in how they viewed the frontiers. Moreover their understandings of other societies would have had an impact on their relationships with those living on the border regions and their interaction could have affected the manner in which ideas were passed between groups of people.

On one level, the frontiers can be understood as a physical marker such as the border of the Roman empire, or maybe a division between Romans and non-Romans. On a more complex level though, it is often forgotten by those who study the Roman frontiers that they were not simply lines of fortifications, but a complex matrix of people interacting and influencing one another. Since the human element to this study is frequently overlooked, or if it is considered it is done so in a rather simplistic manner such as in terms of the 'Romans' and 'others', it leads to an oversimplification of the understanding of what the Roman frontiers were.

One reason why the term frontier has not been critically questioned until recently is because scholars in the 19th century set a general precedence for the way the subject is examined and understood. The study was introduced by scholars attempting to define the meaning of Roman frontiers via how they understood other frontiers such as the American West, or the Imperial British frontier in India (Whittaker 1994: 1-10). Basically, all of the frontiers studied in the 19th century were defined as a boundary between the civilised world and the barbarian others (Whittaker 1994: 2). The American frontier was not seen entirely as a division between people, but rather "the meeting place between savagery and civilisation" (Turner 1893; Whittaker 1994: 5), whilst the British frontier was a division between the civilised and the barbarian (Whittaker 1994: 5). French scholars defining the Roman frontiers saw them not only as natural division such as mountain ranges or rivers, but as Gautier stated in the context of the southern mountains in Algeria, as being used by the Romans to demarcate their territory with what lay beyond as "*un autre monde*" (1952: 211-12; Whittaker 1994: 4). This 'other world' was made up of people who were described by Gautier to have been uneconomical and uncontrollable. Two issues are brought out through these examples. The first is the assumption that the Romans were somehow of the same mind-set as those who were stationed and fighting on the 19th century frontiers. The second is an ethnocentric view that places the Romans in a completely opposite, and in the 19th century scholars' definition, more civilised position than that of the indigenous population located on or near the frontiers. Their descriptions of the frontiers are also structural in nature, in that they point the Romans as viewing the people living beyond the frontiers as completely 'other'. In some respects it is likely that the Romans did view other societies as radically different, as Hadrian's biographer states his wall in Britain was built to divide the Romans from the barbarians: "*qui barbaros Romanosque divideret*" (SHA. *Hadr.* 11. 2); but in other respects the archaeology, as shall be described in the following chapters, denotes the possibility that such oppositions were not that strong. The soldiers' views might also not have been so diametrical because many of them would have come from areas beyond the borders and again would have had a different world-view. Therefore, the 19th century descriptions may be anachronistic in this definition, as the term is defined in an embedded view of binary opposition that has developed out of more recent frontier expansions.

Nineteenth century imperial views are still an inspiration for many frontier scholars. One would expect such attitudes and ideas to be implicit in earlier studies of the subject, and indeed such ideas are notably demonstrated in the *limes* conference lecture series of the 1950s and 1960s. Unfortunately, however, much of the study has not moved along with recent scholarly methods and interpretation and much of the recent work tends to be similar to that in these early studies (evident in one of the more recent publication of the 1995 *limes* conference already discussed: Groenman-van Waateringe *et al.* 1997). One representative case is a paper on the site of Sewing Shields, a turret, located on Hadrian's Wall. This site has been interpreted as being abandoned by Roman soldiers in the 3rd century, though there is evidence that after its military abandonment it was still being used as a place for metalworking. It is argued that the metal workers were local inhabitants, rather than the soldiers because "the general atmosphere of the site was one of industrial squalor, rather than military neatness" (Allason-Jones and Dungworth 1997: 318), strongly implying an ethnocentric attitude about the Romans being more advanced than the locals who were somehow incapable of doing things in the ordered manner of the military. This assumption automatically rules out other means of interpretation. For example, the metalworking may well have been carried out by a military unit who found the abandoned site an ideal area to work; why it had to be done in an area of "military neatness" shows assumptions made about the soldiers in comparison to the locals. There is an idea that the native population in the north of Britain was somehow even less 'sophisticated' than the native population in the south of Britain (Webster 1969) and this has had a direct effect on the way scholars have divided the archaeology of the Romans and the natives. Even Whittaker, who points out this ethnocentric attitude in frontier studies, does not escape viewing them in the same manner. He says that the empire stopped where it did because those who lived beyond might not have been capable of supporting an army, pointing out that they were almost too poor to fend for themselves, let alone the Romans. Since these people are regarded as being poor, Whittaker argues that they were beyond the scope of the Romans to civilise (1994: 97, 113-4, 123-4). Such perceptions stultify many efforts to understand the more complex situation of how the Roman soldiers interacted with other groups of people and understood their frontier zones.

Elton (1996: 3), rather than arguing for a definition of the term frontier, points out that the frontiers are abstract because there were a number of overlapping zones within the line of fortifications constituting four groups of people: Roman soldiers, Roman civilians, local natives and barbarians. Within each group described by Elton other boundaries could be found that defined different aspects of the culture. The boundaries he mentions are religious, political, social, ethnic, linguistic, economic and military (1996: 3). These could, but did not have to, coincide. Perhaps rather than asking why the expansion of the frontiers slowed down in their movements, the main question should be, what interaction was taking place on the frontiers that might have dictated the soldiers' lifestyle?

3.3 Roman Views of the Frontiers

In an attempt to move away from these more traditional studies, it is necessary to try to understand how the Romans perceived the frontiers and those societies that lived on them. For the Roman view, Dyson argues that during the republican period "Rome was a society of frontiers" (1986: 7), meaning that the Romans did not understand their empire to have permanent boundaries. The fortifications where the soldiers stopped were only temporary and would be used as starting points for the next campaign to expand their territory. Whittaker (1994: 11) disputes this arguing that even though the Romans probably did perceive their empire as never-ending, paradoxically they were also committed to having visual limits in their society. Statues of Janus, a Roman god with a face on both sides of his head, were used to guard exits and entrances concurrently, and to define territory boundaries. Boundaries to buildings are marked by elaborate doorways dividing the outside world with that of the home (MacMahon 2003). Officially laws existed for demarcating land. The intangible contradiction of expansion and borders is expressed in their mythology, manifested in the symbolism of the two gods, Iuventas and Terminus, who were associated with Jupiter and personified expansion and boundaries of law and order respectively. To simplify a complex situation, Iuventas is symbolic of expansion into areas that have not been affected by Romans, whilst Terminus represents Roman order and control on an area that has been added to the empire. Thus it is not physical boundaries, but boundaries created in areas that are practising Roman law that are important. The dichotomy, according to Whittaker, demonstrates how expansion cannot be approached without providing some form of administration through laws (1994: 10-11). Yet, this description does not consider the attitudes of the native people living around the frontier territory, as Whittaker assumes that the Roman laws were adopted by all groups and were understood in a Roman manner. Even in areas that were technically under Roman control, it is clear that some native populations in Britain did not always adopt a Roman lifestyle. This is seen with their continued use of Iron Age-style round houses (Clarke 1999; Hingley 1999). Perhaps Roman laws did not prohibit people, in some cases, from living in the lifestyle to which they were accustomed and their views of boundaries might have differed from that of the Romans.

It is obvious in contemporary literature that there was a belief in Roman society that they controlled the known world. Before and during Augustus' reign one of the main objectives of Rome was to attempt to conquer the known world. Support for this is seen in Augustus' *Res Gestae,* where he states that he conquered more territory and brought it under Roman control: "I extended the territory of all those provinces of the Roman people, on whose borders lay people not subject to our government": *"omnium provinciarum populi Romani quibus finitimae fuerunt gentes quae non parerent imperio nostro fines auxi"* (*RG* 26). The idea of *imperium* without limits is also apparent in Roman poetry. In the *Aeneid*, Virgil mentions *"imperium sine fine",* or an empire without an end (1. 278). The poetry of Tibullus, a late 1st century BC elegiac poet, proclaimed the glory of a never ending Rome in his fifth poem, where he mentions Romulus not yet forming an eternal walled city, *"Romulus aeternae nondum formaverat urbis moenia"* (5. 23). Livy, for example, asked, "who could question a city founded on eternal growth": *"Quis dubitat quin in aeternum urbe condita"* (4. 4. 4). These imply temporal longevity rather than spatial expansion and they support the idea that most Romans, at least in the late republic and early 1st century AD, could not imagine a boundary to their empire, or a limit to the time in which their empire was to survive (Whittaker 1994: 11). Whether these sentiments were honestly felt by the majority of people is open to question because these works were most likely written with a political bias.

Moreover, Whittaker argues that the Romans basically understood everyone to be a Roman citizen. Regions outside the Roman world were viewed to hold people living in an area that was awaiting Roman law and order, but at the same time believed the area and the people to be somehow part of the Roman empire (Whittaker 1994: 20). If this is a fair statement of the Roman perception of the frontiers, then it shows that perhaps things were not visualised in a strict oppositional manner - civilised:uncivilised, familiar:other.

3.4 Why were Boundaries Created?

Having established that the Romans, at least in the 1st centuries BC and AD, perceived their empire to have no boundaries, one can then ask why there were boundaries and more importantly why they stopped where they did? Mann argues that the army did begin to slow their attempts to expand their territory and areas of control in the 2nd century, and the lines of military advance became smaller and even complacent lines of fortification, unlike the situation in the 1st century (1974: 512). One explanation for the instigation of this change in attitude might have come very early on when Varus lost three legions in the Teutoburg forest in AD 9 to an attack of Germanic groups lead by Arminius. This disaster was an awakening to the Romans that they were not invincible. After the event Augustus warned Tiberius not to continue his expansion across the Rhine, by saying that the empire should be left within its boundary stones, *"addideratque consilium coercendi intra terminos imperii"* (Tac. *Ann.* 1. 11). It is more likely that Augustus had not intended for Tiberius to stop his campaigns entirely; rather, it is possible that he wished for him to wait a short time to allow for the situation to calm down, and then proceed with the expansion. In spite of the warning of Augustus, Tiberius sent Germanicus into Germania, and later Gaius, Claudius and the Flavians led campaigns near, or across the Rhine. In the Flavian period fortifications were constructed on the eastern side of the Rhine, but the expansion was not as ambitious as it had been during the reign of Augustus. There was no longer a move to go as far as the Elbe. Fortifications were constructed in more substantial materials of stone and concrete, rather than wood and turf, indicating a greater permanency to them and ultimately the frontiers. In spite of this, the borders of some of the frontiers were moved even farther to the north, in the case of Britain and Raetia in the 2nd and 3rd centuries. Even though movement might have been slower in the 2nd and 3rd centuries than in the 1st century there was still a desire to expand the outer edges of the empire.

Mann argues that the soldiers were forced into becoming settled because they were not continually encouraged to go on campaign. Nonetheless, there were battles being fought in different areas of the empire, so it is more likely that each emperor concentrated on specific regions, allowing for others to remain peaceful. It also seems likely that as the Romans gained a better awareness of the size of the continents of Asia and Africa, they began to see the improbability of their aim, causing the frontier lines to acquire increasing definition (Mann 1974: 512; Whittaker 1994: 85-97).

Economic and social changes are other reasons that might have contributed to the frontier becoming permanent (Whittaker 1994: 85-97). Whittaker believes that many of the frontiers correspond to the limits of cultivation. Clearly the supply of food is very important to any army. Even though there were supplies delivered to the soldiers from throughout the empire, it can be expected in an age when travel was unpredictable that the army would have needed to be in an area where food and supplies were easily available in case of an emergency. Whittaker points to the Antonine Wall in Britain where he feels that the natives within the region were not able to produce enough supplies for the soldiers, causing the army to return to Hadrian's Wall (1994: 97). Yet, as mentioned earlier, this is somewhat of a coloured point because Whittaker implies that the societies beyond the wall were too poor to support the Romans. In fact, there is plenty of evidence for extensive cereal cultivation during the Iron Age in northern Britain and southern Scotland (Topping 1988; van der Veen 1992). Whittaker also states that travel was difficult, but contrary to this statement the Romans imported goods to all areas of the empire. It is true that travel could be unpredictable, but with a good system of roads and shipping, the importation of items was not impossible. Furthermore, when the army originally moved into unknown territories that were to become part of the empire, not all populations they encountered were agrarian societies, some for example relied more on gathering and hunting for their food supply. The army could not have relied on these societies for food, so they would be dependent upon their own importation of items, along with hunting and gathering until their settlements became more established (Wells 1995: 173). At the same time the soldiers had to be adaptable and in some ways independent from the supply system of the empire to survive. With this consideration in mind, simple supply and demand economics becomes questionable as a main factor in the slowing of frontier expansion. Obviously food supply could have been a factor, but not the single factor for why there was a development of the frontiers.

Watson argues that another reason for the military slowing down may be that the soldiers themselves were not moving far from their homes when they joined the army. Initially both the auxiliary and legionary soldiers were expected to serve for 25 years moving with their units to wherever their presence was required (Watson 1969: 134-5). Often in the 2nd and 3rd centuries auxiliary soldiers did not move from one station to another and they became quite settled. Sometimes when they were asked to move, after having established a 'life' in their fort, problems arose within the units, who did not wish to transfer from their home areas (Saddington 1997: 493). The legionary soldiers were originally recruited from Italy. Later, however, the men were selected from veteran colonies and other areas in the empire, possibly making the soldiers' movement, in some cases, only a short distance from their birthplace. Following their service, the legionaries were encouraged to settle in veteran colonies. Instead, it seems that many were likely to inhabit areas near their fortresses because they had acquired wives and families (Watson 1969: 134-5). Their sons might then have been recruited into the same units, and it is possible that in some cases they would not travel far from their families in order to serve in the army.

The immobility of the army appears more obvious in the case of the auxiliary troops. The names of auxiliary units were primarily taken from the area where the unit originated, but as the soldiers retired they too, like the legionaries, often settled and married women from the regions of their fortresses. If they had sons who joined the army it is believed that they would have served in the same unit as their fathers'. In spite of this, troops did relocate, as is evident with the Batavians moving into the fort of Carrawburgh on Hadrian's Wall in the 3rd century. Mann argues that the names of the units stayed the same, but the ethnic background of the troops differed from that of the original unit (1974: 515-6). Yet, it is possible that the children of the auxiliary soldiers were taught to maintain some of their parents' original cultural traditions, so the ethnic background might have changed, but many of the practices and customs could have been maintained and passed on through the generations. Roxan has looked at military diplomas to see what happened to soldiers after they retired and noted that some soldiers returned to their homes and others stayed near their units (1997: 483-6). What is interesting about this is that if those who returned home had sons who joined the auxiliary troops, then they may have been placed in the same units as their fathers, and the ethnic background of the units might have stayed moderately the same, rather than the unit slowly undergoing a process of Romanisation. Further evidence for soldiers keeping their own identity is in the style of uniforms worn in the third century, that were of 'foreign' dress and this might have helped to denote their ethnic group (James 1999: 19, 21-3). There is the possibility that the background of the units changed through time as new soldiers joined the original unit, but it does not mean that the soldiers would have adopted a Roman lifestyle. Some scholars admit that the soldiers did find it necessary to interact with non-military and non-Roman peoples in the area, this tends only to be viewed for its economic possibilities (Hanson 1989: 58; Okun 1989: 2).

3.5 The Status of Auxiliary Soldiers

For the Roman military, Barrett and Fitzpatrick (1989) note that it is all too easily assumed that Roman authority was the dominant force; and therefore, it is generally only the Roman point of view that is studied, since it is believed to have been forced onto native cultures. The problem is further enforced by the distinct division between Romanists who will not always consider the archaeology of contemporary Iron Age societies, because it often falls under the field of prehistory, and is therefore perceived to lie outside the field of Roman studies (Barrett and Fitzpatrick 1989: 9).

Cultural variation within the army's auxiliary units can be examined and compared because they consisted of groups of non-Roman citizens, who were placed in units according to their homeland, such as a cohort of Gauls. As discussed above, the auxiliary soldiers are often defined as less 'civilised' than those in the legions. The legions are seen as having soldiers more versed in the Roman way of life because they came from Italy and the "more civilised provinces of Gaul and Spain" (Scullard 1979: 71). This opinion is consistent with Cunliffe's thoughts on the auxiliary soldiers. He states that the auxiliary soldiers were made up of bands of rampaging Celts who were in need of Romanisation; a process that would raise their status when they returned home to their own societies (1989: 126-7). The use of auxiliary soldiers is believed to have cost the empire nothing because the soldiers had the acceptable job of learning to act like Roman citizens (Drummond and Nelson 1994: 189; Watson 1969: 15). Saddington argues that in order for these soldiers to be controllable they had to be Romanised to stop any problems that might occur (1997: 496). At the same time, he points out that many were allowed to maintain their ways of fighting (1997: 493). The assumption is that these units can only be civilised if they adopt a Roman life-style. Yet, by allowing them to keep their traditional fighting techniques somehow implies, to me at least, that the more 'barbaric' aspect of fighting could be retained because that is what these soldiers were thought to be good for. There is also the possibility that some problems were avoided by allowing auxiliary groups to keep their command structures, as is suggested by Tacitus, who implies that the Batavians went to Britain without trouble (Tac. *Hist.* 4. 12). This statement provides some evidence that the Romans were probably not, as a matter of course, turning their auxiliary soldiers into homogeneous units.

3.6 How Did Native Populations View the Roman Soldiers?

Another way to examine perceptions of the frontiers is to look at the archaeology of the native settlements to determine the frequency of interaction occurring and how the natives understood the Romans. By understanding the indigenous acceptance, or rejection of Roman aspects, one can possibly learn if there was a Roman tolerance for people to live in their own ways. It is only recently that examinations have started to be undertaken looking into the views of the native cultures towards the Romans. before this any interaction was generally looked at in the one-sided terms of Romanisation. As mentioned in Chapter 1, any form of colonial interaction is not a simple process of diffusion between an active donor and a passive receptor; cultural influence is an active, motivated and creative process. Colonial interaction must be looked at from the standpoint of the social and cultural logic of the indigenous cultures with their proper institutions and their complex histories (Dietler 1995: 90). When examining both parties, natives and colonists, it is important to try and understand how they were linked in networks of interaction. Any interaction between different groups of people is driven by different logics of social action and interest that produce continual transformations in the regional structures of power (Dietler 1995: 91). This means that different groups will interpret actions differently and if one aspect of a culture is adopted it tends to be adapted to fit a different set of understandings (c.f. Sahlins 1985).

Besides Romanisation, another term used by scholars is 'acculturation', meaning the total acceptance of one culture's influence and ideas by another. This idea is employed as a method of demonstrating how native cultures would have gladly acknowledged a Roman way of life because it was more 'civilised'. Unlike the term Romanisation, the approach of the term acculturation looks at the other culture, but in a very limited view. The problem is that it assumes that one aspect of a society will be adopted with complete understanding; however, any society, if it chooses to adopt a specific aspect of another's determines the end product of the specific aspect by adapting it to fit their beliefs (Woolf 1998: 14-15). It also assumes a development of the less civilised society into something more civilised (Webster 1999). There are likely to be different patterns of change with regard to different spheres of activity. Some aspects such as means of subsistence might be accepted more rapidly in societies, but cultural values might only be accepted and adapted in a much slower manner (Shennan 1996: 290). To change the understanding of Roman interaction, Barrett and Fitzpatrick suggest the abandonment of cultural blocks such as Roman and native, along with the concept of acculturation and its evolutionary assumptions, and to try and understand the ways in which varied cultural values penetrated the routine existence of all people (1989: 9). This idea is repeatedly made in more recent scholarship; however, it is difficult to do away with these terms because they are useful in helping us organise our data, thoughts and interpretations. Perhaps a way around it is to refer to as many different possibilities as one can: Roman native, soldier civilian, non-Roman soldier, male, female, etc. and recognise that identities can be fluid and contextual.

Archaeological case studies do not always show an immediate acceptance of the Roman way of life. For example, communities living in the area around the fort of Newstead in Scotland retained their native lifestyle, perhaps because they did not perceive the Roman way of life to be as orderly or superior as theirs (Clarke 1999). Another instance, already mentioned, is seen on the Roman frontiers of Africa, where it is argued that gaps were left in the lines of fortifications to allow for transhumant groups to pass through the frontiers without problems (Raven 1993: 13, 77). This North African lifestyle was not disrupted, but at the same time the large gaps in the lines of fortifications did give the Romans some control over where the groups could move. It could be questioned who actually dictated the gaps; was it the Romans attempting to maintain some control, or were they left where it was common for the groups to move? Either way, it seems as if there was no, or very little, disruption to their way of life. Furthermore, there are examples from Roman Spain that show that some of the indigenous groups were maintaining aspects of their traditional culture and not incorporating Roman aspects when they came into contact with them. The areas of Lusitania, Galicia and Cantabria have archaeological evidence that supports the fact that people were continuing to worship their own gods, speak their own language and build structures in their own styles (Curchin 1991: 181-6). Ideas of Romanisation or acculturation seem inappropriate in these instances. If the indigenous cultures were choosing to continue to live in their own manner, can it imply that they rejected other aspects of Roman life, such as medicine? Taken further, could such processes have affected the way certain units of auxiliary soldiers from these areas might have accepted or rejected Roman-style medicine?

3.7 The Relationship between Military and Civilian Cultural Differences

To extend beyond the structural matrix of bipolar opposition that is often used to understand interaction, cultural anthropologists are concerned with how specific aspects of a society are handed down and transmitted from one group to another. Social theory is now being considered more in both anthropology and archaeology to understand what the causes and consequences of a particular social aspect might have been on a group of people and how the transmission of ideas could have occurred (Shennan 1996: 284). Giddens points out that human understandings of their culture can only be articulated in some cases, but much of what we do is at a practical level of consciousness and we know how to take part in our way of living without thinking openly about it (1984). To simplify this, one can use a specific case in western culture by looking at why it is common to shake hands when people meet. The obvious and immediate answer would be politeness, but this does not completely answer the question, why shake hands? These practices are learned, but are never totally explained. By observing how we shake hands it is possible to learn about the cultural proxemics (the study of personal space) and what is acceptable and not. Even though this is an example for anthropologists studying living groups, one can use the same theories when studying the material remains of a culture. Attitudes towards the ill and medicine can be shown by comparing the archaeological remains in their context, and by making such observations social practice can be observed by the archaeologist interested in ancient medicine (Chapter 5).

As it has been pointed out there were many types of interaction occurring on the frontiers, and these events could have had an effect on the way medical treatment was provided to the soldiers. Understanding a specific culture is a complex matter. Sometimes in archaeological studies cultural variation is only used to denote differences in material goods such as types of ceramics, or architectural styles based on who made or used them. Of course there is a danger in giving a particular artefact, burial and building type a specific ethnic identity because one group might have borrowed certain aspects from another (Jones 1997: 132-4) – pots do not equate with people. It is important to try and learn more about how the cultures being studied worked and understood themselves, and the relationship with their material remains. Since one is attempting to understand how a specific culture worked, anthropologists (and archaeologists are placed in this category, since archaeology is a discipline clearly related to anthropology) break up aspects of the culture into symbolic systems, folk models, mental structures and language to gain some understanding of how a specific society functioned (Shennan 1996: 284; Woolf 1998: 12).

Cultural beliefs and aspects would have been learned and carried over in the military zone, as a result of the overlapping of the many boundaries mentioned by Elton. For medical treatment there is no direct evidence of civilians influencing military doctors, though medical specialists were aware of non-Greek and Roman health care. Soranus, as mentioned earlier, provides information about how newborn infants were treated in Germanic and Scythian cultures:

> "*Μετὰ δὲ τὴν ὀμφαλοτομίαν οἱ πολλοὶ τῶν βαρβάρων, ὡς οἱ Γερμανοὶ καὶ Σκύθαι, τινὲς δὲ καὶ τῶν Ἑλλήνων εἰς ψυχρὸν ὕδωρ καθιᾶσι τὸ βρέφος στερεοποιήσεως χάριν καὶ <τοῦ> τὸ μὴ φέρον τὴν ψύξιν, ἀλλὰ πελιούμενον ἢ σπώμενον ὡς οὐκ ἄξιον ἐκτοφῆς ὂν ἀπολέσθαι.*" (Sor. *Gyn*. 2. 12. 81).

Perceived boundaries did not eliminate medical information from passing into Roman scholarship. Varied beliefs could have been introduced to, or at least been familiar to, military doctors. The description of different bodily practices and treatments could also have been a means of propaganda. It is common for one group of people to define other groups as inferior by their medical and bodily practices (here one only needs to think of comments made about the bathing habits of foreigners). Often the treatment of the body or mind is used to demonstrate inferior traits of others, even if these are simply myths. In spite of the perceived inferiority of different medical practices by Roman and Greek writers, it is possible that some doctors could have adopted or adapted the medical practices they might have learned by being stationed in different regions of the empire. This could allow for the possibility of different treatments and sympathetic medicine to move between fort and frontier. As mentioned, the latest find from Stanway, dating to the era of the Roman conquest, has possible divining rods that could have been used in medical practice. Not known to occur in 'Roman' medical kits from later dates, it is these rods and the shape of the medical tools that provide us with more information about the culturally specific nature of later Iron Age medical treatment in the southern part of Britain. Again the instruments from Colchester show a possible merging of ideas. The surgical instruments found with the burial are similar to Roman designs of medical instruments, but they also have characteristics similar to Iron Age instruments from other areas and some are unique. The surgical knives have blades shaped similar to those found on Roman scalpels, but the knife handles are unusual and may be based on local designs (Crummy 2002: 51; Jackson 1997: 1,473), indicating possible Roman military and native interaction with concern to medical practices.

Civilian help might have been employed, especially if doctors or hospitals were not available in fortifications. Although we are not aware of military doctors making use of civilian medical treatments, we do know that civilians did care for wounded or ill patients, as described by Julius Caesar during the Civil War. He mentions how on campaign some sick and wounded soldiers were left behind in friendly villages to be cared for by the local inhabitants:

> "*Caesari ad saucios deponendos, stipendium exercitui dandum, socios confirmandos, praesidium urbibus relinquendum necesse erat adire Apolloniam*" (*BC*. 3, 78. 2).

Caesar also reported one of his commanding officers, Labienus, doing the same thing during his African campaign:

> "*Labienus saucios suos, quorum maximus numerus fuit iubet in plostris obligatos Hadrumentum deportari*" (*BA*. 21).

If this were the case, than soldiers might have learned new ways of treating illness and wounds and introduced these to healers or doctors in their homelands, Roman doctors and/or military doctors, helping to diversify medical practices within the Roman world.

3.8 A Review of the Military Events

The development of the frontiers and the actions that occurred on them could have been a contributing factor, along with cultural variations, in the way in which medical treatment was provided to the soldiers on the frontiers. Although the evidence for the history of the frontiers is readily available, a brief account of the major events for each area in this study is presented here to acquaint the reader with a working background of the important developments in each frontier from the reign of Augustus to the mid-3rd century AD. The mid-3rd century seems the most beneficial time to end this examination because it was a period of upheaval and change in the control and organisation of empire and the army. Although Britain remained fairly peaceful during the 3rd century, the frontier provinces of the Rhine and Danube were plagued with incursions from groups of people who lived beyond the rivers. The problems were finally resolved in the 4th century with a rearrangement in the military and government. Not only were the frontiers administered differently, mainly from an offensive to a defensive point of view. There were also changes in the organisation of the army, which can be seen its supply system for example (e.g. Baker 1995), and it is likely that there was an effect on how medical treatment was offered.

Since this is intended to be a very brief introduction to the history of the frontiers, specific details about the development and history of separate fortifications will not be presented. However, information about the units and dates of occupation is provided in Appendix 1, Part 1. This more specific information will also be useful in making comparisons with the frontiers and units in the proceeding chapters.

3.8.1 Germania (Appendix 1 and Figs. 1)

Combined, both German provinces have a greater number of fortifications than any of the other frontiers being examined. The historical development of Germania is complex and riddled with conflict. It was originally a single province, but at the end of the 1st century it was divided into two provinces by the emperor Domitian. Germania Inferior ran from the North Sea at the mouth of the old Rhine to the fort at Sinzig in modern Germany. Germania Superior, at its farthest expansion eastwards, ran from the fort at Andernach to the Raetian border near Lorch (Schönberger 1969: Fig. 1).

During the campaigns of Drusus there was some construction of fortifications beyond the line of the Rhine on the Lippe river. The fortifications of Haltern, Oberaden, Beckinghausen, Rodgen, Holsterhausen and Anreppen were built to help with the movement towards the Elbe (Wells 1972: 165-221). Following the Varian disaster in AD 9 the forts on the Lippe were abandoned and the troops settled on the west bank of the Rhine.

Tiberius was warned by Augustus not to extend the boundaries of the Rhine (Tac. *Ann.* 1. 11). Clearly though, this advice was not strictly followed because Germanicus led campaigns beyond the river in AD 15 and 16. The legionary fortress at Strasbourg (Argentorate) was constructed and one was built at Windisch (Vindonissa). To support these fortresses a number of auxiliary forts were also built along the Rhine (Maxfield 2002: 147; Schönberger 1969: 151). In total Tiberius had eight legions stationed along the Rhine, four in what would become Germania Inferior and four in the future Germania Superior.

Germany became more volatile when the Batavians revolted on the lower Rhine in AD 69. Vespasian defeated them in the same year and following the attack he reorganised the frontier. Four legions were stationed on the lower Rhine. The auxiliary forts were reconstructed in stone, making them permanent and stronger to attack (Haalebos 1995: 5). Upper Germany had not escaped incursions either, as the Mattiaci attacked Mainz. To combat further invasions, auxiliary forts were constructed on the Taunus beyond the Rhine on the Main (Maxfield 2002: 148). Furthermore, Vespasian shortened the distance of travel and communications between the Rhine and the Danube. To do this he constructed a road that ran from Strasbourg through the Black Forest to the banks of the Danube near Tutlingen (Drinkwater 1983: 57; Maxfield 2002: 148; Millar 1967: 112).

When Domitian became emperor he inherited a number of problems on the Rhine. During his first visit to Germany he was made aware of a possible uprising by the Chatti, who were preparing to cross the river. The emperor launched a successful campaign in either AD 82 or 83 to help quash any possible movement towards the frontiers. His campaign was of vital importance because it enabled him to strengthen the Roman presence beyond the upper Rhine by constructing a string of auxiliary fortifications on the Taunus and Wetterau between the Main and Lahn rivers some 30 miles east of the Rhine (Jones 1973: 79-80).

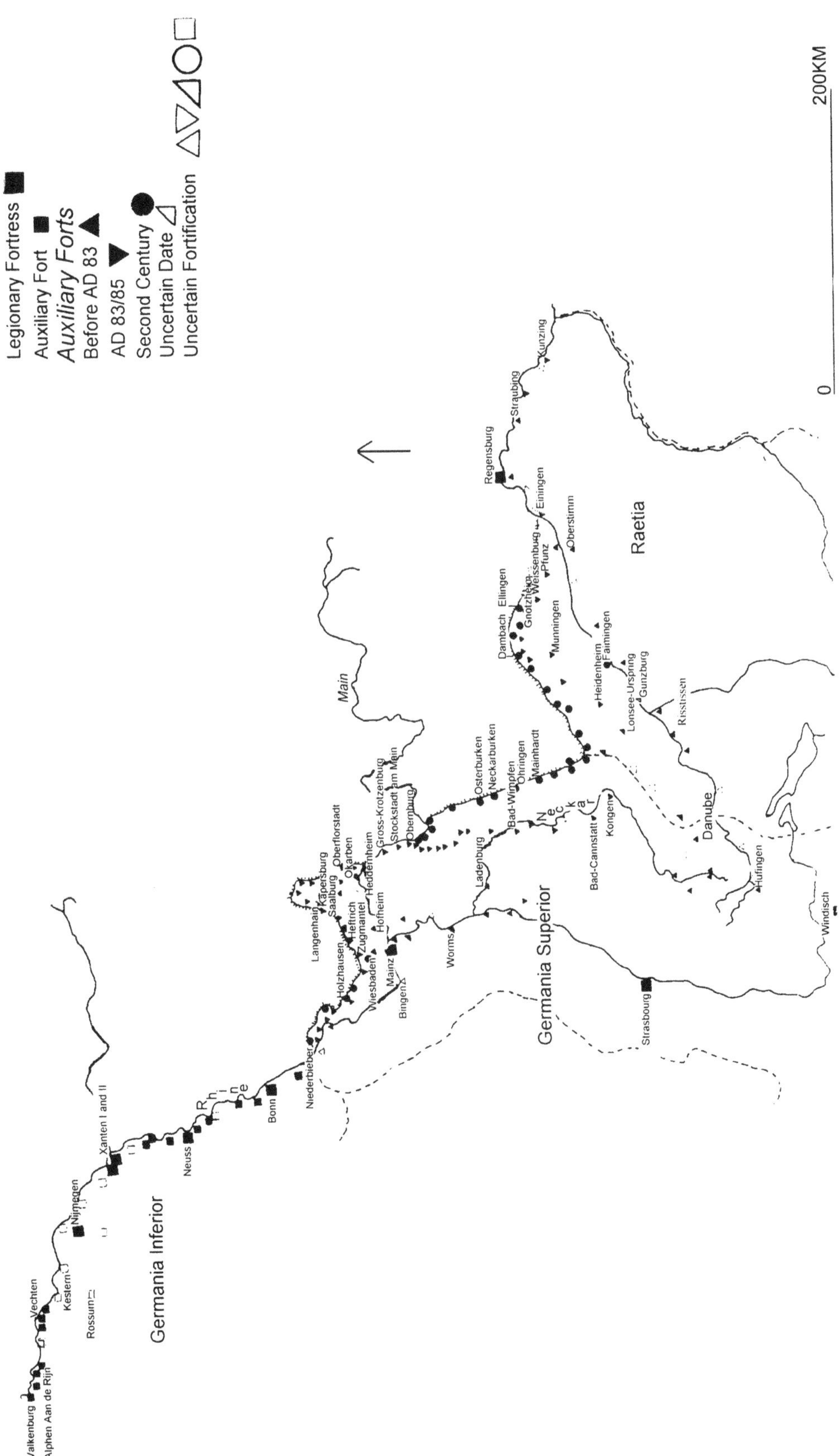

Fig. 1. Map of the frontiers of Germania Inferior, Germania Superior, and Raetia. After Schönberger 1969: Fig 20.

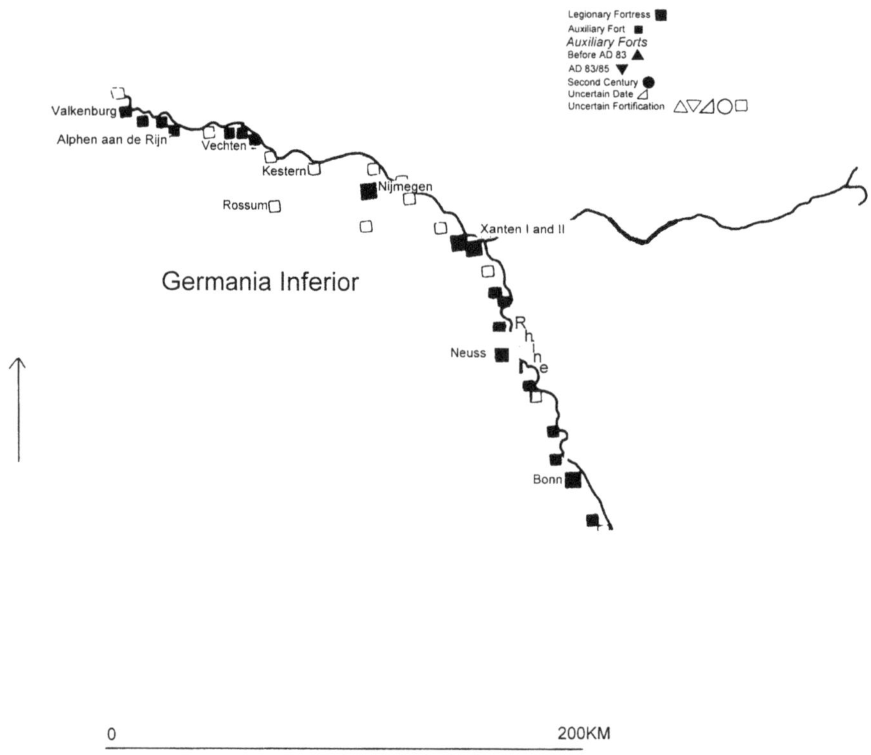

Fig. 2. Map of the frontier of Germania Inferior. After Schönberger 1969: Fig. 20.

Included in his construction, Domitian reinforced the forts with a line of wooden watchtowers and stone forts, creating a more visible frontier (Maxfield 2002: 153; Millar 1967: 112). In order to gain greater control over the area he divided Germany into two provinces (Figs. 2 & 3), which could, therefore, be governed separately. Domitian's victory was soon overshadowed by a revolt in AD 89 by L. Antonius Saturninus, the commander of both legions at Mainz. After this, Domitian abolished the use of double legionary fortresses throughout the empire (Schönberger 1969: 158).

Trajan created the Odenwald Limes in the upper Rhine, which was a military road guarded by observation towers on the river Main. Ten small forts were constructed beginning at Worth and running southwards to the Raetian border at Lorch. (Maxfield 2002: 155-6; Fig. 3). Eventually, except for Friedburg in the Wetterau, all of the auxiliary forts behind Trajan's line were abandoned and the military control, except for the legions, was limited to a long narrow strip on the outer edge of the frontier (Maxfield 2002: 156-7).

Antoninus Pius was the last emperor to advance farther into Germania Superior. He set up 12 forts beyond the Neckar river that ran in a line south to the Raetian Limes (Fig. 3). The fortifications were constructed of stone, expressing the intention that they should be permanent (Schönberger 1969: 167-8).

In AD 213 the Alamanni invaded for the first time, and in 233, during the reign of Severus Alexander a major Alamannic invasion was directed at Upper Germany and Raetia. The frontier was restored by Maximinus Thrax, but in AD 260 lands east of the Rhine and north of the Danube were abandoned for the original Julio-Claudian frontier (Maxfield 2002: 165-6).

3.8.2 Raetia (Appendix 1 and Fig. 4)

Raetia was an alpine province located in what is now the Austrian Tirol, southern Bavaria and the northeastern corner of Switzerland. Raetia was a fairly peaceful province that played an important role as link between the Rhine and Danube. In 16 BC Drusus and Tiberius conquered the Raeti and the Vindelici, two tribes that occupied this region:

> "*At. Ti. Caesar quam certam Hispanis parendi confessionem extorserat parens, Illyriis Delmatisque extorsit. Raetiam autem et Vindelicos ac Noricos Pannoniamque et Scordiscos novas imperio nostro subiunxit provincias*" (*Vell.* 2. 39.3).

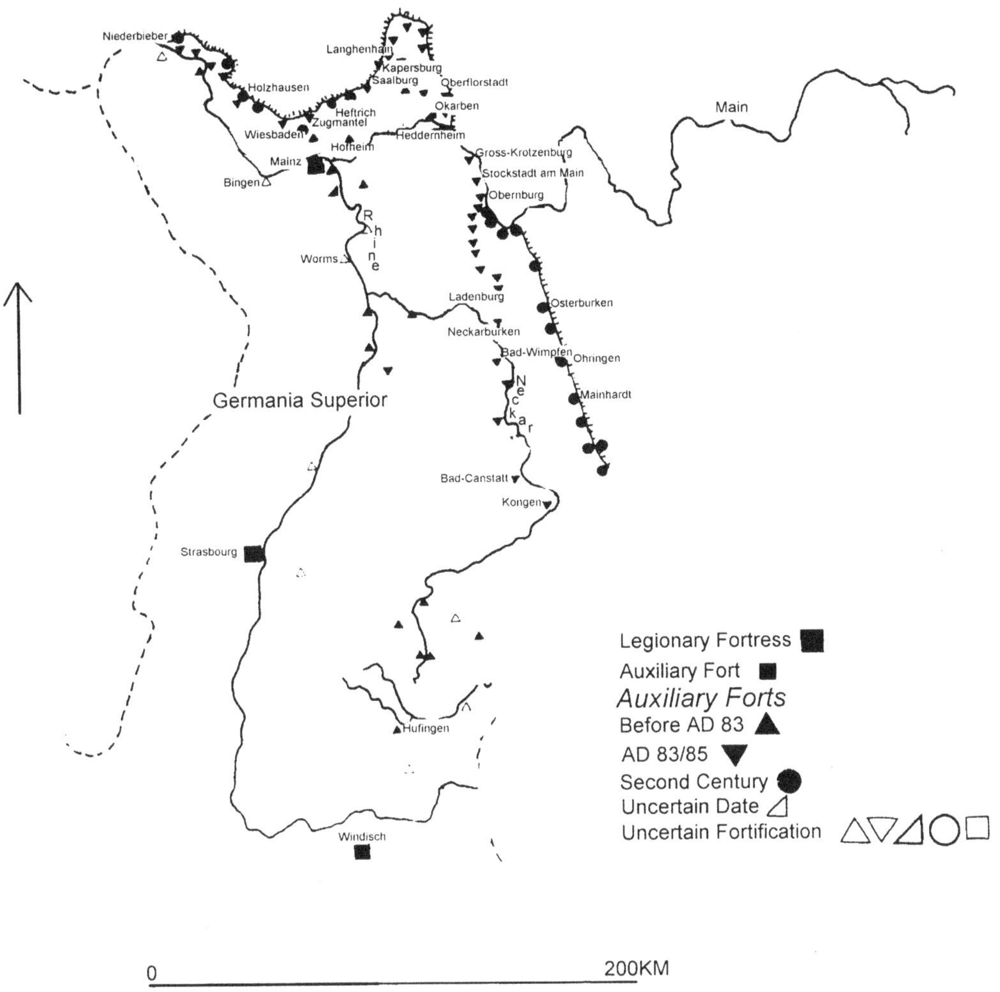

Fig. 3. Map of the frontier of Germania Superior. After Schönberger 1969: Fig. 20.

It is thought that during the campaigns of Drusus in this region two legions were stationed at Augsburg-Oberhausen; however, a fortification has never been found, only a large number of military accoutrements were found through dredging in the river Inn, indicating some form of military presence (Schönberger 1969: 145). Little occurred in the province until the time of Claudius, who was responsible for changing the government from one of native alliance to provincial rule. Claudius realised its importance as a link between the Rhine and the Danube rivers and sought to place the area under Roman control (Whittaker 1994: 348). In order to organise a communication system, he moved all of the auxiliary troops that had been previously scattered throughout the province to a road along the southern bank of the Danube (Cook *et al.* 1979: 784; Maxfield 2002: 147).

During the Flavian period military movement beyond the Danube increased the size of the province. Auxiliary forts were constructed by Vespasian on the road that ran from Strasbourg to the Danube (Whittaker 1994: 46). Domitian created a larger province by moving the troops north of the road into the Swabian Alb, where he had a new military road guarded by auxiliary forts constucted (Maxfield 2002: 154, 159; Whittaker 1994: 46). Hadrian reinforced the Domitian's defences by building a wall of stone with watchtowers attached to it, the *Teufelsmauer*, north of the military road (Maxfield 2002: 159-60).

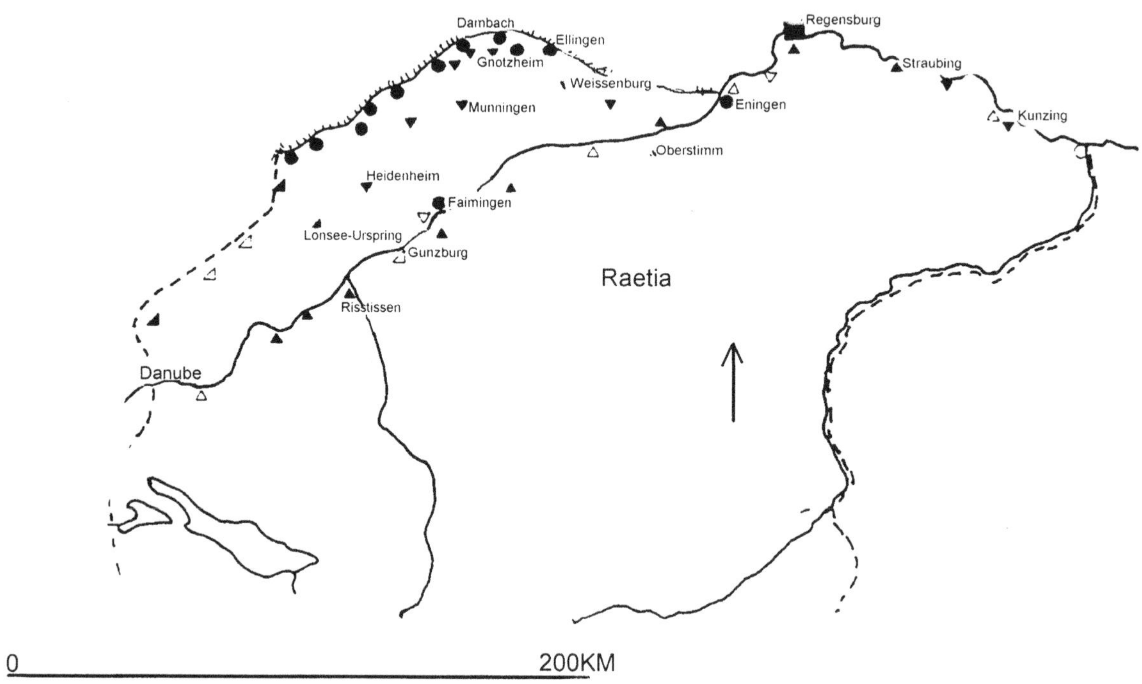

Fig. 4. Map of the frontier of Raetia. After Schönberger 1969: Fig. 20.

The final change to Raetia was made during the Marcomannic Wars, during the reign of Marcus Aurelius. The security risk created by the groups of people living north of the Danube caused Marcus Aurelius to have the first and only legionary fortress constructed at Regensburg (Maxfield 2002: 164; Millar 1967: 115; von Elbe 1974: 322). After a legionary fortress was built the commander of the unit was given the duty of governing the province. The Antonine boundaries of Raetia were maintained until the mid-third century when attacks by the Alamanni forced the soldiers to return to the southern bank of the Danube (Maxfield 2002: 190-2).

3.8.3 Noricum (Appendix 1 and Fig. 5)

The province of Noricum, created by Augustus, was located to the east of Raetia (*Vell.* 3. 39.3; Cook *et al.* 1979: 211) in what is now Austria with its northern border on the Danube. Noricum was overrun by the Pannonians and Noricans in 12 BC. Rather than making it part of the Roman empire, when P. Silius Nerva conquered the Noricans he allowed them to live as a dependency of Rome:

"*Καὶ οἱ Παννόνιοι τήν τε Ἰστρίαν μετὰ Νωρίκων κατέδραμον, καὶ αὐτοί τε πρός τε τοῦ Σιλίου καὶ τῶν ὑποστρατήγων αὐτοῦ κακωθέντες αὖθις ὡμόλογησαν, καὶ τοῖς Νωρίκοις αἴτοι τῆς αὐτῆς δουλείας ἐγένοντο*" (Dio Cassius, 54, 20. 2; Cook et al. 1979: 348).

During Claudius' reign the province was changed, like Raetia, from a native alliance to provincial rule, governed by an equestrian *praefect* (Whittaker 1994: 44). Since there were few incursions in the province there was a sparse military presence with fewer forts in comparison to other provinces. The geography of the Danube in western Austria also helped to protect Noricum. In the section of the frontier between Passau and the Wachau much of the Danube flows in a narrow steep-sided valley that would have made crossing difficult on both sides (Maxfield 2002: 175). The eastern section of Noricum, between the Wachau and the Wienerwald, faced the Tullnerfeld, located north of the river. This was a heavily populated area that was home to the Marcomanni. Because the Marcomanni were a possible threat, and the river was easier to ford in this area, five auxiliary forts were constructed in a 31 mile (50 km) stretch (Maxfield 2002: 174-6). In order to man these new forts, troops from the interior of Noricum were moved to the outer line on the Danube (Alföldy 1974: 66, 147).

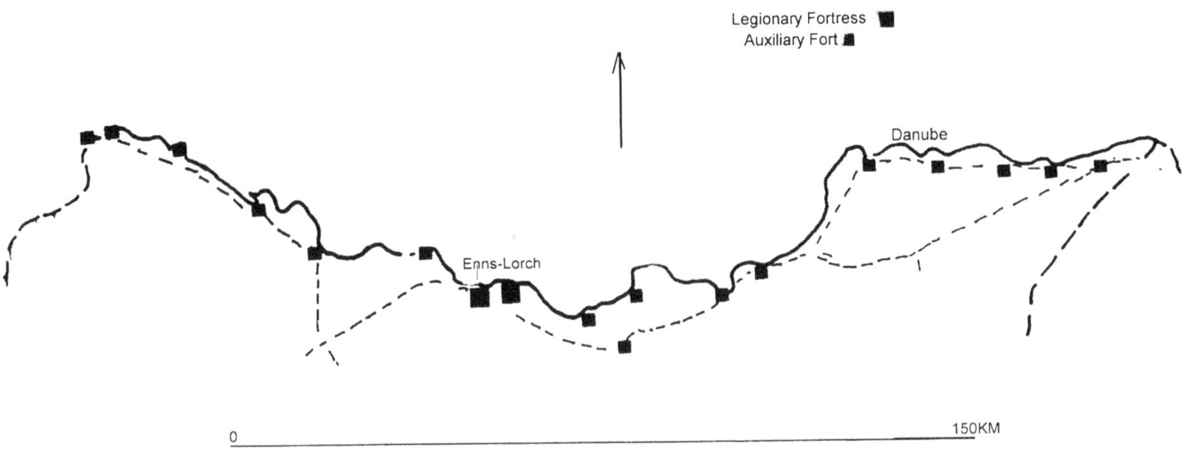

Fig. 5. Map of the frontier of Noricum. After Alföldy 1974.

There were most likely nine auxiliary forts occupied during the reign of Hadrian (Alföldy 1974: 144). The province remained peaceful and there are no recorded invasions during the 1st or early 2nd centuries. It only held the strength, in auxiliary troops, of roughly one legionary unit. The troops probably helped to police the area and protected the transportation of supplies.

The first threat came to the area during the Marcomannic war when both the Marcomanni and Quadi crossed the Danube into Pannonia and proceeded into Noricum. Marcus Aurelius had to protect Noricum as it was particularly close to the Italian border. In 171 he had a legionary fortress constructed at Albing to house the first legion to occupy Noricum, *II Italica*. Albing, however, was built in a low-lying area near the confluence of the river Enns and the Danube and flooded frequently. The legion was transferred to slightly higher ground at Lauriacum before the end of Commodus' reign (Alföldy 1974: 165-6). The commander of the legion then became the *legatus Augusti pro praetore* or governor of the province. The next invasion into the province was not made until the mid-3rd century (Alföldy 1974: 159, 202).

3.8.4 Pannonia (Appendix 1 and Fig. 6)

Like Noricum, Pannonia was also overrun in 12 BC, and Tiberius was forced to fight for four years before he was able to gain some control of the area. Pannonia was made into a province in AD 9 when it was separated from Illyricum (Maxfield 2002: 174). In the later reign of Tiberius or under Claudius a legionary fortress was constructed at Petronell (Carnuntum), which was also established as the capital of the area, and the first unit to be stationed at the site was the *Legio XX Apollinaris* (Móscy 1974: 40). At the same time, auxiliary forts were built at Brigetio (Szóny) and Aquincum (Budapest) (Maxfield 2002: 175). Pannonia was located in what is now eastern Austria from just west of Vienna, to the south of Hungary on the Danube.

Few changes were made to this province until the reign of the Flavians. During this time more auxiliary forts were added to the Danube frontier to strengthen it, especially since the Dacians were beginning to become a threat to the middle and lower Danubian provinces. It seems that watchtowers were also constructed towards the end of the 1st century (Maxfield 2002: 178).

Trajan fought two Dacian wars and when he had secured Dacia as a province he found that the Iazyges, a group that inhabited the Hungarian plain in the non-Roman territory between Dacia and Pannonia was a threat to the province of Pannonia. In order to maintain security in the province, he divided it into two: Pannonia Superior and Inferior, enabling the governor of Pannonia Inferior to keep a closer watch on the Iazyges. The new province of Pannonia Inferior, beginning at the Danube bend in modern Hungary and running southwards to the border between Hungary and Serbia, was governed by a praetorian legate. Pannonia Superior, which occupied the western section of the original province, was governed by a consular legate. For better protection Trajan added more legions to the front line in Pannonia Superior at the fortresses of Brigetio and Vindobona (Maxfield 2002: 178). Only one legion was stationed in Pannonia Inferior at the fortress of Aquincum (Maxfield 2002:182; Zsidi 1995: 14-5).

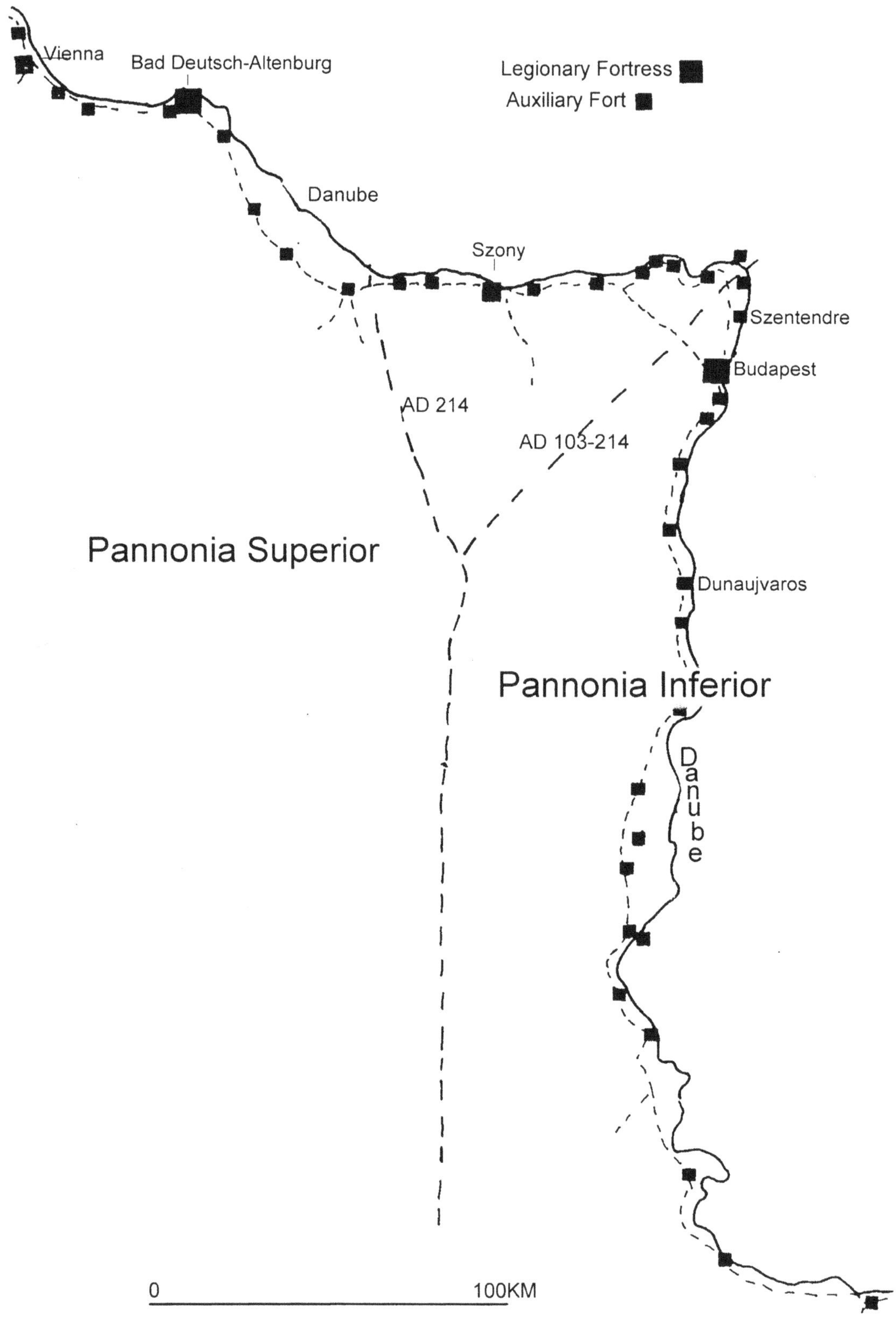

Fig. 6. Map of the frontiers of Pannonia Superior and Inferior. After Mócsy 1974.

In the mid-2nd century, during the reign of Marcus Aurelius, a string of watchtowers was also built on the frontier of Pannonia Inferior because of the Marcommanic wars. Groups of 'Gothic' people invaded the lower Danube in the mid-3rd century, followed by incursions during the later part of the century on the middle Danube by the Marcomanni, Quadi and Sarmatae (Maxfield 2002: 187; Millar 1967: 115-6).

3.8.5 Britannia (Appendix 1 and Figs. 7 & 8)

In this study the main area of discussion relating to Britannia will concern Hadrian's Wall, although there were other frontier lines of military forts in the province of Britannia such as those in Wales and the Antonine Wall in Scotland. The Welsh frontier ran from Chester to Caerleon close to the present day border between England and Wales. It also had a line of auxiliary forts running east to west across the centre of Wales, and a row of forts on the north and south coasts of Wales (Jarrett 1969).

There was much disruption after the Claudian invasion of Britain in AD 43. However, it was not until the Flavian era that more visible lines of fortifications began to appear in the province. In c. AD 84 Domitian sent Agricola north into Scotland, and construction began on small military posts and the legionary fortress at Inchtuthil. He defeated the Caledonii in a decisive battle at Mons Graupius (Scullard 1979: 45-6). The campaign in Scotland, however, was cut short by an unexpected Dacian attack on the Danube. At the time Domitian found it necessary to leave three legions in Britain and relinquish the newly gained territory in Scotland.

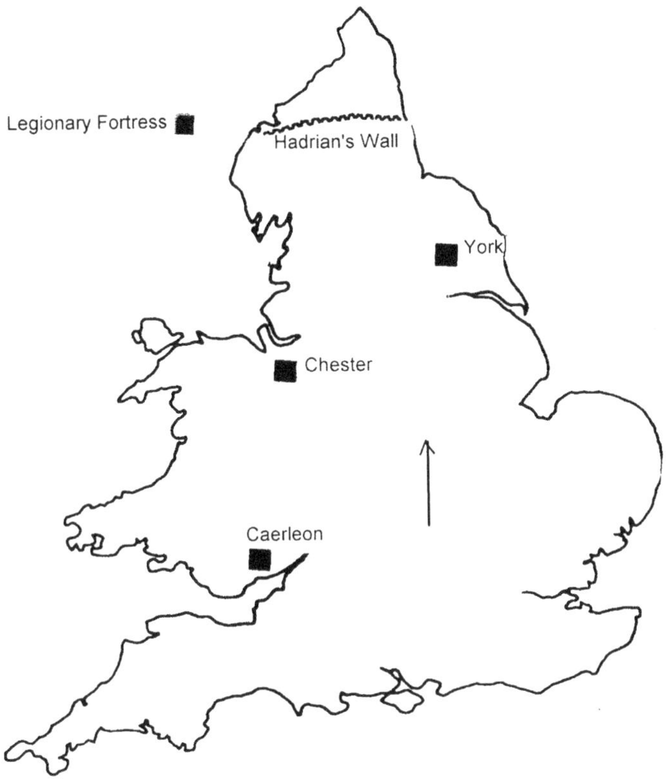

Fig. 7. Map of the legionary fortresses in Britannia.

Thus, Domitian sent troops from Britain to defend the Roman territory on the Danube (Breeze 2002: 201). When the Dacian campaign ended, the legions returned to Britain and were stationed at Caerleon, Chester and York (Scullard 1979: 46; Breeze 2002: 201-5). These three fortresses remained the permanent legionary posts in Britain.

When Trajan came to power there was an increasing threat from the Dacians that caused him to abandon Roman auxiliary fortifications in southern Scotland in order to keep Britain secure. He fortified the Stanegate road that ran from Corbridge to Carlisle, with watchtowers and auxiliary forts. He strengthened the legionary fortresses and had them rebuilt in stone in the early 2nd century (Breeze and Dobson 1991: 16-26).

Hadrian consolidated the British frontier and built a wall across northern Britain. Roughly 9,500 men would have served on the Wall. Initially it seems that Hadrian's Wall was intended to be similar to his fortification in Raetia where forts were left behind the wall, in this case on the Stanegate road. However, forts were constructed on the Wall soon after its construction began. The plan was to have a tight network of forts set about a half day's march apart from one another that would be used to control the key strategic points along the Wall (Webster 1981: 122). The Wall frontier also had a number of outpost forts, located to its north.

The remainder of the 3rd century continued to stay fairly peaceful in Britain. At the beginning of the

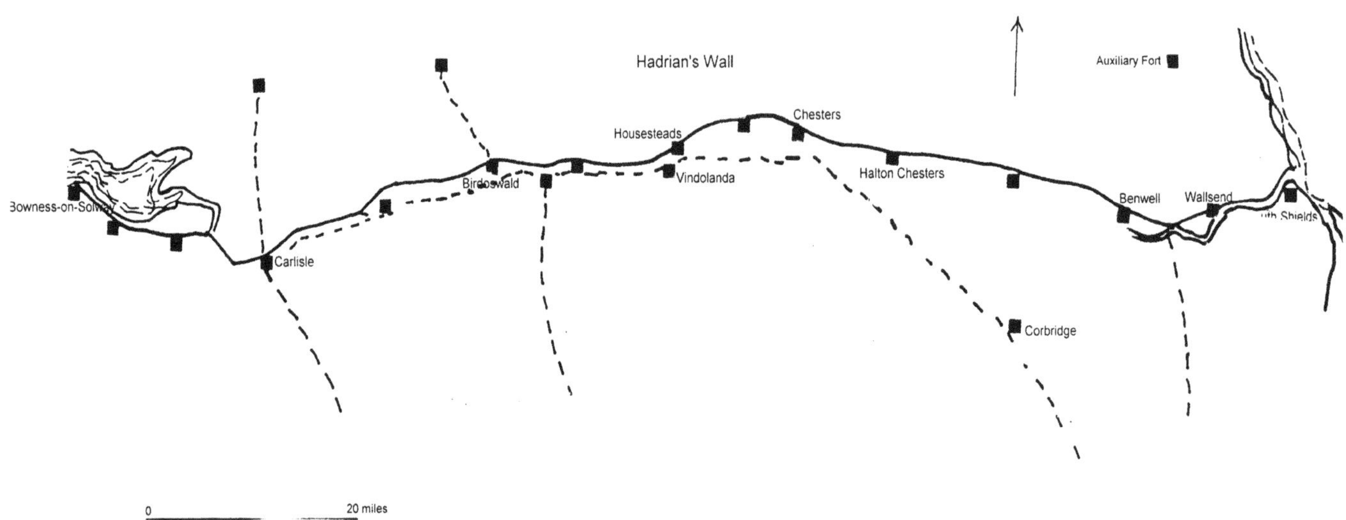

Fig. 8. Map of Hadrian's Wall. After Breeze and Dobson 1991: Fig. 9.

4th century the province was faced with threats from Saxon attacks. Hadrian's Wall, however, remained the northern frontier until Roman rule ended in Britain in the beginning of the 5th century (Scullard 1979: 65-6).

3.9 CONCLUSION

To understand the medical system of the army one must be aware of the development of each frontier and their differences. Their various natures of construction would have affected the interaction that took place between the military and local inhabitants. In order to understand the medical system of the army, one must be aware of both issues because they can play an important role in how medical care might have been affected and organised.

CHAPTER FOUR

LITERARY AND EPIGRAPHIC EVIDENCE RELATING TO ROMAN MILITARY MEDICINE

4.1 INTRODUCTION

One of the main concerns of the preceding three chapters was to explain why and where there is a need to approach Roman archaeology, especially that of military medicine and the frontiers, with an increased use of anthropological and interpretative methods commonly used in other fields of archaeology, such as historical, colonial and prehistoric. This methodology shall be employed in this and the following chapters, not only as a means of signifying the complexities of Roman military medicine, but, more importantly, to ask specific questions about the different influences, such as military incidents and the background of the units, that might have contributed to the means by which medical care was distributed to soldiers. Since inscriptions mentioning doctors are one of the main sources of information used by scholars attempting to 'make sense' of military medicine, they shall be examined before discussions are made about the relationship of artefacts (specifically medical tools) to military medicine. The prime concern for most scholars who have examined the extant epigraph remains is to discern the meanings of the various titles given with the term *medicus* and how a system of medical care might have been structured in the army (Davies 1969a & b; 1972; 1989; Domaszawski 1908: 45-7; Haberling 1910: 4-10; Nutton 1969; Penn 1964; Richmond 1952; Scarborough 1968; Wilmanns 1995a & b). These interpretations then used, rather uncritically, as a framework for understanding the rank of medical personnel, and this is then applied to the army as a whole (Davies 1969a & b; 1972; 1989; Jackson 1993: 83; Richmond 1952; Wilmanns 1995a & b). Because of this, it is necessary to reconsider the foundation on which the assumption is based.

This chapter begins with a discussion of previous scholarship on the literary and epigraphic material concerning the expectations of the soldiers' health, the prescribed ranks of the doctors and the organisation of the medical care system. Following this, comparisons of the literary remains from the different provinces, unit types and auxiliary groups with the name of their unit's home will be made to see if the evidence supports earlier arguments, or if it challenges our current understandings of the organisation of medical care in the army.

4.2 RECRUITMENT

The primary literature related to recruitment is an ideal place to begin a discussion on the potential soldier's first contact with the Roman army and possibly its medicine. Although only fragmentary descriptions remain about the topic, scholars have tried to tie together an accurate picture of how the system of recruitment was arranged (Davies 1969a: 202-22; Watson 1969: 39; Wilmanns 1995b: 44-6).

Vegetius (c. AD 383/450?) a late Roman writer, provides us with the most information on the subject. The work of Vegetius is not wholly reliable because he was writing two centuries or so after the end of the period in question and he borrowed from numerous authors who described the army in the early empire. Some problems with his work could be that he was either describing practices in the army whilst he was alive that were different to those in the principate or he may not have understood or correctly interpreted what was written before he wrote his treatise. Nonetheless, with caution, his work must be considered. He first presents a detailed description of the type of person he felt made a desirable candidate for the army before any mention is made of the recruitment process. Men from temperate climates were considered to be the ideal candidates for soldiers because they possessed the best qualities of people from both the warmer and colder climatic regions of the empire. People from warmer areas were thought to be of greater intelligence, but had less blood and, therefore, lacked the steadiness and confidence to fight. Whilst those who were living in the colder climates were considered to be less intelligent, but had the abundance of blood and readiness for war. Consequently, the finest soldiers were expected to have the mental ability to be disciplined during training and battles, along with a capacity for fighting:

> "*Omnes nationes, quae uicinae sunt soli...amplius quidem sapere, sed minus habere sanguinis dicunt ac propterae constantiam ac fiduciam comminus non habere pugnandi,...Contra septentrionales populi, remoti a solis ardoribus, inconsultiores quidem, sed tamen largo sanguine redundantes, sunt ad bella promptissimi. Tirones igitur de temperatioribus legendi sunt plagis*" (*Mil.* 1. 2-3; Davies 1969b: 209).

Cato believed the best recruits were raised on farms: "*At ex agricolis et viri fortissimi et milites strenuissimi gignuntur*" (*De Agri Cultura.* proem. 4), and it is possible that Vegetius adopted this idea from him since he also states that individuals from the country were better suited for training than persons from urban areas: "*De qua parte numquam credo potuisse dubitari aptiorem armis rusticam plebem...*" (*Mil.* 1. 3; Davies 1969b: 209). Both writers were convinced men more familiar with hard work and the outdoors would find it easier to assimilate to the harsh training of military life, whilst those who were not accustomed to strenuous outdoor living would find the experience difficult. The possibility exists that these ideas may have been passed down throughout the centuries.

On the other hand, recruiting officers who were from different regions of the empire might have carried with them their own beliefs about who would make a suitable candidate for the army. Since soldiers were enlisted from many regions in and around the empire there is an indication that these ideas were not always followed. It seems more likely that those who wished to join the army were chosen on the results of an entrance examination known as the *probatio*. Our understandings of the requirements to pass the *probatio*, are insufficient at best (Watson 1969: 39). According to Herodian there were three points of physique a recruiting officer should examine most closely during the *probatio*: age, height and suitability of health, as he notes the emperor Antoninus Pius mustering young men into their ranks on certain occasions so he could examine these three aspects (4. 9. 5; Davies 1969a: 212; Watson 1969: 39). While discussing the life of the emperor Maximinus, Herodian states that Maximius was recruited into the army because of his size and strength

> *"ἐν ἀκμῇ δὲ τῆς ἡλικίας γενόμενος διὰ μέγεθος καὶ ἰσχὺν σώματος ἐς τούς ἱππεύοντας στρατιώτας καταταγείς" (6. 8. 1. 2).*

Herodian's work provides a general idea of what the *probatio* might have consisted of, but he does not explain how these aspects were examined and what the exact specifications were, as no indication is presented about what constituted his idea of appropriate size and strength. Therefore, we must turn to other sources to try and piece together the possible specifications for enlistment, if Herodian is correct.

Height is the only component of the *probatio* for which exact standards have been mentioned in the classical sources. The minimum height set for entrance into the Roman army was originally five feet ten Roman inches, with six Roman feet or over being the ideal height of a recruit:

> "*Proceritatem tironum ad incomam scio semper exactam, ita ut VI pedum vel certe V et X unciarum inter alares equites vel in primis legionum cohortibus probarentur*" (Vegetius, *Mil.* 1. 5; also mentioned in the *Codex Theodosianus* 7. 13. 3).

The standard height was lowered during the reign of Valentinian in the late 4th century to a minimum of five feet seven Roman inches since the number of recruits was diminishing and because more frequent skirmishes created a need to maintain a large army (*Codex Theodosianus*, 7. 13. 3).

Age is more difficult to determine because no precise figures are given in any extant source. Inscriptions can be used to show the ages of soldiers during their recruitment. Wilmanns mentions a study by Scheidel (1995b: 46 note 105) who says that 75% of the inscriptions mentioning ages of recruitment range between 17 and 20, implying that the age of recruits did not have to be as standardised as height, but the ages are still fairly specific nonetheless. According to Vegetius, who quotes Sallust, adolescents were considered to be the ideal age for army selection because their bodies were nimble and they were at an age when they were willing to learn more than those who were slightly older and had more set ways of thinking:

> "*Adulescentes legendi sunt, sicut ait Sallustius nam simul ac iuventus belli patiens erat, in castris per laborem usum militiae discebant*" (*Mil.* 1. 4).

Since there does not appear to have been a minimum or maximum age it is conceivable that a person could choose the time when he may have felt that he was physically and/or mentally prepared to join the army.

The physical examination is the most problematic element of the *probatio* to determine because no exact stipulations, if there were any, survive in the literature about how the examination was executed, what the expectations of a healthy body were, or even how thorough an examination might have been. From the evidence of an Egyptian papyrus it might be suggested that soldiers were examined, at least in some cases, for distinguishing features, marks or scars on their body, that could be used for identification in case the soldiers fell in battle (*POxy* 1022=CPL III; in Davies 1969a: 222):

[C.] Minicius Italu[s C]elsiano suo sal[u]tem.
Tirones sexs probatos a me in coh(orte) cui praees in numeros referri iube ex
xi kalendas martias: nomina eorum et icon[i]smos huic epistulae subieci .
Vale frater karissim[e.

C. Veturium Gemellum, Annor(um) xxi, sine i(conismo),
C. Longium Priscum, Annor(um) xxii, i(conismus) supercil(io) sinistr(o)
C. Iulium Maximum, Annor(um) xxv, sine i(conismo)
[.] Lucium Secundum, Annor(um) xx, sine i(conismo)
C. Iulium Saturninum, Annor(um) xxiii, i(conismus) manu sinistr(a)
M. Antonium Valentem, Annor(um) xxii, i(conismus) frontis parte dextr(a)

[C]. Minicius Italus to Celanus, Greetings
Give orders that six recruits who have been approved by me in the cohort under your command be included in the ranks from Feb. 19. I append this to the letter their names and descriptions.

C. Veturius Gemellus	21	no distinguishing features
C. Longius Priscus	22	scar on left eyebrow
C. Julius Maximus	25	no distinguishing feature
[.] Julius Secundus	20	no distinguishing feature
C. Julius Saturninus	23	scar on left hand
M. Antoninus Valens	22	scar on right side of forehead

POxy 1022=CPL III

Since this fragment records marks on the body it might be suggested that, in this unit at least, there was some interest in certain physical aspects of the solders' or prospective soldiers' bodies as a means of identification. In order to make a note of the marks, there might have been a superficial assessment of the soldier's physique. One must also consider the possibility that no examination was given and the recruit simply might have been asked if he had any distinguishing features or marks.

Another papyrus fragment from Egypt (*POxy* 39; Davies 1969a: 211) signifies that a test for vision might also have been part of the physical examination:

Ἀντίγραφον ἀπολύσεως ἔτους ιβ Τιβερίου Κλαδίου Καίσαρος
Σεβαστοῦ Γερμανικοῦ Αὐτοκράτορος, Φαρμοῦθ(ι), κΘ, σεσημ(ειωμένης).
ἀπελύθηι [ὑ]πὸ Γναίου Οὐεργιλίου Καπίτων[ο]ς τοῦ ἡγεμόνος
ἀμφοτέρων
Τρύφων Διονυσίου γέρδιος, υπο <κε> χυμένος ὀλίγον βλέπων,
τῶν ἀπ' Ὀξυρύγχων τῆς μντροπόλ(εως).
'Επεκρίθ(η) ἐν Αλεξανδ(ρεία)
'Επεκρίθ(η) ἐν Αλεξανδ(ρεία)
'Επιπκέκριται ἐν Ἀλεχανδ(ρειά)

Copy of a release dated and signed in the 12th year of Tiberius Claudius
Caesar Augustus Germanicus Imperator, Pharmouthi
Discharged by Gnaeus Valerius Capito, praefect of upper and lower Egypt to
Tryphon, son of Dionysus, weaver, with weak sight owing to a cataract
Of the metropolis of Oxyrhynchus.
The examination was conducted in Alexandria
The examination was conducted in Alexandria
The examination was conducted in Alexandria

POxy 39

There is disagreement about whether the person being discharged was a soldier or a civilian: Davies believes that the papyri was a military discharge (1969a: 211); Jackson states that it is military as he feels it is evidence of an eye examination being given during recruitment (1996: 2229); Watson suggests that it is civil (1969: 41). No matter if the situation is military or civil, the letter implies that people were examined for problems concerning vision. Nevertheless, there is nothing specific about whether eye-tests were a routine procedure, or only available when a problem was noticed. One would expect that eyesight was an especially important issue for recruitment into the military, and examinations were made throughout the soldier's military career. Yet, this is the only fragment that mentions the possibility, and it seems most likely that Tryphon was a civilian, since he is on a list of the men from the city of Oxyrhynchus rather than being associated with a military unit. Even though this fragment is mentioned frequently in literature concerning military medicine, one cannot say more than the fact that it hints at the possibility of eye examinations in the army.

Vegetius puts forward more possible suggestions about what the recruiting-officer should concentrate on when making the physical examination. The officer was advised to:

> "*Sit ergo adulescens Martio operi deputandus vigilantibus oculis, erecta cervice, lato pectore, umeris musculosis, ualentibus brachiis, digitis longioribus, ventre modicus, exilior clunibus, suris et pedibus non superflua carne distentis sed nervorum duritia collectis*".
>
> "look hard at the face, eyes and entire confirmation of the limbs, to choose an able soldier. The person chosen should have alert eyes, a straight neck, broad chest, muscular shoulders, strong arms, long fingers, small stomach, slender buttocks and calves and feet that are not swollen by surplus fat, but firm with hard muscle." (Veg. *Mil.* 1. 6; Milner Trans)

Milner thinks the suggestions Vegetius provides here are contrived and supposes the criteria for the selection of soldiers was based on the selection of cattle for stock breading because no other literary source presents such precise details. Other sources tend to simply mention the words *statura* and *robur* rather than offering a precise description of the exact specifications that were to be looked for (Veg. *Mil.* note for 1. 6 page 7 number 3). A statement made by Frontinus reports that Pyrrhus remarked to his recruiting officers that it was up to them to choose the big men, but Pyrrhus would make them brave: "*tu grandes elige, ego eos fortes reddam*" (*Strat.* 4. 1. 3; Davies 1969a: 213), illustrating that the physical selection might have incorporated an examination of stature. Again no information is given about the standards that were expected.

According to Vegetius, those who passed the initial selection were then expected to take a second examination that tested their stamina in physical activities. This second test was suggested to have taken place because some recruits may have appeared stronger than they were, or those who might have appeared somewhat weaker may have been more suitable than originally expected:

> "*Sed non statim punctis signorum inscribendus est tiro delectus, verum ante exercitio praetemptandus, ut, utrum vere tanto operi aptus sit, possit agnosci*" (Veg. *Mil.* 1. 8).

This second exam, unlike certain aspects of the *probatio*, is only attested in Vegetius, so Milner is unsure if it ever really existed (1. 8, page 9, note 2). Though it seems as if it should have been part of the exam because soldiers had to be physically capable of training and performing daily duties.

It is difficult to determine whether Vegetius' statements are correct, but it seems likely, depending on the recruiting officer, that some would have considered these aspects when choosing men for the military. On the other hand, even if Vegetius' ideas of how a soldier was chosen do not correspond with the criteria of the recruiting officer, his statements along with the other sources mentioned imply that there was more to the selection of a recruit than height and age.

The description of the ideal body provided by Vegetius seems to conform to the archetypal classical model, if compared with the Greek sculptures of Polykleitos' as described in his *Kanon*, where the body is to be symmetrically balanced (Pollitt 1972: 107-8). This body type is not only represented in Greek depictions, but also in many imperial Roman sculptures from the first two and a half centuries AD, which draw upon the classical Greek tradition. It is seen in sculptures of Roman emperors depicted wearing armour, such as the statue of Augustus from Livia's villa at Prima Porta (Lawrence 1972: 256-7). The representation of soldiers on Trajan's column are also idealised and illustrated with toned muscular bodies (Lawrence 1972: 273). Since the artistic depictions of soldiers' bodies fit the description provided by Vegetius it is possible that the writer's ideas originated from what he saw in the artwork surrounding him. Even though 4th century artwork differed in style from that of the 1st and 2nd centuries, many of the earlier monuments would have been visible. It is likely that active members of the military would have had the body type described by Vegetius, if they carried on with their daily exercises, so he may have discussed what he saw in the military rather than with the recruits.

One must not forget that the Roman officers would not have originated from the same areas of the empire, and they might have brought different ideas or understandings from their society about the ideal recruit. For example, some might have been looking for maturity, or the mental preparedness to fight, whilst others might have concentrated on the physical aspects of the men being examined. This idea is simply a suggestion because there is no literature that mentions this, and it is difficult to assess what the ideal body of people from the provincial areas would have been. Much of the artwork of the provinces and of the soldiers is somewhat 'block-like' or more abstract in form, taking the Adamklissi monument from Dacia as an example (Ramage and Ramage 2000: 198-9, figs 6.17 and 6.18). Provincial art is not always intended to be strictly representative as it is sometimes schematized, which makes a reading of its meaning more difficult. This difference in style may reflect variations of concepts about the body throughout the empire.

A modern example of variation in ideal bodies is seen in the female body. In western societies the ideal female body is depicted on fashion models, who are tall and thin, but in reality few women fit this expectation. In contrast, oriental women, for example, theoretically should be petite. These ideals are not only culturally specific, but are historically constituted. Seventeenth century European art frequently depicts voluptuous women, far from the image of today. Furthermore, women in the European middle ages starved themselves for religious purity and females living in the Victorian era saw an emaciated body as being associated with social superiority (Counihan 1999: 102). Perceptions of an ideal body can change not only from place to place, but from era to era and conform to the social ideologies of the time.

In spite of all these fragments the only certainty is that there was some form of entry requirement in the Roman army, height being the one aspect that appears to have been uniform. Age and physical stature, on the other hand, cannot, at this point, be said to have been standardised.

4.3 Is there Evidence for Soldiers' Health being Maintained?

Once a person was recruited, it would be expected that their health would have been maintained to keep them fit and healthy. In order to impede illness Vegetius describes how preventative measures were taken by the army to maintain a soldier's health. Consideration was given to the environment in which the soldiers lived; the salubriousness of the fortification's location was probably as important as its strategic position: *"loci salubritas eligatur"* (Veg. *Mil.* 1. 22; Davies 1989: 209-12; Jackson 1988: 37). Weather was another factor that concerned Vegetius because he believed, as seen in the medical literature of the time, that heat and cold contributed to health and he suggested precautions for the construction of fortifications. For areas with ample sunlight and heat he recommends tree cover, although in some areas of the frontiers, such as Africa, there may have been a problem complying with this instruction. For cold and damp places a good reserve of firewood is recommended:

> "*Locis, ne in pestilenti regione iuxta morbosas paludes, ne aridis et sine opacitate arborum campis aut collibus, ne sine tentoriis aestate milites commorentur"* (Veg. *Mil.* 3.2).

More importantly, Vegetius stresses that an adequate supply of untainted water was one of the most desirable means of maintaining health, believing that pestilent water was the major cause of disease. Marshes were to be avoided because the tainted waters were comparable to poison that could infect an entire unit:

> "*Nec perniciosis vel palustribus aquis utatur exercitus; nam malae aquae potus, veneno similis, pestilentiam bibentibus generat"* (*Mil.* 3. 2; Johnson 1983: 36).

In support of this, and possibly where Vegetius gained the idea, is a statement by Onasander, who wrote during the reign of Claudius. In discussing the building of a palisaded camp Onosander argues that it must be in a location that is not too marshy, nor damp as rising vapours and rank smell could bring disease:

> "*Τά γὰρ τοιαῦτα ταῖς ἀναφοραῖς καὶ ταῖς ἀπὸ τῶν τόπων δυσωδίαις νόσους καὶ λοιμοὺς ἐμβάλλει στρατεύμασι, καὶ πολλῶν μὲν ἐκάκωσε τὰς εὐεξίας, πολλοὺς δὲ ἀπώλεσεν, ὥστε μὴ μόνον ὀλίγον, ἀλλὰ καὶ ἀσθενὲς ἀπολείπεσθαι στράτευμα"* (The General 8.2).

It is attested in the archaeological evidence that attempts were made by Roman soldiers to avoid water becoming tainted. Cisterns, wells and aqueducts were constructed in and around fortifications (Johnson 1983: 202-6, 208-10). Plumbing has also been found by archaeologists to have been an important feature in the construction of many fortifications (Johnson 1983: 209). Latrines were constructed with a drainage system that flushed bodily waste outside the fortification. They were usually built against a defensive wall, allowing for the drainage to be close to the exterior of the structure, rather than waste to be flushed through the entire site (Johnson 1983: 211-14). Bathing facilities were also commonly located within or nearby fortifications and fresh water was brought into these structures, by aqueducts, springs or rivers (Johnson 1983: 204-6, 209, 210-11). Even in civilian life environmental conditions were important to Roman constructions. Vitruvius mentions placing rooms in houses according to the season that they were to be used so people could receive the best air, shade or sun, depending on what was necessary for their health (6. 4. 1-2). These suggestions were a consideration for the Greeks, as well. One of the Hippocratic writers (Decorum XV) states that the location of the bed of a sick person should be placed in an area according to the season and type of illness. Some illnesses required breezy conditions in which to be cured, whilst others required covered areas. The Hippocratic writer, like Onosander, suggested avoiding malodorous areas because smells can encourage, or aggravate an illness:

> *" 'Εσκέφθαι δὲ χρὴ καὶ τὰ περὶ ἀνακλίσεων, ἅ μὲν αὐτῶν πρὸς τὴν ὥρην, ἅ δὲ πρὸς τὰ γένεα· οἱ μὲν γὰρ αὐτῶν ἐς εὐπνόους, οἱ δὲ ἐς, καταγείους, καὶ σκεπινοὺς τόπους· τά τε ἀπὸ ψόφων καὶ ὀσμῶν, μάλιστα δ' ἀπὸ οἴνου, χειροτέρη γὰρ αὕτη, φυγεῖν δὲ καὶ μετατιθέναι."*
>
> "The bed also must be considered. The season and the kind of illness will make a difference. Some patients are put into breezy spots, others into covered places or underground. Consider also noises and smells, especially the smell of wine." (Trans. Jones Decorum 15)

It is with the issue of health and the environment that one can compare the modern western understanding of health care with that of the Romans. As westerners we are aware that a clean environment is conducive to good health; however, the treatment of an illness in accordance to certain weather conditions and situating architectural structures to the season is something not considered in most modern western medical thought; although exceptions are made in alternative medical treatments. This aspect is mentioned frequently in Roman and Greek literary sources. Archaeologists have not compared buildings, rooms in buildings or even the layout of fortifications to see if there is any evidence of the Romans and soldiers applying rules relating to the positioning of buildings and rooms for reasons of health. Such a study would involve not only comparing the layout and aspect of a structure, but it would require understanding the purpose of a specific room or building. This might sound a simple task, but there are problems with the identification of structures in fortifications and of rooms in buildings (Chapter 6). Only when more thorough studies of room function are made can this task be undertaken by archaeologists, who could then make comparisons of fortifications in different areas of the empire to see if all units used the same rules when constructing fortifications and buildings. Such a study would further scholars' understandings of how health care was incorporated into the daily lives of those living in the Roman empire.

Besides the prophylactic measures suggested for construction, exercise was recommended not only for training, but also as a means of preserving health. Exercise in armour was thought to be better for soldiers' health than a visit to the doctor, so the infantry and cavalry were advised to train on a daily basis, and they were even expected to do so during inclement weather; although, they might have performed indoors or under some form of covering (Veg. *Mil.* 1. 9, 1. 10, 1. 19), perhaps in a basilica such as that found at the baths at Caerleon (Zienkiewicz 1986). Their exercises also involved plenty of manual labour, which would have contributed to their physical fitness. Overall, soldiers were advised to be frequently involved in the felling of trees, carrying burdens, jumping ditches, swimming in the sea or rivers, marching at full step or even running in their armour and with their packs (Veg. *Mil.* 1. 9, 1. 10, 1. 19). In his manual, Vegetius states that Augustus and Hadrian expected the infantry and cavalry to proceed with a march three times a month. The infantry was commanded to advance ten Roman miles at the military step, armed and equipped with all their weapons and then retire to camp with parts of the march being completed at a brisker running pace:

> *"Praeterea et vetus consuetudo permansit et divi Augusti atque Hadriani constitutionibus praecavetur, ut ter in mense tam equites quam pedites educantur ambulatum; hoc enim verbo hoc exercitii genus nominant. Decem milia passuum armati instructique omnibus telis pedites militari gradu ire ac redire iubebantur in castra, ita ut aliquam*

intineris partem cursu alacriore conficerent" (*Mil.* 1. 27).

Discharges were given by doctors to soldiers whose suffering prevented them from continuing with their military career. A specific military example is noted for a group of soldiers from Vindobona (Vienna) who were dismissed because of ill health (P. Rainer 165). A military diploma from Bulgaria was given to a group as an honourable discharge because they had sustained injuries in a battle (CIL XVI 10 of 70 mart 7). The *Codex Iustinianus* states that men released from the army on grounds of ill health after serving 20 years were entitled to the official privileges granted to veteran soldiers (5. 65.1 AD 213 in Campbell 1994: 204). The seriousness of the discharge is demonstrated in the *Codex* by the fact that those who had been dismissed would not be given the opportunity to return to the army once a doctor had judged them seriously ill (12. 35 (36) 6 in Campbell 1994: 204). That doctors were able to discharge soldiers on grounds of ill health is a demonstration that precautions were taken in the army to keep the seriously ill or wounded from becoming a burden to the unit, and it would allow for soldiers to recover properly. In spite of all the possible suggestions for preventative measures, soldiers still fell ill, or became wounded, so the question is what is known about how these soldiers were cared for?

4.4 Who might have Provided Medical Care to the Soldiers?

If a soldier became ill medical treatment was supposed to have been provided to him for free (*S.H.A.* Aurelian 7.8). The question raised by this statement is who were the people providing the medical treatment? One of the most common views of military doctors is that the majority were of Greek origin (e.g. Boon 1987: 54; Johnson 1983: 159 and to some extent Salazar 2000: 79). Since some of the first doctors to be recorded in Italy who did not follow the local medical traditions were Greek, there is an opinion that the majority of doctors in Rome had to be Greek. This is also expected to be the case in the Roman army (Callies 1968). When looking at the names of military doctors on inscriptions, using Wilmanns' prospopography (1995b: 141-252) some have Greek names, but not all of them do. Some have Latin names, and others have a combination of names in both Greek and Latin. From the comparison it does not seem that there are any dates that specifically apply to when doctors with Greek or Roman names were more common in the military. The doctors with specific types of names do not seem to have been associated with a particular area within the empire either. From the 93 inscriptions mentioned by Wilmanns there is no doctor with a particular cultural background that was particularly favoured over another in the Roman army. There is also no indication that the legionary or auxiliary units favoured a doctor with a specific background. For example, units stationed in the city of Rome, where one might expect more doctors with Greek names, had doctors with Latin names (e.g. CIL VI 37194=ILS 9071, CIL VI 2532=ILS 2093, CIL VI 2594, CIL VI 179, CIL 31145+p.3069).

It is also advisable not to judge the ethnicity of the doctors by their names because they may have had a Greek name and culturally envisioned themselves to be Roman, as they might have lived in Rome or in a Roman style. A modern example of the difficulty in using names as a cultural indicator can be seen in American names. Being American I have what is often termed as an Ellis Island name, one where the surname was changed upon entry into the United States. I do not have a true Ellis Island name because my surname was not changed until about a century after that side of the family emigrated. My surname, Baker, is anglicised, yet its origin is German. My German ancestors emigrated from Hamburg to Philadelphia in 1751 and kept the name Becker until they converted from Lutheranism to Catholicism in the 19th century, the conversion of religion was made because a Becker married into a Catholic family, and we assume the name was changed by my ancestors to sound more American. Moreover, the German side of the family has been in America longer than the Italian, Irish, English and Dutch sides. As a family we would associate ourselves more with our Italian and Irish ancestors because these were the countries where four of my great grandparents were born and their languages were spoken by my grandparents. Yet, although I might say I am Italian, Irish, English, Dutch and German, I have no real contact with these places. Ultimately I consider myself American - an American living in England - which further complicates my identity because I do not consider myself to be British in spite of having lived in the country for almost ten years. My personal experience, or identity crisis, exemplifies the complex issues in a name; a person's identity is not always dependent upon their name or the place they inhabit. Only two inscriptions from the frontiers in question have the home of the doctor inscribed on them, and their homes are not representative of their names. There is one with a Greek name, Zosimus, but his home was Ostia (Appendix 2, number 10). Whether he considered himself Greek or Roman is not certain, nor is the form of his medical practice. It seems that since he took the Roman title *medicus* he might have operated in a more Roman style of healing, but one must be careful when saying this because the doctors may have spoken Latin, but possessed non-Roman understandings of medical treatment. Another doctor named Aemilius Deciminus worked in Adium near Brigetio in Pannonia Superior, but came from Germania Inferior (Appendix 2, number 22). He has a Latin name, but it can be questioned whether his home area dictated his medical thinking. Since most inscriptions do not have the home of the doctors written on them, one cannot determine their place of origin. It may be said that not all doctors were Greek, and that one cannot judge the sort of medical traditions they followed because of their names.

It has already been shown in Chapter 2 that medical care was provided to Roman soldiers, and more evidence has come to light in the form of a writing tablet from Vindolanda (Bowman and Thomas 1991: 93-4). The tablet is a daily strength report for the first cohort of Tungrians that lists soldiers who were available for their daily duties and those who were absent. The report (Inv. No. 88/841 period I dital) was found in the pre-Hadrianic area of Vindolanda, located in a ditch in the west defences of the earliest phase of the fort. The ditch appears to have been filled by AD 90/92 and would probably reflect the situation at Vindolanda a few years after the departure of Agricola (Bowman and Thomas 1991: 62, 66; Bowman and Thomas 1994: 93-4, 98). The heading of the report contains the date, the unit's name, the commanding officer's name and the total strength of the unit. Following this, it displays a list of the numbers of soldiers absent from the fort, followed by a total of those who remained in the camp. Of the remaining soldiers there is a roster of those who were unfit for duty listed in categories according to the reason for their absence. Fifteen men were recorded as sick (*aegri*), six were listed as wounded (*vulnerati*) and ten as having eye problems (*lippientes*), leaving 265 men to perform routine duties in the camp (Bowman and Thomas 1991: 66-9; 1994: 93-4). It might be implied from the tablet that there was some form of separation of soldiers in accordance with their illness, since it is curious why those unfit for duty were divided into three groups. One possibility for this division is that there were different doctors available to treat people placed in these three groups. In support of specialists, Galen does mention an eye doctor having been associated with a naval unit (Appendix 2, number 40), so it is possible that a specialist might have worked at Vindolanda. Another suggestion may be that the division corresponded to places where the different groups were being treated, and rather than having different doctors the patients were excluded from certain areas on account of their problems. Another possibility is that the divisions meant both the doctor and places for treatment were different for each group of patients. It must also be considered that this division might have been the means by which the Tungrians categorised illness in accordance with their particular beliefs and understandings of illness and its treatment, and such a division was not applied in all of the units across the frontiers.

It is clear from the inscriptions that there were several types of doctor and supplementary medical personnel in the Roman world. Although the evidence for them is variable, scholars such as Davies and Wilmanns have attempted to discern some form of structure to the rank and organisation of the doctors (Davies 1969b; 1972; 1974: 306-7; Wilmanns 1995 a & b). It seems that medical care in each fortification was the responsibility of the tribune or the *praefectus castrorum,* an official, junior in rank to the commanding officer and responsible for the logistics of the legion (Davies 1969b: 84; 1974: 306; 1989: 212; Wilmanns 1995a: 75-7). According to Vegetius the position of *praefectus castrorum* carried the responsibility of providing care for the sick and being in command of the *medici* (*Mil.* 2. 10). The *Digest of Justinian* also mentioned that one of the jobs of the *praefectus* was to inspect the sick (49. 16. 12. 2 Trans. Watson). However, it is the medical personnel below the *praefectus* whose positions are not clearly understood, as their rank and status are not described or only briefly mentioned in the ancient sources, or on inscriptions. It appears that the camp commander was responsible for the doctors and making sure that medical care was provided to the soldiers.

The doctors mentioned most are those who were placed on the list of *immunes* quoted in the *Digest of Justinian* under the laws on military matters by Tarrutienus Paternus (L 6, 7; Watson Trans; Davies 1969b: 84; 1974: 306-7; 1989: 212). The *immunes* were soldiers designated with special tasks that allowed them to be dismissed from regular duties, yet they did not benefit from a higher rate of pay, receiving the same rate as the *munifex.* The medical personnel listed as *immunes* were the *optiones valetudinarii, medici, capsarii* and *qui aegris praesto sunt* (those who were responsible for the sick). The list also shows that doctors recorded along with a large category of other specialists, such as architects, veterinarians, arrow makers, carpenters, stonemasons and librarians. Because there may appear to be some form of ranking to the list of doctors, it is easy for modern scholars to make the assumption that ranks were inflexible in the Roman army. However, Wilmanns points out that rank in the Roman army was more variable and complex compared with modern military groups (1995b: 53).

The persons holding the title *optiones valetudinarii* have been interpreted to have been in charge of the administration of the hospital and those who worked within it (Davies 1969a: 84). It is not even certain if this person did anything medical, except for possibly running the hospital, perhaps being someone more like an administrator. Inscriptions mentioning this position have only been found in legionary fortresses (Wilmanns 1995a: 117-19), and for the area covered in this study they have been found at Bonna and Aquincum (Appendix 2, numbers 1, 25, 26). Outside the area of study, one inscription was found in Rome (CIL VI 175) and two in the legionary fortress at Lambaesis in Africa (CIL VIII 2563; CIL VIII 2553). Wilmanns mentions an inscription for an *optio convalescentum* that was found in Lugdunum for a cohors urbana (1995b: 117; CIL VI 1057). Perhaps this position was similar to the *optio valetudinarii*, but it could literally mean a person in charge of those regaining strength or recovering, whilst the other seems to be in charge of running the hospital. It may be that the cohors urbana, an urban unit, did not have a hospital, and therefore would not have needed an *optio valetudinarii*. Perhaps rather than ordering supplies for the hospital, the *optio convalescentum* ordered supplies for the doctors who used them on the patients in a number of places, such as the barracks or even the doctor's 'office'. Maybe they arranged for the ill soldiers to stay with someone in the city to convalesce. Since the only known *optiones valetudinarii* are from legionary fortresses it might be suggested that the medical organisation in these places needed more administrative staff because of the higher number of people living within them (Wilmanns 1995b: 117). *Valetudinaria* are known to have existed, but whether they existed in all fortifications is not clear. Obviously if units did not have a *valetudinarium* there would be no need for someone to run it. It is also possible that a person was not needed to run every *valetudinaria*, which could also explain the small numbers of inscriptions mentioning the *optio valetudinarii*.

The *capsarii* are believed to have been responsible for the care of minor injuries and cleaning wounds because the name refers to a box or *capsus* that was used to hold bandages (Davies 1969b: 83; Wilmanns 1995b: 122). Trajan's column has a depiction of a man in armour helping to bandage a wounded soldier, and the scene has been the source of much debate. It is often argued that it is a representation of a *capsarius* (Davies 1969: 84; Jackson 1988: 132; Wilmanns 1995b: 135). However, Scarborough maintains that it is not a doctor because the person is wearing armour, and this he feels is proof that there was no systematic medical care available to the soldiers, except the help of other soldiers (1968: 254). One could probably expect that anyone helping soldiers while in the midst of battle would probably be wearing armour to avoid being injured themselves. Wilmanns, on the other hand, says that *capsarii* were so commonly known that anyone would have recognised one on the column (1995b: 135), yet, they might have also recognised the figure as a soldier helping the wounded. There is some evidence that soldiers knew first aid. Dionysius of Halicarnassus mentions that soldiers knew how to bandage themselves because sometimes they did it to avoid active duty "*κατεδήσαντο γὰρ αὐτῶν οἱ πολλοί τοὺς ὑγιεῖς χρῶτας ὡς τραυματίαι·*"(IX. 50. 5), and this is proof to Scarborough that the depiction is of a soldier (1968: 254). Whatever the depiction on Trajan's column might be, there are still inscriptions surviving from auxiliary, legionary and *numerus* units that mention the *capsarii*. Overall the *capsarii* were probably minor doctors or medics, but their work is deemed important enough to allow them to be excluded from the regular duties of a soldier. Wilmanns argues that they were part of the medical corp (*Sanitätsdienst*) (1995b: 74; 1995a: 173) that consisted of minor doctors who were more likely to have worked with the auxiliary units. She believes that the auxiliary groups would probably not have needed as many *medici* because there were fewer people stationed in the forts (1995a: 174). In spite of her argument they do appear in all types of units, including a *collegium* from the legionary fortress at Lambaesis (CIL VIII 2553). Since some units seem to have numbers of them, rather than one, it may be that their jobs were somewhat like modern nurses. King argues that in the Greek medical tradition, nursing would have been the job of the doctor as a means of controlling his or her patient, or rather the control of the care (1991: 19). However, in the army where there were more people it is possible that a nursing position, if that is what it was, might also have been useful in units with large numbers of soldiers where extra help would have been necessary.

The duties of the persons designated as those who care for the sick may have been as simple as feeding and comforting the sick, possibly suggesting that their medical knowledge was minimal (Davies 1969b: 84; 1974: 306-7; Wilmanns 1995b: 55). There is no further supporting evidence for this position, but there is a papyrus fragment of a letter from a soldier named Terentianus apologising to his father for not having been in touch because he along with the entire unit had suffered from an outbreak of food poisoning because they consumed rancid fish (P. Mich 478 in Davies 1971: 130). In an earlier letter to this one, commented on by Davies, Terentianus apparently told his father that he had to be fed by others (1971: 130). This could have been performed by the person mentioned on the list of *immunes*, who may have been employed only to help when the need arose. It is also possible that the person mentioned in the letter was simply another soldier who was not ill and helping the doctors.

The *medici* are the most common type of doctor mentioned on inscriptions; yet the duties of the *medici* are difficult to describe because there are a number of discussions by medical writers such as Galen and Celsus who tell of different expectations of doctors. To complicate the situation further, some doctors have titles added that differentiate them from the standard *medicus* such as *ordinarius, miles* and *duplicarius*. The standard *medici* inscriptions are found throughout the empire in both military and civilian contexts. As for their careers in the military, Davies and Wilmanns believe that they could have served various lengths of time, and there does not seem to have been a set number of years a person was expected to remain in the military as a doctor as there was for soldiers (Davies 1969b: 83-6; 1989: 214; Wilmanns 1995b: 85). The length of time spent in the army would allow for more training and possibly for more security regarding payment, as, unlike civilian doctors, army doctors were guaranteed a salary (Wilmanns 1995b: 101).

The *medicus ordinarius* is noted on inscriptions throughout the frontiers and according to both Davies and Wilmanns may have the same rank as a centurion, believing the word *ordinarius* is synonymous with the title centurion (Davies 1969b: 89; Wilmanns 1995a: 175-6; 1995b: 80-8). Davies also states that in a general context an *ordinarius* had a higher status than the average medical orderly (Davies 1969b: 89). It is possible that these soldiers had a permanent position in the army and made it a lifetime career, giving them the title (Davies 1989: 214), which might be supported by one inscription of an *ordinarius* from Lambaesis who was an octogenarian (CIL VIII 18314). Nonetheless, Nutton notes that there is no indication as to what the rank actually meant (1969: 268). The four known *ordinarii* on the western Roman frontiers have been found in fortifications of the three types of units: legionary, auxiliary and *numerus* (Appendix 2, numbers 7; 18; 22; 39). This particular rank of doctor may have existed in other regions of the empire, but there is no evidence to suggest that it did, which might indicate that perhaps this was a position particular to the military on the frontiers. Since the *ordinarius* is attested from a variety of units it seems that the calibre of medical care did not differ between units, but at the same time it need not indicate that there was a standard organisation of care across the frontiers.

The rank and role of the *miles medicus* is not entirely understood. Only two are known of from the area of study (Appendix 2; numbers 2, 32), and there is another possible example from Poetovio (Appendix 2, number 23), an interior military colony in Pannonia Superior. According to Nutton there is the possibility that the soldier was proud of being both a soldier and a doctor so he maintained both titles placed on his tomb, or that he was a soldier who had gained medical training whilst in the army (1969: 267-8). Since the general term *medicus* was on the list of *immunes* there might be the possibility that a *miles medicus* was made exempt from regular duties because he was a doctor who gained his training as a soldier. Davies suggests it was a medical orderly who possessed the basic knowledge and skill with the art of healing (1989: 214). Perhaps the person holding this position performed the daily duties of a soldier, but was only employed as a doctor when there were high numbers of casualties. A *miles medicus* is recorded on an inscription at Iversheim, a legionary kiln works near Bonn (Appendix 2, number 2; Wilmanns 1995b: 77). It might be that he was mainly a soldier who had medical training and was sent out to do the same work as the others at the kiln, but in case of an emergency he could then take on the role of a doctor and be made exempt from his regular duties until the situation had passed.

There are other types of military doctors mentioned on inscriptions, but not in the frontier areas concerned, providing an even stronger suggestion that there were variations in medical care between unit types and areas of the empire. Domaszewski argues that urban units and units stationed in Rome had *medici* with higher positions, as they were placed along with officers and senior commanders on inscriptions (1908: 15, 26). This may be comparable to the Praetorian Guard being the highest order of soldiers because of their close proximity to the centre of the empire. If Domaszewski is correct, urban military doctors might have been of higher rank, and he suggests that they were probably of a higher standard because of this. His argument is typical of a core-periphery understanding that the centre of the empire was somehow more sophisticated, with aspects of life of a higher quality than those on the frontier (Webster 1999: 24-5). However, the location of the doctors does not imply quality, nor does it imply rank, as those who were stationed on the frontiers might have been equal to or better than their counterparts in Rome.

Rather than seeing the doctors in the urban units as being of higher calibre and having a higher rank, it seems more plausible that they served the needs of their unit. There are three types of medics listed on inscriptions from urban military units not found on the frontiers thus far: *medicus castrensis, medicus clinicus* and *medicus chirurgicus*. The *medicus castrensis* is mentioned twice: in a unit of *equites singulares* from Rome (CIL VI 31,172), and the other was from a cohort stationed in Lugdunum (CIL XIII 1833). The title translates literally to camp doctor. The rank is not clear, but if the physician was a camp doctor perhaps it means that he was in charge of all the other medical care in the troop. There are two other types of medics only found in urban units. A *medicus clinicus* was also listed as belonging to the Praetorian Cohort in Rome (CIL VI 2532). This position was thought by Davies to have been a doctor who specialised in internal ailments (1969b: 87; 1989: 214). Rome was a large city and could probably support a specialist, so it may be that the *clinicus* was living and working with civilians in Rome, but also worked for the army. Another specialist associated with the Italian troops was the *medicus chirurgicus* (*AE* 1945: 62), probably a doctor who specifically performed surgical operations, or at least that is what seems likely to have been his or her main concern.

Furthermore, there is also evidence for other types of specialists, few of which have been found in the epigraphic and literary evidence of the western frontiers and some of the positions might not have been entirely medical. An eye-doctor is mentioned in Galen as being attached to the *Classis Britannica* (Appendix 2, number 40). A possible administrative position was the *seplasiarius*, who was responsible for ordering ointments. Wilmanns does not believe that they were medical (1995b: 123), but the term is rather ambiguous and there is the possibility that the *seplasiarius* did order ointments used in medical treatments, so the existence of the position shall not be ruled out entirely. One inscription was found at the legionary fortress in Mainz, and perhaps, similar to the role taken by the *optio valetudinarii*, the *seplasiarius* was acting as extra administrative help in a unit of many people and ordered ointments for both medical and non-medical needs. Another administrative position recorded was the *librarius*. The person holding this title looked after the paperwork for the entire unit rather than for a single part of the fortification, such as the hospital (Davies 1989: 212). It is probable that a smaller unit might have depended upon the *librarius* for ordering medical supplies, rather than an *optio convalescentum, valetudinarius* or *seplasiarius*.

There also seemed to have been veterinary specialists in the army. Since veterinarians are not concerned with the health of the people stationed in the unit, it is pointless to mention them in detail here. However, a horse doctor, not known in any other unit, is mentioned on an inscription of a cavalry unit stationed in Egypt (IGRR I 1373). This may be a further indication that army units were provided with the choice of deciding which type of medical care they desired, or needed.

The descriptions of the types of doctors presented above are mainly those given by Wilmanns and Davies. However, the descriptions and understandings of the positions are tenuous, as there is very little available evidence, besides the pay scale, to understand the rank of the doctors, if there was one. Moreover, there is much ambiguity about whether some of the positions were medical, such as with the *seplasiarius*. Even though scholars present interesting interpretations about what the titles might have stood for, their explanations do not bring us closer to supporting the belief that there was a single system of medical care throughout the army. It seems that there is actually more evidence to support differences within the medical care system, as the various titles of *medici* and healers are fairly random in their placement.

4.5 Medical Education

One might also not expect a uniform system of medical treatment in the army because medical education was not standardised at that time. Since there was no standardised medical education in the Roman world or regulations over education anyone could set him or herself up as a practising doctor. Information about the different ways one could learn the skills of healing is, again, only available in fragmentary accounts. One manner in which people could become doctors was through an apprenticeship (Drabkin 1944: 336-7), which is supported by Martial, who describes students travelling with doctors to observe patients. He found some to be bothersome, as he says that when he was feeling ill, the doctor's visit with his hundred students made him feel worse due to the students touching him with their cold hands, presumably to gain experience:

> "*Languebam: sed tu comitatus protinus ad me venisti Symmache discipulis centum me tetigere manus Aquilone geltae non habui febrem, Symmache, nunc habeo*" (5. 9).

Another possible means for gaining a medical background was for students to visit *auditoria* specifically set up for medical training. According to the author of the *Scriptores Historia Augusta* on Severus Alexander (44. 4): *auditoria*, perhaps meaning schools, were available for the study of the arts, including medicine, "..*Medicis...salaria instituit et auditoria decrevit*" (44. 4). The location of the *auditoria* was not described in the text, but it might be presumed that the author was referring to places in the larger cities and on certain islands.

The island of Kos and the city of Alexandria were known for their medical 'schools'; however, not every person intending to be a doctor would have received their training in these places.

Anatomical study, as discussed, was difficult at certain periods in Greek and Roman times because there were debates over the ethical issues of practising dissection and vivisection on humans. Celsus believed that dissection of bodies was advantageous; however, he did not agree with vivisection (*de med.* Proem. 40-44). Romans did have some knowledge of human anatomy because dissection and vivisection were practised during the Hellenistic period in Alexandria, and some doctors would have had access to these studies in libraries. The Romans, on the other hand, were not practising dissection on humans and they had many unanswered questions about how the body functioned. According to Galen military doctors were sometimes fortunate because they could dissect the bodies of fallen enemies, and he comments on a specific instance where this was done to Germanic warriors.

> "*κατὰ γοῦν πολλὴν σχολὴν οἱ ἀνατομικώτατοι τῶν ἰατρῶν ἐπισκοπούμενοι τὰ μόρια τοῦ σώματος, ἐν πολλοῖς ἐσφαλμένοι φαίνονται διόπερ οὐδ' οἱ βουληθέντες ἀνατέμνειν σῶμα πολεμίου Γερμανοῦ τεθνεῶτος ἐπὶ τοῦ κατὰ Μάρκον Ἀντωνῖνον πολέμου πλέον ἠδονήθησαν τι μαθεῖν τῆς τῶν σπλάγχνων θέσεως*" (2. 385 K,).

Scarborough believes this statement is an indication that military doctors were not trained until they entered the army, and their reliance upon fallen enemies attests to a lack of proper training and knowledge of human anatomy (1976: 74). However, it is possible that Scarborough is too stringent, as doctors may have been trained, but simply wished to gain a better understanding of the physiology of the body.

Furthermore, the study of medicine was complicated by the fact that the field was divided into different areas. Celsus informs us that the study of medicine was divided into three main areas - dietetics, drugs and surgery:

> "*Iisdemque temporibus in tres partes medicina diducta est, ut una esset quae victu, altera quae medicamentis, tertia quae manu mederetur*" (Cels. Proem 9.5; Jackson 1995: 192).

This is repeated by Galen:

> "*... τό τε χειρουργικὸν λέγω καὶ φαρμακευτικόν, καὶ διατητικόν, καὶ μάλιστά γε τὸ κατὰ χειρουργίαν ἀμφοτέρων τῶν ἄλλων*" (13. 604 K).

It may be that these three areas were studied by many people who intended to become doctors or that some doctors only studied one of these areas. To support this uncertainty over the way specialisms were divided Baader (1967: 233-4) mentions that Galen described a number of other specialists, such as those who were interested in eye diseases, ear disorders, dentistry, throat operations, hernia, anal complaints, fever, dieting and hydrotherapy (On the Parts of Medicine 1.3. 2-1, translated from the Arabic by Lyons; Baader 1967: 233 note 64).

For surgical experience, it was recommended in the Hippocratic work on the *Physician* (9. 219 L) for doctors to join the army because they would have a greater opportunity to observe injuries and to learn how to treat them through surgery:

> "*ξυμβαίνε δὲ τὰ τοιαῦτα πλειστάκις καὶ ξυνεχέστατα περὶ τὰς ξενικὰς στρατιὰς γίνεσθαι.*"

Both Celsus and Galen also mentioned the skills a doctor and surgeon was to have. According to Celsus:

> "Esse autem chirurgus debet adulescens aut certe adulescentiae propior; manu strenua, stabili, nec umquam intremescente, eaque non minus sinistra quam dextra promptus; acie oculorum acri claraque; animo intrepidus; misericors sic, ut saniari velit eum, quem accepit, non ut clamore eius motus vel minus quam necesse est secet; sed perinde faciat omnia, ac si nullus ex vagitibus alterius adfectus oriatur."

> "surgeons had to be youthful, or at any rate nearer youth than age; with a strong and steady left hand as well as right; with vision sharp and clear, and spirit undaunted; filled with pity, so that he wishes to cure his patient, yet is not moved by the cries to go too fast or less than necessary; but he does everything just as if the cries of pain cause him no emotion" (7 Proem. 4, Trans. Spencer).

Galen suggested that "practitioners should merely be equipped with all the necessary drugs, foods, drinks and instruments to meet anything that might happen to the patient, it is their duty to foresee anything that might happen to the patient" (*de opti med. cogn.* 2, 6 Trans. Iskandar). Both explain that doctors had to be intelligent and skilful as well as caring, yet one can never be certain how much of this was adhered to.

An ambiguous picture is therefore given about medical education and divisions within the art. When doctors or healers who were trained outside the Roman medical sphere encountered doctors with what we would consider Roman medical training, it is likely that they would have seen different styles of practice, developed through a variety of methods of learning. Such distinctions, it is conjectured, may have made others wary of Roman medicine, reinforcing their faith in their own medical practices, which can tentatively be implied in the initial names of the units adopting the use of medical inscriptions. Moreover, if healers in other societies appropriated certain aspects of 'Roman' medical practices from one doctor, what they learned might not have been practised by another who had a different type of training.

4.6 A Comparison of Medical Inscriptions from the Northwestern Frontiers

Having established that we have a very imprecise picture of how the doctors were organised, if they even were, it is now necessary to examine the inscriptions mentioning medical personnel from the western frontiers to ascertain more specifically whether certain units or particular areas were receiving more, or different, care in contrast to others. Although the sample of inscriptions is small, it provides a point on which to start such an investigation. There are only about 93 military inscriptions in total (this number is from Wilmanns' interpretations), but there is much that can still be said about the topic. The inscriptions are mainly from altars, tombs and unknown fragments that were found in a number of areas both within and around the fortifications. The inscriptions that are known may not be representative of the original number or distribution. There are a number of possible reasons why the numbers of inscriptions in the archaeological record are low: many might have been re-used; inscriptions might only have been set up by people or units that had more money or had more of a tradition for erecting inscriptions than others. Wood was sometimes used instead of stone, which does not survive well in the archaeological record. Sometimes the legions are thought to have had more inscriptions, but in the case of medical ones a number of legionary units in the area of study: Vienna, Nijmegen, York, Caerleon and Xanten - do not have medical inscriptions and many of the other fortresses only have one or two. Perhaps there was not a great tradition for medical inscriptions, or perhaps it was simply the preference of the unit or the doctor as to whether these were set up. Whatever the reason for the small number, this should not be a deterrent in attempting to ask new questions. It is possible that patterns can begin to appear even with a limited amount of evidence.

Overall there are 42 medical inscriptions from the area of study (Appendix 2); however only 32 of these are definitely military. The remaining ten inscriptions mentioned might be military: one of these (Appendix 2, number 42) will be discussed in chapter 6; three are not in the area of study, but have some bearing on the arguments (Appendix 2, numbers 4, 23, 41); and the others (Appendix 2, numbers 14, 15, 16, 17, 40, 41) might have a relationship with the military and will be discussed when necessary. There are variations in the number of inscriptions between the frontiers. Of those relating to identifiable military doctors and medical staff, three were found in Germania Inferior (Appendix 2, Table A1); Germania Superior has nine (Appendix 2 Table A2); Raetia one (Appendix 2, Table A3); Noricum one (Appendix 2, Table A4); Pannonia Superior two (Appendix 2, Table A5); Pannonia Inferior 12 (Appendix 2, Table A6) and Britannia has four (Appendix 2, Table A7). There is an obvious difference between the numbers of inscriptions that have been found in each of the provinces, and to attempt to understand why this might be a few comparisons must be made. The first is to see if there were specific types of doctors or medical staff only found in specific areas or units. Of the medical personnel the *medici* are the most commonly mentioned on the inscriptions. Thirteen are mentioned for the legions (Appendix 2 numbers 6, 11, 12, 19, 21, 24, 27, 28, 29, 30, 33, 36, 37), and five are definitely known from auxiliary units in the area of study (Appendix 2, numbers 3, 8, 9, 10, 38). There is one inscription that might have been associated with an auxiliary unit in Germania Superior (Appendix 2, number 14), but it was found in Italy, and the doctor is mentioned as having worked in two units. It has been placed under Germania Superior on account of Wilmanns' interpretation. Its exact date is not known either, but it is given one tentatively to the 2nd century (1995b: 194-6). Without knowing the exact location of the units given on the inscription, or an exact date of when this doctor worked for the units, it is impossible to say exactly where the unit was stationed at the time the doctor worked for them. Importantly though, this inscription indicates that doctors were able to move to different units whilst they served in the army. From this comparison the evidence shows that the *medici* worked in a range of units on the frontiers of Pannonia Inferior, Noricum, Germania Superior and Inferior and

Britannia. Pannonia Superior is the only province that does not have an inscription of a *medicus*.

The *medicus ordinarius* appears in all types of units. For the legions, one was found near Brigettio in Pannonia Superior (Appendix 2, number 15) and in Regensburg (Appendix 2, number 22). Wilmanns argues that another was found in Regensburg (Appendix 2, number 17), but there is so little of the inscription surviving that one cannot be too sure if it referred to a *medicus ordinarius*. As for other units, one was found in the auxiliary fort at Housesteads (Appendix 2, number 39) and another at the *numerus* fort of Niederbieber (Appendix 2, number 7). As the number of inscriptions for this type of doctor is less than the common *medicus* perhaps it was, as has been suggested, of higher rank, or simply not common in the army. Since inscriptions for the *medicus ordinarius* appear in a couple of provinces, it does not seem to be specific to one area. Even though more appear in the legions, it is not specific to them, indicating that whatever the rank of the doctor might have been it was not exclusive to the legions.

Two inscriptions relating to the *miles medicus* are known from the area of study. One was from Aquincum and the other was found at the kiln works at Iversheim near Bonn (Appendix 2, numbers 2, 32). There is potentially one from Poetovio, a veteran's colony, that has an inscription mentioning a *medicus miles* (Appendix 2, number 23). This person had also worked for a legionary unit, so perhaps he too was a soldier who only helped to cure people when there was a need of extra help.

The *capsarii* are found on legionary inscriptions (Appendix 2, numbers 13, 20, 31), auxiliary inscriptions (Appendix 2, numbers 34, 35), and on one from the *numerus* unit of Niederbieber (Appendix 2, number 7). Wilmanns states that this is the one that would be more prevalent in the smaller units (1995a: 173; 1995b: 73), though this does not account for the presence of *capsarii* inscriptions from three of the legions. These epigraphic remains are only known from Germania Superior, Pannonia Inferior and Superior and Africa, possibly suggesting that *capsarii* were restricted to specific areas, or units that considered them a necessary component of their medical staff.

The *optiones valetudinarii* are only known from legionary inscriptions (Appendix 2, numbers 1, 25, 26). Since they are not found in the auxiliary units it might mean that the position was only needed because of the larger number of people living in the fortresses. Inscriptions relating to these are only known from Pannonia Inferior and Germania Inferior.

The information provided by the comparison of the inscriptions suggests that there were no differences over which type of units received health care. The auxiliary, legionary and *numerus* groups, from the limited inscriptions, appear to have had a fairly equal calibre of doctors offered to them. The legions have evidence for a wider variety of medical staff than the other two types of units. With the exception of the ten inscriptions from Aquincum, the numbers of inscriptions per legionary fortress is fairly equal, usually one or two in number, to that of the auxiliary units.

As mentioned above, the numbers of medically related inscriptions vary between the frontiers. In the case of Raetia and Noricum inscriptions only appear for the legionary fortresses that were constructed after the Marcommanic Wars and none appear in the auxiliary units from the two provinces. The other province that does not have inscriptions associated with the auxiliary units is Pannonia Superior. In these three provinces it is possible that there were medical personnel stationed at the auxiliary units, but no inscriptions remain if they were even erected. It is also possible that the limited evidence of medical inscriptions from this area suggests that medical care was not provided in the units, or if it were, it was not the Roman style medicine scholars expect to be found in all fortifications, but something based on the cultural background of the unit. In Raetia and Noricum it may be that the military events of the Marcomannic war prompted the introduction of medical inscriptions, or Roman medical treatment, into the two provinces.

Germania Superior has the highest number of inscriptions and the greatest number of fortifications with inscriptions. This might be because overall it has the largest number of military installations in the area of study, and since it was one of the more active military areas, units might have had found it necessary to employ doctors. Britannia and Germania Inferior are fairly equal in their numbers of epigraphic material. From this general observation one can say that the arguments provided by Wilmanns and Davies about how the system of medical care was organised do not apply to the military as a whole. There are differences in the numbers of inscriptions between provinces, which might be a result of the number of fortifications per province. Provincial variations also appear in the types of units associated with medical inscriptions. Some provinces only have inscriptions from legionary fortresses, whilst Britannia has more from auxiliary forts and the numbers are fairly equal between units in Germania Superior. Thus the results of this comparison may indicate that there was not a standard organised system of medical care. The medical care offered to the units seems to have been fairly equal in the types of doctors working in the different types of fortifications: legionary, auxiliary and *numerus* units, for example *medici ordinarii*, thought to be of higher rank, were found in all three units. Yet, each province varies with respect to one another in the fortification types that had medical personnel and in the numbers of staff.

4.7 Are the Dates of the Inscriptions Indicative of any Patterns of Standardisation?

There might be the possibility that the dates of the inscriptions can provide more clues about why differences occur between the frontiers and units. Overall, the inscriptions date mainly from the mid-2nd and 3rd centuries AD. Very few of these can be dated precisely. For the frontiers, the inscriptions from Pannonia Inferior date to the 2nd and 3rd centuries, Pannonia Superior to the late 1st or early 2nd centuries, the inscriptions of the doctors from Noricum and Raetia date to the late 2nd century after the legionary fortresses were constructed. The inscriptions from Germania Superior range from the 1st to the 3rd centuries. Wilmanns argues that the higher numbers of inscriptions dating from the 2nd and 3rd centuries is an indication of an acceptance of Romanisation (1995b: 133-4). If there was a vast acceptance of Roman style medical treatment it seems that a wider variety of units would have had doctors referred to on inscriptions, especially if the units were becoming permanently settled in certain areas, as do those from Germania Inferior. Britannia's inscriptions date to the 2nd and 3rd centuries. In general, the dates span the times when the frontiers were becoming more settled, as Pannonia Superior's line did not advance after the early 1st century and the inscriptions date to that period, whilst the remaining frontiers were either created or became more permanent in the 2nd century. Those that date to the 1st century are from Germany and Pannonia Superior, regions that were fortified earlier, and the fortresses from which they come - Carnuntum, Mainz, Bonn and Vindonissa -played important roles in the early development of these frontiers. Thus, it is possible that the events of the time would have affected when and where the inscriptions were erected. Nonetheless, even during the 2nd and 3rd centuries, when more inscriptions appear, many units have no epigraphic evidence of medical care, further suggesting variations within the units and the provinces.

One can also ask whether a specific time period might be associated with the popularity of a certain type of doctor. The dates of the inscriptions for the *medici, medici ordinarii* and the *optiones valetudinarii* range from the early 1st to the 3rd centuries, so these positions were not distinctive to a specific period in time. Inscriptions of the *capsarii* and the *miles medicus* have a smaller date range - the early second 2nd to the 3rd centuries. Perhaps they became more common when the military was becoming more settled and they could have been employed as extra help when necessary. In general though, it seems that most doctors were available to all types of units from very early on in the imperial period. Although there are more inscriptions from the legionary fortresses that date to the 1st century, this may be on account of the auxiliary units not being as established in fortifications as early as the legions were (Mann 1974: 510).

4.8 Cultural Variations amongst Auxiliary Units

Since there are variations within the numbers of inscriptions per province one should consider other possible reasons for this besides date and events. Here is an opportunity to ascertain whether the number of medical inscriptions is directly correlated with the total number of inscriptions from each province or not. This will help determine whether the variation in the occurrence of medical inscriptions is a product of the overall inscription frequency or survival, or represents real variability in the provision of medical staff. A sample of just under 1,000 inscriptions was taken from a random selection of auxiliary forts to test the commonality of both medical and non-medical inscriptions. Only a selection was chosen and only from auxiliary units because it would have been impossible to locate all the inscriptions for every fort in all the provinces concerned; some inscriptions are not published, others are in obscure publications, or published two or three times. By restricting the collection of information to the CIL and RIB references a solid and reliable sample of inscriptions could be obtained (Table 4.1). The sample contains forts that have and do not have inscriptions relating to medical personnel.

TABLE 4.1: RATIOS OF MEDICAL INSCRIPTIONS TO NON-MEDICAL INSCRIPTIONS

PROVINCE	MEDICAL INSCRIPTIONS	NON-MEDICAL INSCRIPTIONS	RATIO OF MEDICAL TO NON-MEDICAL INSCRIPTIONS
Pannonia Inferior	2	59	1:29.5
Pannonia Superior	0	10	0:10
Noricum	0	42	0:42
Raetia	0	62	0:62
Germania Superior	3	345	1:115
Germania Inferior	1	60	1:60
Britannia	2	375	1:187.5
Totals	8	953	1:119.1

A random selection of forts was chosen from: **Pannonia Inferior** - Ulcisia Castra (CIL III 3638-3444, 10574-10578), Intercisa (CIL III 3326-3339, 10301-10325), Vetus Salina (CIL III 3340-3341, 10326-12332); **Pannonia Superior** - Schwecht (CIL III 4555-4664); **Noricum** - Melk (CIL III 5660-5670, 11804-11813), Traismaur (CIL III 5653-5659, 11794-11803), Comagena (CIL III 5650-5652, 11793); **Raetia** - Heidenheim (CIL III 5929-5932), Eining (CIL III 5935-5941, 11942-11958), Pfünz (CIL III 5918-5918b, 11926-11941), Epfach (CIL 5773-5784, 11887); **Germania Superior** - Obernburg (CIL XIII 6619-6628, 11772-11773a), Osterburken (CIL XIII 6566-6591, 11766-11769), Groß-Krotzenburg (CIL XIII 7408-7420), Saalburg (CIL XIII 7444-7492), Heddernheim (CIL XIII 7330-7391), Stockstadt (CIL XIII 6629-6657, 11774-11798), Schlossau (CIL XIII 6503-6511), Neckarburken (CIL XIII 6489-6495), Canstatt (CIL XIII 6437-6447), Lopodunum (CIL XIII 6414-6425, 11739-11741), Rotweil (CIL XIII 6350-6357), Worms (CIL XIII 6212-6260); **Germania Inferior** - Valkenburg (AE 1975: 634), Roomburg (CIL XIII 8823-8826), Katwijk aan Zee (CIL XIII 8827-8828), Fectio (CIL XIII 8810-8819), Durnomagus (CIL XIII 8520-8528), Rigomagus (CIL XIII 7785-7820); **Britannia** - Binchester (RIB 1028-1040), Birdoswald (RIB 1872-1929), Carvoran (RIB 1775-1842), Housesteads (RIB 1576-1631), Carrawburgh (RIB 1520-1563), Chesters (RIB 1520-1563), Benwell (RIB 1327-1325), Wallsend (RIB 1299-1311).

First of all, from the information that could be gathered in the sources, it is noticeable that the distribution of fortifications with inscriptions varied greatly. There were higher numbers with inscriptions in Germania Superior and Britannia, whilst Pannonia Superior had a smaller number. With this sample three provinces do not have medical inscriptions from auxiliary forts - Pannonia Superior, Noricum and Raetia. The auxiliary units in these provinces do have other inscriptions, yet their numbers were generally lower. Taking an average of one medical inscription per 119 inscriptions, more significant are the high percentages of medical inscriptions from Pannonia Inferior and Germania Inferior. There is a relative scarcity of medical inscriptions from Britannia. Germania Superior fits the expected average. In general what is implied from this study is that there is no easy correlation between the number of medical inscriptions with the total body of epigraphic material. The reason for this could include a differential use of materials - certain kinds of inscriptions being made in wood others in stone across different areas - or different traditions for making medical inscriptions in the military. Provincial customs no doubt relate to the production of inscriptions being made. Other reasons may be that each province, or unit was permitted to dictate how they wished to organise their medical care. The amount of archaeological excavations that have taken place also differs between areas, along with the size of the frontiers and the number of forts, which could contribute to the discrepancy in numbers.

Not only do numbers differ, but one can test whether there might have been units from specific areas that were more likely to have erected medical inscriptions in stone than other units. Since the legions do not give a name of origin they cannot be used to make such a study; however, the auxiliary units that had the name of their homes can be examined for such an inquiry. One might argue that the auxiliary units might have become culturally more Roman throughout time (Mann 1974: 515; Watson 1969: 144), but this is based on the assumption that groups would have wished to become increasingly Romanised, gradually shedding all of their original cultural identity (Cunliffe 1989: 126-7).

Another question that must be considered is whether there were differences in the types of auxiliary units that might have evidence for medical treatment. There are a number of different varieties of auxiliary units: cohorts of infantry, *alae* or cavalry units, *cohors equitatae* a mixture of infantry and cavalry soldiers and special groups of archers all of which were in groups of either 500 or 1,000 soldiers. Before continuing, it must be made clear that there is no intention in this study to assume that each auxiliary unit consisted of a homogeneous group of soldiers from the same area with the exact same cultural practices and understandings. It is clear from inscriptions that there were different cultural groups within a single unit. From Britain the *cohors Tungrorum* has three altars (RIB 2100, 2107 and 2108) dedicated by groups from other areas of the empire. However, since it is difficult to determine cultural composition within a unit from the archaeological material, the unit names represent the securest means by which to gain an understanding of the make up of these groups, and hence explore culturally determined variations in medical practice. Table 4.2 shows where the units with inscriptions came from originally. There are eight inscriptions in the sample from auxiliary forts, along with one from the numerus fort of Niederbieber that has two types of medical personnel mentioned on it. The tablet from Vindolanda (Bowman and Thomas 1991: 62, 66; Bowman and Thomas 1994: 93-4, 98) discussed above mentions the sick, and it can be inferred from this that there might have been a doctor at the fort. Thus the table below lists the forts with medical inscriptions, the type of doctors, and the name of the unit. One inscription, possibly from Germany, mentions two units' names and is included in the comparison.

TABLE 4.2: INSCRIPTIONS RELATING TO UNITS FROM A KNOWN PLACE OF ORIGIN

FORT	PROVINCE	MEDICAL PERSONNEL	UNIT TYPE	UNIT NAME	PROVINCE OF ORIGIN
Ulcisa Castra	Pannonia Inf.	Capsarius	Cohors (1000) Sagittarioum	Syrorum	Syria
Dunaújváros	Pannonia Inf.	Capsarius	Cohors (1000) Sagittarioum	Hemesenorum	Syria
Niederbieber	Germania Sup.	Capsarii	Numerus	Exploratum Germanicorum	Germania
Niederbieber	Germania Sup.	Medicus Ordinarius	Numerus	Exploratum Germanicorum	Germania
Groß-Krotzenburg	Germania Sup.	Medicus	Cohors (500)	Vindelici	Noricum
Obernburg	Germania Sup.	Medicus	Cohors (500)	Aquitanorum Civium Romanorum	Gaul
Osterburken	Germania Sup	Medicus	Cohors (500)	Aquitanorum	Gaul
Valkenburg	Germania Inf	Medicus	Cohors Equitata	Gallorum	Gaul
Binchester	Britannia	Medicus Ordinarius	Ala	Hispanorum	Spain
Vindolanda	Britannia	?	Cohors (500)	Tungrorurm	Gaul (Belgica)
Housesteads	Britannia	Medicus	Cohors (1000)	Tungrorum	Gaul (Belgica)
Unknown	?	Medicus	Ala	Indiana Gallorum	Gaul
Unknown	?	Medicus	Ala	Astorum	Spain

From the table above it is obvious that the majority of different auxiliary types are represented in the inscription record. Two *cohortes milliaria sagittariorum*, or units of archers had *capsarii* in Pannonia Inferior. A *cohors milliaria* from Housesteads had a *medicus ordinarius*. Two *cohortes quingenaria* and two cavalry units were represented with a doctor each. As already mentioned, the *numerus* unit had *capsarii* and a *medicus ordinarius*. Since there does not seem to be any distinction between unit types, the implication is that there was probably no discrimination over which units were to receive medical attention; generally supporting the idea of Nuttons' that all types of soldiers had medical care offered to them. Nonetheless, the small numbers of inscriptions could variously imply either that all units were not receiving treatment, or that they were but did not have a tradition for making inscriptions, or possibly that they had other means of health care that was not Greek or Roman and they did not call their doctors by Latin or Greek titles. This last probability is also in need of further consideration, and will be examined more thoroughly with the archaeological remains of medical tools in the following chapter.

If one looks at the auxiliary units with inscriptions, the majority of the doctors were in units from areas in Gaul. Of the sample of 12 inscriptions two were for Syrian units, one was for a unit from Germany, two were from Aquitania, two from Gaul, two from Gallia Belgica, two from Spain and one from Noricum. In addition to this sample is a writing tablet from Vindolanda (Bowman and Thomas 1991: 62, 66; Bowman and Thomas 1994: 93-4, 98). Although the number is small, it is curious that the majority of troops with evidence for Roman medical inscriptions come from different areas of Gaul. In comparison, the units in forts from throughout the area of study without medical inscriptions or evidence relating to medical care (Appendix 1 part 2) have auxiliary units from other areas of the empire not mentioned on Table 4.2. Thus, perhaps one could say that Gallic troops had more of a tradition for making inscriptions, but this would be too simple an argument. The reason is that when one examines the *corpora* of inscriptions it is noticeable that inscribed stones appear throughout the empire regardless of the unit's origin. Perhaps those from Gaul either adopted Roman medicine and incorporated it into their units, or adopted Latin titles for their healers.

4.9 Contact between Military and Civilian Populations

One avenue that might show movement of medical ideas from military to civilian populations involves looking for evidence of Roman military doctors caring for civilians. There is also the chance that perhaps civilian healers might have been called into Roman fortifications to provide assistance. For the first part of the question, reference can be made to a burial inscription from Dacia, erected for a legionary doctor (Appendix 2, number 41). This seems to indicate that the doctor might have been given civilian honours by people living in the nearby *municipium*. Perhaps this was done because he had helped the local civilian population when they were in need of medical assistance. Many soldiers had wives and families who would have required medical assistance from time to time. Such contacts could have been a means for maintaining good relations between military and civilian groups. It could also be a method for a military doctor to learn more about the ailments of women and children, a skill that could be used by doctors who wished to practise civilian medicine after their service in the army was completed. There is not much to support the idea of doctors working after their service in the army except for the statement by the Hippocratic writer (On the Physician 9.219 L) saying that doctors should join the army to gain more surgical experience. Whether this advice was followed in Roman times is not known. It is, however, a possibility that some doctors would have wished to practise after working in the army.

Despite the obvious reasons for why a military doctor might have cared for civilians there is little solid evidence to support this. Possible support for this is three inscriptions of doctors from the civilian areas located around fortifications (Appendix 2, numbers 4, 16, 21). These are from Carnuntum, Bingen and Vetera. The inscriptions were found in close proximity to the fortifications, perhaps indicating that they relate to military doctors who had set up monuments outside the fort, as there is a military inscription of a doctor from Aquincum that was found outside the military zone (Appendix 2, number 31). There is a problem with the location of these: many reports do not state whether the inscriptions were found *in situ,* and it is possible that the inscriptions were originally placed on the inside of the fortifications and could have been moved at some point. Alternatively, the doctors could have been non-military personnel who were available to help the army when necessary. One interesting point is that where there are inscriptions for civilian doctors, or rather inscriptions of doctors that do not mention a military unit found outside fortifications, there are no, or very few, inscriptions for military doctors from within the fortifications. Vetera and Bingen have no other medical inscriptions from the fortifications themselves, but do have them from outside the structures (Appendix 2, numbers 4 and 16 respectively), whilst Carnuntum has one inscription from the settlement outside the fortress (Appendix 2, number 20) and it has the *spolia* of an inscription mentioning a *capsarius* found built within the wall of the so-called hospital of the fortress (Appendix 2, number 21). Since the doctors on these inscriptions refer to themselves as *medici* it suggests that their style of medicine was Roman, and perhaps those who inhabited the civilian settlements of Carnuntum and Vetera had more of a Roman lifestyle, Vetera being a military settlement and Carnuntum a civilian capital. As for the inscription near Bingen, it may be that the doctor also helped with the nearby legionary fortress at Mainz. Perhaps this doctor was influenced by Roman style medicine and treated civilians in a Roman manner as he called himself a *medicus,* though it must be remembered that even though a

Latin term is used it is also possible that the doctor had other means of practising medicine that might have been learnt through their own society.

For economic reasons it is clear that contact was frequently made between the civilian and military societies (Wells 1999). Simply because they traded with each other does not indicate that local inhabitants would have accepted Roman medical treatment, in fact they may have rejected it. Moreover, certain groups in the military may have had their own doctors and would not have wished to call upon local practices of medical treatment. Although Caesar states that soldiers on campaign were left in friendly areas when they were wounded one does not know what sorts of treatments were offered to these soldiers. Overall there is insufficient evidence to say whether military doctors cared for civilians or vice versa.

4.10 CONCLUSION

Even though no specific conclusions can be made about medical care in the Roman military from the evidence of inscriptions alone, one thing that is clear is that there is not enough evidence to support the current belief in a standardised system of medical care. The possibility must be entertained that medical traditions varied between military units. Some may willingly have accepted Roman style medical treatment, but others may, as part of a means of retaining aspects of their original cultural identity, have brought various 'indigenous' medical traditions with them. However, from the comparison of auxiliary units with medical inscriptions a pattern does seem to have emerged that units from Gaul might have adopted Roman style medical care to a greater extent than other units. Since the number of inscriptions is low, archaeological evidence of surgical instruments must be looked at in conjunction with the epigraphic remains in order to explore whether there were either provincial or more specific cultural variations within Roman military medicine.

CHAPTER FIVE

NEW PERSPECTIVES ON THE MATERIAL CULTURE OF MEDICAL INSTRUMENTS IN RELATION TO THE ROMAN ARMY

5.1 INTRODUCTION

Examinations of material remains in relation to their context, associated finds, and depositional practices can provide excellent opportunities for expanding our understanding of past societies, both where there is sufficient historical documentation and where there is not. In order to enquire further about the possibility of how military events and provincial and cultural variations might have affected the organisation of medical care on the frontiers, this chapter comprises a comparison of the medical instruments found at fortifications on the frontiers concerned. The instruments can be studied to ascertain who was being treated - soldiers only, or possibly civilians. Inferences can be made into the deposition of the instruments and might demonstrate attitudes towards items relating to the body and illness; for example, whether they were expendable, something to be carefully curated, or whether through use they might have become 'polluted', thus determining the ways in which instruments were disposed of; and on a more general level this might provide some indication about how doctors and medical care were perceived through the eyes of the soldiers.

5.2 WHAT IS A ROMAN MEDICAL INSTRUMENT?

Roman medical tools have been described and discussed through the methodology of typological comparisons, which mainly consist of lists of instruments with brief descriptions of their appearance and their intended functions as discussed in the classical sources. The archaeological interpretations of these tools are limited because rarely do these studies address issues pertaining to their deposition, contextually related finds, gender and possible variations of their uses in different areas of the empire (e.g. Bliquez 1981a; 1994; Bliquez and Oleson 1985; Braadbaart 1994b; Jackson; 1990; 1994b; 1995; Künzl 1983; 1996; 2002: 51-53; Milne 1907). In order to undertake this study the traditional classical archaeological approach could not be used, because it generally relies on descriptions and typological discussions of material culture, but makes little use of the context and deposition of the material remains as a main source for interpreting the past. Additionally, in studies of classical medicine the archaeological material is frequently tied to the literary sources. As Salazar (2000: 230) says in her book on the literature of war wounds in antiquity:

> "In addition to the literary evidence, there is also a fairly large amount of archaeological evidence. Although on its own this material would be open to numerous, contrasting, conjectures, it can be used along with literary evidence and in comparison with it."

To be fair, Salazar is not a trained archaeologist; yet her statement is consistent with the general belief in classics, as discussed in the introduction, that material remains are somehow secondary to the literature, and even if the two demonstrate opposing points of view, as Salazar says they sometimes do, she still insinuates that without literary sources to support the material remains there is little point in interpreting meanings from artefacts. The narrowness of this approach is obvious because the literature does not tell us everything about past societies, and it seems fair to say that even as a source of material culture literature is open to just as many "numerous, contrasting conjectures". Furthermore the literature is seen as the only context in which the material culture can be ascribed a meaning; however, if material remains are examined within their own context (their location and associated finds) more can be understood about the functions, meanings and role in social practices of finds (for a more detailed discussion see Baker 2002a; 2004). Many parts of the Roman empire do not have much in the way of a literary record, as even extant epigraphic sources only provide us with glimpses into the structures and thoughts of these societies. It is the archaeological material that must primarily be relied upon to gain insights into provincial Roman life.

The instruments that have been identified are only those that scholars have recognised by comparisons with the classical texts, which presents a one-sided understanding of the medical tools. We see the medical writer's point of view, but each writer will often have a different view of how a tool can be used, providing us with various functions for the instruments. One cannot say whether the tools were used in the same manner by all doctors; it would seem most plausible that they were not. Contextual studies of the medical instruments and comparisons of their associated finds have so far not been made to see if the Romans, or people living in the provinces, had any other types of medical instruments that are not mentioned in the so-called rational medical texts.

Künzl (1986a: 30) states that archaeologists concerned with studying Roman medical instruments must continue with typological identifications. A reason for this is because not all of the medical instruments mentioned in the ancient sources have been identified in the archaeological record (Künzl 1986a: 30; Jackson 1990: 7; 1994a: 168). One should not ignore the fact that typological studies have supplied us with information about possible ways the tools were intended to be used in certain medical situations. However, these recent typological identifications have, unintentionally, hindered the possibility of making other examinations into the understanding of Roman medicine by setting prescriptive classifications and forms of analysis on the medical instruments. Although the ascribed classifications help us to organise data, they may only have some approximations to past realities. Thus, the divisions are modern classifications that are then transferred directly onto our understanding of the past. Deetz has argued that:

> "modern artefact typologies allows for controlled comparisons between collections from different sites. But such classifications are entirely formal, and arrived at, by necessity, independently of what the makers of the objects perceived as different types. With the rich documentary materials of historical archaeology, such classifications are not only sterile exercises, but are potentially very mis-leading" (1977: 13).

Miller maintains that archaeologists try to make the artefacts fit very concrete forms, which served one function only, when it is more likely that they have a multiplicity of meanings and purposes (1994: 406). One example of how the single definitions of a medical tool's function has potentially mislead scholars into ascribing an incorrect function to a tool is apparent in the identification of some scalpels found in a structure identified as a *fabrica* on the Bonner Berg near Bonn (van Driel-Murray and Gechter 1984: 62). Much evidence for leather working has been found in this structure, and it is quite possible that the application of the scalpels found within were used to work leather, rather than being employed on people. Jackson notes this as well when discussing the tools found in the so-called surgeon's grave at Bingen. Some tools seem to be carpentry tools, that could also be bone-working instruments. He puts forward suggestions that they could be both, or the doctor could have needed carpentry tools to make splints and other apparatuses (2002: 89). Thus the modern identification of these as surgical tools need not exhaust the range of functions they were employed as. There is also the likelihood that such artefacts could have changed their meaning and function throughout their 'life span', at one point being ascribed a medical function and another time perhaps a non-medical function.

Jackson provides a convincing argument that the tools are well-designed to perform medical procedures, such as male and female catheters. The latter are excellent examples of instruments made to conform with the anatomy of the body (2002: 89). One must consider this point when discussing the medical function of some tools. One dreads to think of the consequences of the tool shaped for a male body being used on a female and vice versa. Nonetheless, one cannot rule out the possibility that some doctors might have found tools very useful for some procedures we would not consider.

More recently scholars have classified medical instruments into three groups: toilet, surgical and surgical/toilet (e.g. Braadbaart 1994a & b; Kunzl 1983; 2002: 51; Jackson 1990; Riha 1986). These modern typologies might not be an indication of how the Romans and others would have categorised them. If one looks at the literary texts that describe the use of the implements there are no distinctions made between the different types in accordance to modern categories, as they all seem to be described equally. Archaeologically, they are rarely found in sets of one particular type, with the exception of the artistic representations of boxes of scalpels (Salazar 2000: 239-47). In this instance, however, it is a single type of tool, rather than a particular classification that is depicted. Rather than continuing with this tradition, the data derived from instruments used in this study was not divided into these categories, simply because they are too strict. For example, scalpels are generally placed in the category of surgical instruments, but they might have been used for preparing medicines, or cutting bandages, and as shown above they could also have had functions not related to medicine. The identification of surgical/toilet instruments is also not without problems. They are often relegated to being considered somehow less important by modern scholars for providing evidence of medical treatment, possibly because their design is often more simple than some of the 'designated' surgical instruments and because they are found more frequently in the archaeological record. Yet, they are described by Celsus and Paul of Aegina, for example, to serve functions in a number of complicated surgical procedures, just like the tools we have designated as being strictly surgical.

The one modern category of instruments not considered in this examination was that of toilet implements. These were not considered because they tend to imply personal use, rather than having been used by a doctor on a patient. Although, it is possible that they may well have been used by doctors as a medical tool. Though they generally tend to be associated with personal hygiene and were not considered, even though personal hygiene was an integral part of Roman health care. It was the doctor's treatment that is of concern for this study, not personal treatment; although its importance cannot be denied in the study of medicine. Objects not considered here include chatelaines (sets of nail-cleaners, ear probes and tweezers attached on a ring) and tweezers that measured under 6 centimetres in length and if they had a round hook for attachment to a chatelaine. Usually those found suspended on a loop are defined as having a personal use; however, even these could still be used in the treatment of ophthalmia (Bliquez 1988: 50-1). The identification of tweezers for personal hygiene and forceps for surgery are again based on modern definitions of their functions. There is nothing in the Latin or Greek sources that describes their difference, but modern interpretations generally define tweezers for personal use as less than 8 centimetres long (Bliquez 1988: 50-1), whilst forceps, instruments that measure 10 centimetres or more, are defined as surgical tools. In general this study only uses instruments of 6 centimetres or more, but it is also possible that even these forceps were used for personal hygiene rather than surgery.

Another problem with the use of these categories is that the instruments are regularly taken out of their archaeological context when they are recorded, and published in separate classes. Rarely are other objects mentioned that were found with them, artefacts that may shed greater light on our understanding of medical practice. Such frustrations are aired for many aspects of Roman archaeology, as Allison (1997: 78) has discussed with problems in her work on room contents in the houses of Pompeii. She found her study hindered by the lack of information in the finds catalogues because objects had been divided into distinct categories without contextual information. The omission of such information in any study, and specifically with medical instruments, leaves one with less of an understanding of original material associations - that is of what combinations of objects might have been employed in medical treatments, and objects that might have been considered a necessary part of the rituals of healing. (The term ritual does not necessarily have to be magical or religious, just a practice that is similar from one time to another, which can be a process that mediated between different states of being including illness and health [Turner 1974].) In support of ritual, or 'irrational' aspects in Roman medicine, archaeological evidence of sanctuaries, amulets and altars to medical gods indicate that they were either used in conjunction with 'rational' aspects, or 'rational' medicine was not always trusted or even practised. The two aspects were enmeshed within one another and not considered separate as they are today. Thus certain objects occurring with recognised medical tools might have served a function in the ritual of medical practice that has yet to be understood. It also becomes problematic when the context is known, but not considered to be of much importance. This might be the case with a cupping vessel from the Roman fort at Zugmantel that is argued by Künzl to be 16th or 17th century because of its design; however it was found in a Roman context, in celler 77 of the site, and it is argued to be a stray find (1984/5: 31). Here the logic of classification overrides the archaeological evidence. If the date of the artefact is correct, we must question how it was placed in a sealed Roman context. But if we consider the fact that is was found in such a context one can ask a number of questions. Did the Romans have other types of cupping vessels of which no other examples survive? Is it possible that the indigenous population of the area, or culture of the soldiers living in the fort developed their own cupping vessels that did not conform to the Roman designs with which we are familiar? Even though it is possible that the identification is correct, the archaeological context should not be relegated to a secondary status. One should also ask what was happening at Zugmantel in the 16th century in order for the artefact to find its way into the Roman site?

Objects found in tombs with identified medical tools might begin to shed some more light on the full range of medical beliefs and practices. The burial from Stanway, Essex (Jackson 1997: 1471), already discussed, has identifiable surgical instruments along with pottery, a gaming board with gaming pieces and iron 'divining' rods. The instruments were found on the game board, in close proximity to the rods; perhaps these two objects might have had an important 'ritual' aspect to the medical treatment offered by the doctor. Künzl's study of medical instruments found in tombs mentions other finds buried with medical tools, but he does not consider their possible functions in the ritual of medical practice (1983). Some of these finds are rather unusual, such as three Neolithic stone axes (Künzl 1983: 57), a cuttlefish bone (Künzl 1983: 59) and an iron bell (Künzl 1983: 79). It can be speculated that in certain areas these items might have been used as charms, or tools that were integral to medical treatment. While the medical texts give one perspective on treatment, the material culture can be used to establish culturally determined behaviour and to ask what other practices people are expressing through their objects. It is possible that we do not have a strong understanding of what other items were important to Roman medical practitioners, or in treatment outside the context of Rome, non-Roman style medicine.

Aiming to approach the subject of medical tools, this study has its limitations in the fact that very little contextual information of the material culture is available from the museum records and publications, information that could help expand on our knowledge of different Roman medical tools and practices. Thus, only the instruments that have already been identified as such and are similar to those found in Italy, especially Pompeii, were considered in this work as a means of determining the spread of some aspects of Roman medicine.

5.3 Manufacture of Instruments

Before comparing the instruments something must be said about their manufacture and distribution to facilitate our understanding of their trade and distribution. The distribution of the instruments could have affected the way medical knowledge was spread and how implements were used.

Like so many aspects of Roman archaeology, there is the assumption that any object that appeared to be Roman was based on a standardised design that was centrally produced. For example, Samian ware was manufactured in Gaul and distributed throughout the empire. A recent study of material culture from military sites in Germany has shown that people living in *vici* were fabricating items for soldiers in the styles the soldiers requested. Therefore, manufactured goods that appear Roman, were not necessarily made by Roman groups (Wells 1999 145-6). Some items found at the military sites also had native influences incorporated into them from both the people making the objects and the soldiers who had requested them, such as pottery and metalwork (Wells 1999: 145-6). Wells has noticed that Germanic societies were becoming more 'Roman' and Romans on the provinces more 'Germanic' (1999: 226). Other evidence for interaction where Roman soldiers were using local items can be seen in Germanic ceramics found in the fort of Zugmantel on the Rhine frontier (von Usler 1934, 1980). The army in Britain also used local black-burnished ware from Dorset. Therefore, the question is who was influencing whom? Objects need not be linked to specific ethnic identities – material culture can be quite flexible – the way it is adapted and used and the functions and the meanings are often entirely re-worked (Jones 1997: 106-8). This means that even if a medical tool is adopted by a group living in a Roman province it might not have been used in the manner Romans from Italy would have understood it.

As far as medicine is concerned, the question of who - meaning a group of people rather than an individual - was making the instruments has not been an issue of much concern. A possible reason for this is that the instruments tend not to vary much in design between provinces, something that became evident in the museum research undertaken for this study. The main concentration of research in this area has been on the practical aspects of how the instruments were made (Healy 1978; Jackson 1990: 10-11). On the whole, there is not a large variety of surgical instruments in the archaeological record. This is probably because in the majority of cases one implement could be used to treat a number of medical problems; the so-called 'doctor's kit' often only contained a few specific types of instruments (Jackson 1988: 114, 2002: 91-2). Certain more specialised instruments, such as syringes, specula and trepanning saws, have been found, usually on their own and not in kits, but they tend to be rare, and might represent treatment by a doctor who specialised in caring for specific ailments or had the money for unusual tools.

It may be that the rare surgical instruments are an indication of a specialist. An example of this is the cremation burial found at Bingen which had a large number of bone working tools including a trepanning saw (Appendix 5, Table A5.25; Como 1925). These instruments were found with more common instruments such as scalpels, hooks and probes. It may be that it was not an uncommon medical set, simply one that has survived because the tools were buried with the person who used them, made them, or perhaps was sometimes associated with the doctor or maker. Since bone-working instruments are not common in the archaeological record it could mean that they were passed down from doctor to doctor, or were recycled.

The types of materials used in the manufacture of the instruments could explain the ease or difficulty in making the instrument, and furthermore could have added to their cost and rarity. Surgical instruments were made with a variety of metals, but copper-alloys are the most common because the metals were easily obtained and simple to work and cast (Healy 1978: 249). The metal was also resistant to rust, which would have lengthened the life of the implement. Other metals such as gold, silver, copper, tin, lead, iron and zinc were also used in manufacturing the instruments. Gold and silver items are scarce, and archaeologists tend to agree that they were either luxury items or used for votive offerings (Healy 1978: 149-50). Some instruments have gold and silver inlay or gold platting to make them more appealing to the patient, or to indicate the status of the doctor or patient; however as Lucian said he would rather have a doctor with a rusty knife than a charlatan with a gold one (Chapter 4; *The Ignorant Book Collector* 29), suggesting that nice-looking instruments did not fool everyone. Iron was used for cautery ends and bone-working tools such as forceps and saw blades. Scalpel blades were made of steel (Appendix 3). It has also been suggested that some metals were used for their healing properties, such as lead tubing for gynaecological instruments (Healy 1978: 246-8). However, there are other instances when it seems as if the maker of the instruments was fabricating them from whatever materials they had close at hand (Jackson 1990: 10). Instruments as seen in Appendices 4 through 10 were sometimes made of bone, especially spoon probes and ear probes. Horn and glass have also been mentioned in the fabrication of cupping vessels (Appendix 3). Albucasis, a 12th century Arabic medical writer, who drew much of his information from Roman and Greek sources, mentions vaginal specula being made out of boxwood (Spink and Lewis 1973), and this could be an indication that perishable materials were used in the construction of instruments and perhaps even explains why some are so rare, such as specula. Therefore, some of the instruments that have been mentioned in the literary sources, but for which we have none or very few extant examples, might have been made in larger numbers, but of perishable materials. Alternatively they might have been constructed of very specific materials that were difficult to obtain, and so made only in small numbers when necessary.

Most of the instruments were manufactured by casting and hammering the metal (Healy 1978: 249-51). The main body of the instrument would have been cast while the finer details in the blades and teeth would probably have been worked into shape by hammering and/or filing. The more complicated instruments such as specula and trepanning saws probably took more time to make and also would have required more skill, so this too could be an explanation for the scarcity of these instruments.

On the whole it seems that the majority of instruments were fairly simple to make, so it must be asked if any metal workers could have manufactured the instruments, or if most had been made in special workshops and ordered by doctors throughout the empire. There is some evidence that medical supplies were ordered for military hospitals. A papyrus fragment of an order form from a military unit in Asia Minor (BGU 1564=Sp 395, papyrus Egypt 138; Campbell 1994: 239), mentions white blankets of soft wool being ordered for the military hospital, so it is possible that tools might have been ordered in this manner as well. The blanket ordered was to be made from wool, a raw material that was probably easily found throughout most of the empire, so perhaps this was ordered on account of a specialised skill involved in its production, rather than lack of raw material. Certain metals could not be obtained in all areas of the empire (e.g. copper and tin), so the metalworkers would either have to order the raw materials to make the objects, or import the goods or recycle. It probably depended on what the manufacturer deemed important to their business, and the demand of instruments from those who were purchasing the tools – soldiers, the army or doctors.

Inscriptions marked on some instruments provide another clue about the manufacturers of the tools (Künzl 1983: 31-3; Künzl 1984). Gostenčnik (1997) has recently examined forceps with the name 'Agathangelus' inscribed on them. This name appears on a number of forceps with a distinctive design throughout the western empire. Gostenčnik has looked for parallels in both the shape and the name to determine where the workshops of Agathangelus might have been located (1997: 147). From her examination it seems that there might have been two workshops, one in Italy and one in Gaul. Although her study focuses only on a few instruments, the stamp implies that some instruments were being made in specific places, and doctors or people were buying them from certain workshops. It is also plausible that the doctors would commission instruments from metal-workers in the area where they served or trained and then take their instruments to wherever they travelled, possibly explaining the various locations of the instruments with the stamp.

Künzl (1983: 33-5; 1984) also argues that styles of decorations might be a means of determining where the instruments were being made. It is apparent that this would be a most difficult task because of all the tools I examined there did not seem to be any typical design from a specific area. However, a more accurate means of determining either the place of manufacture, or at least the place where the raw materials came from would be the employment of metallurgical analysis (Jackson 1990: 10). Once a specific program of metal analysis has been made then perhaps the instruments with decorations can be analysed with more care to see if there are decorations specific for a certain region. Instruments could have been made at the fortifications. Metalworking was routinely undertaken within military sites, and the fortress of Neuss has a room in its so-called hospital that had a high number of instruments, which might suggest a place of manufacture or storage. These instruments are mainly probes (Appendix 4, Table A4.1), suggesting the possibility that only certain instruments might have been made locally, whilst others might have been commissioned from special workshops. Alternatively, the instruments may have been stored or deposited in this building.

There are many ways in which instruments could have been obtained by doctors working within Roman fortifications. Yet, the manufacture of the instruments like so many other aspects of medicine is in need of more study by archaeologists with specialist knowledge of the techniques of metalworking and metal analysis in order to see if there were regional differences in fabrication. This could provide us with a stronger basis on which to examine the possibilities of trade and interaction of medical ideas. It could also be another means of examining the possibility of regional and cultural variations in medical practice.

5.4 Comparison of the Data

All of the instruments gathered in this study are described in the appendices (Appendices 4-10); though to help the reader understand the general functions and appearance of the tool a brief description of the ones discussed in the text is provided in Appendix 3. The collection of data for this examination was not undertaken entirely for its own sake, nor was it the intention to produce a fully comprehensive catalogue of medical instruments on the frontiers. The intention was to generate as large and as representative a sample of medical tools from the military sites as possible in order to examine questions about variations in medical practice. This study constitutes a sample of 1,078 instruments. Table 5.1 below shows the number of instruments found and the percentage of the total for each province.

In itself this comprises a large sample, though it is here broken down to smaller units based on province, unit type and instrument type for the purposes of analysis. Although in some cases the artefact population is small (e.g. in the case of instruments from *numerus* forts), the validity of observation has been treated on occasion by means of chi-square tests; though it should be remembered that statistical significance and archaeological significance are not always the same thing (Fletcher and Lock 1991: 11-12). Archaeological significance is often more dependent upon contextual patterns or perceived significant variations from normal representations (e.g. the apparent overabundance or exclusion of specific finds from an artefact assemblage or site).

There are roughly 226 known fortifications in the area of study. Of the fortifications that have been examined there are 69 known to have produced medical instruments, representing 30.5% of the total (Fig. 9).

Germania Superior has the highest number of fortifications with instruments (26), whilst Noricum has the lowest (one). Noricum may be the lack of archaeological work on military fortifications in comparison with the other provinces. Though, having said this, there have still been archaeological excavations on auxiliary forts in the province, so there may be other reasons for the lack of medical artefacts. This general survey shows that the number of fortifications with a yield of medical instruments is greater in the two Germanias, Britannia and in Raetia. There is a noticeable decline in the numbers on the mid- and lower Danube areas. However, another issue of this comparison is to examine whether the percentages of fortifications with instruments is the same for all of the provinces, given the fact that each has a variant number of fortifications overall.

Table 5.1: Number of Instruments per Province

Province	Number of Instruments	Percentage of Total
Germania Inferior	143	13%
Germania Superior	474	43.9%
Raetia	78	7%
Noricum	30	2.7%
Pannonia Superior	202	18%
Pannonia Inferior	30	2.7%
Britannia	121	11%

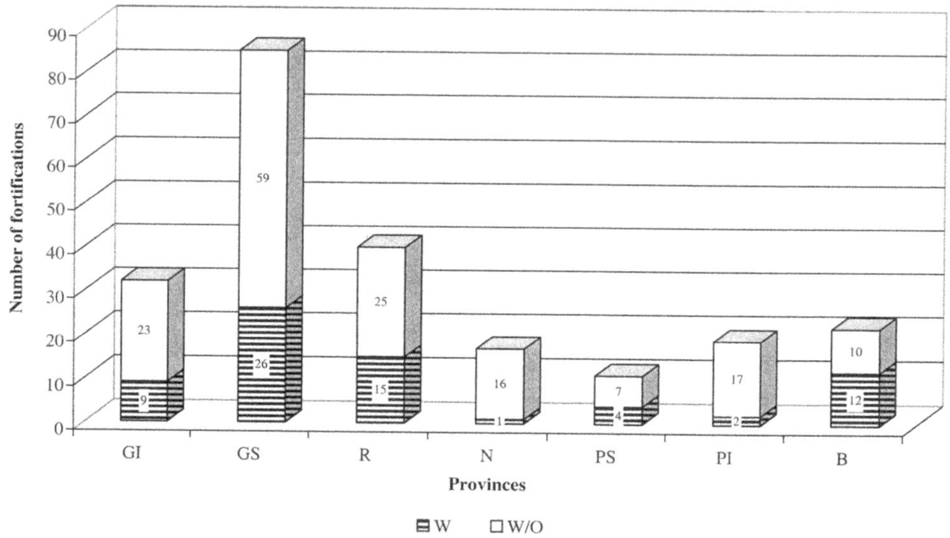

Fig. 9. A comparison of fortification numbers with instruments to those without in accordance with their provance.

This variation according to province between fortifications with or without instruments can be shown to be statistically significant (Appendix 11), illustrating apparently genuine regional differences. There is enough variation to suggest that on a provincial level at least, there is a probability that there were differences in the supply of medical care offered to the soldiers. This provides a hint of the possibility of provincial, rather than centralised, control of the medical care system.

TABLE 5.2: NUMBER OF FORTIFICATIONS WITH INSTRUMENTS

PROVINCE	NUMBER OF FORTIFICATIONS WITH INSTRUMENTS	PERCENTAGE OF THE 226 FORTIFICATIONS
Germania Inferior	9	28%
Germania Superior	26	30%
Raetia	15	37%
Noricum	1	5%
Pannonia Superior	3 (4 with auxiliary fort at Vindabona)	36%
Pannonia Inferior	2	10%
Britannia	12	54%

From here it is necessary to enquire whether there is evidence for differences between the types of units receiving health care, such as the legionary and auxiliary groups. A chi-square test was undertaken (Appendix 12) comparing the number of legionary, auxiliary and *numerus* forts with instruments. The comparison is just significant falling between the 1% and 5% levels. The problematic part of this test is the inclusion of the *numerus* fortifications, because only those in Germania Superior have medical instruments. Therefore, for the *numerus* forts the expected numbers all fall below five, a small sample number (Fletcher and Lock 1991: 63); however, for the legionary and auxiliary fortifications the expected numbers are all above five, so the test for this remains valid. It also must be kept in mind that there are more auxiliary forts in each province compared to legionary fortifications. One would then expect a higher number of auxiliary forts to have instruments compared to the legionary fortresses. However Pannonia Superior and Noricum only have instruments from the legionary fortresses, with the exception of one instrument found at the auxiliary fort near Vindobona (Fig. 10).

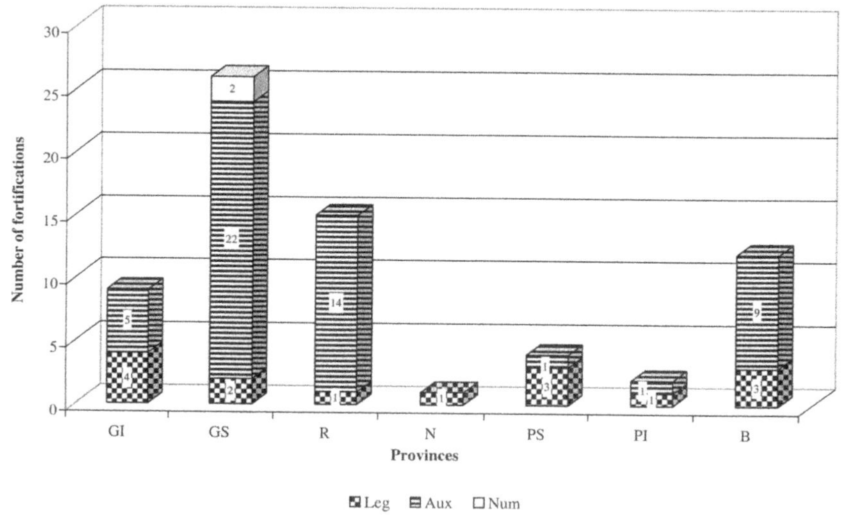

Fig. 10. A comparison of fortification numbers per unit type in accordance with their province

Pannonia Inferior has only one auxiliary fort and one legionary fortress with instruments, so the number is equal. Overall, both the epigraphic (Chapter 4) and artefactual remains demonstrate that the provision of medical treatment was made available to the different types of units from all the frontiers except Noricum and Pannonia Superior. On a percentage basis each province varies greatly with regard to the percentages of auxiliary and legionary fortifications providing evidence of Roman style medical care. For example, the auxiliary forts in Germania Superior make up 84% of the number of fortifications with instruments, whilst they make up only 55% in Germania Inferior. These differences not only suggest provincial variation, but possibly differences within the organisation of each fortification. It is possible that the supply of medical care was under the auspices of the fort commander rather than provincial administration.

Further investigation is made by comparisons of the total number of medical implements per province to see if there is additional evidence for their variations in health care. As mentioned, the total number of implements is 1,078 and they vary considerably between provinces, with Germania Superior having 474 and Pannonia Inferior having 30 (Fig. 11).

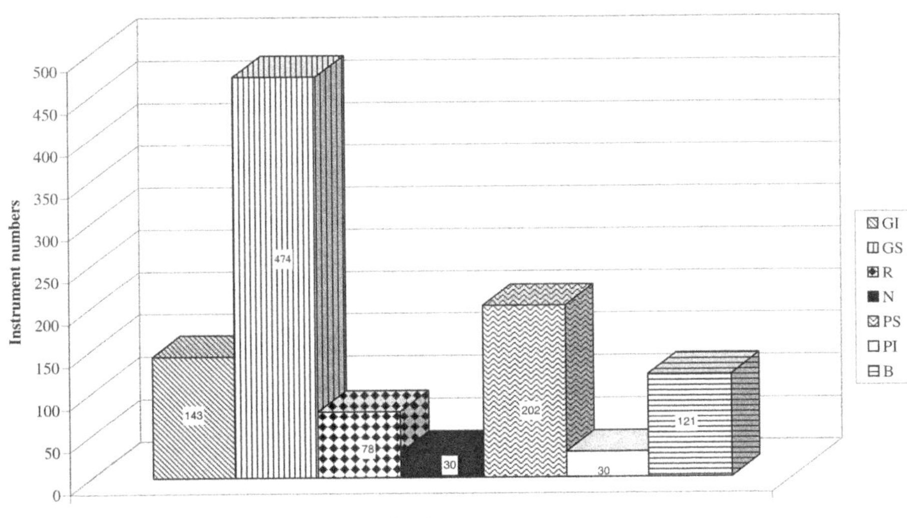

Fig. 11. A comparison of the total number of medical instruments per province.

At first it might be assumed that this difference is accounted for by the amount of excavation that has occurred at each site, yet some have seen similar amounts of excavation, but with varying numbers of medical instruments being recovered. For example, 326 instruments were found at Vindonissa compared to 38 at Caerleon. At the same time some sites have seen little or no excavation because of their location, under medieval towns and modern urban centres, and this might account for the low numbers of artefacts from some sites, such as York and Mainz. Carnuntum and Vindonissa (Appendices 5, Table A5.2 and Appendices 8, Table A8.1) have a far greater number of instruments than other fortifications, showing that the difference in the instrument numbers per province can be affected by a few fortifications. Yet, to present a broad idea of the numbers of instruments: Germania Superior has 474; however 326 of those are from Vindonissa, otherwise making the number 148, which is still the highest number in comparison to other provinces. This sample has been subject to a chi-square test (Appendix 13) comparing the total number of instruments per province according to unit type. Again there are low numbers of instruments from the numerus forts, but the auxiliary and legionary fortifications have produced enough to be valid for the test. Even with this discrepancy the test shows significant variations between numbers of instruments per unit type and province, as the chi-square value falls well below the 0.1% level, again demonstrating that there is a significant difference in the evidence for medical care between the frontiers.

When examining the total numbers of instruments found in each type of unit, the legionary fortresses have a greater amount of material evidence, except in Britain and Raetia where the auxiliary forts have higher numbers of implements. In Pannonia Inferior the numbers of instruments are the same between the one legionary and one auxiliary unit (Fig. 12).

One reason to account for the higher number of instruments in the legionary fortresses might be a larger population living in these structures. It is likely that most legionary fortresses had a population of 4,000 to 5,000 more soldiers and military staff than the auxiliary forts (Johnson 1983: 17-26). As for those provinces with a higher number of instruments in the auxiliary forts, one explanation might be the greater number of fortifications. The higher numbers of instruments from the fortress of Vindonissa might be explained by conditions of survival, as a large number of instruments were found in a waterlogged deposit known as the

Schutthügel (Fröhlich 1910: 126-9). Carnuntum's high numbers might be explained by the lack of precise provenance for many of the instruments: many could have been found in the civil settlement surrounding the fortification and possibly from the auxiliary fort in the region. Nonetheless, these are somewhat superficial explanations for the differences.

Fig. 12. A comparison of instrument numbers per unit type according to province.

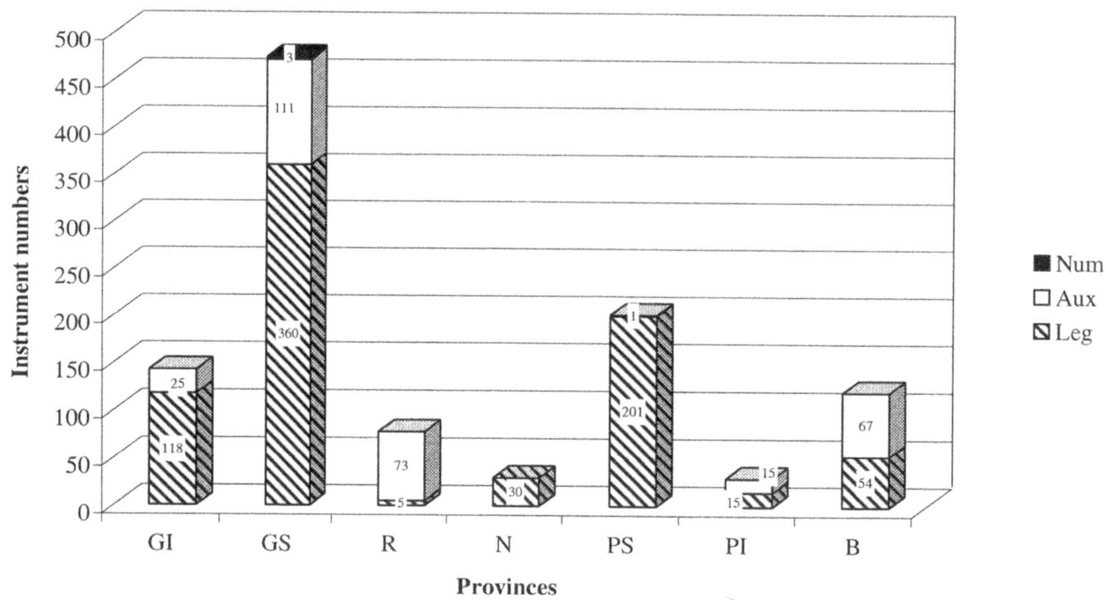

The differences in the numbers of instruments per frontier and unit might also be accounted for by the military events that occurred in each province. Raetia and Noricum were peaceful provinces until the Marcomannic wars (Chapter 3), and they did not have legionary fortresses constructed until after this event. Significantly, in Noricum the only medical evidence comes from this later time, both through inscriptions and finds. As for Raetia, many of the auxiliary forts have a small number of instruments; some of these also date to after the Marcomannic wars. The provinces that had the most warfare appear to have the highest numbers of instruments overall. Pannonia Inferior, however, is the exception to this as it was important to the Dacian campaign of Trajan and the Marcomannic Wars, so why there are not more instruments recorded, if the military events are an instigating factor for medical treatment, is surprising. Another inconsistency into possible expectations can be seen in the comparison of the German provinces with a substantial amount of medical remains and Pannonia Superior with rather little. Both were placed close to rather volatile groups of people and Pannonia Superior was also affected by the Marcomannic Wars, so it may be expected that medical care would be well represented in the archaeological record; however evidence for it is only found in the legionary units. It is possible that this was the case in some provinces and not others, but the two Pannonias do not follow the suggestion, so one must look to other explanations.

5.5 Specific Instrument Comparisons

From the study of inscriptions we have seen that certain categories of doctor are found in different unit types, but are only located in specific provinces. For example, evidence for the *medicus ordinarius* was found in all three unit types examined, but only in a few provinces: Britannia, Germania Superior, Raetia and Pannonia Superior. The sample of inscriptions is too small to make any secure statements about whether this was the case or if these doctors existed in other provinces and were simply not recorded. This pattern can be tested further by juxtaposing specific instrument assemblages with unit types and provinces. It cannot be determined through the instruments whether a *medicus ordinarius* or *capsarius* for example were using the tools, but it can be tested whether there is evidence for certain types of instruments being used in specific areas more than in other places. Generally, Table 5.3 shows that certain types of instruments are far more common than others: spoon probes, spatula probes, ear probes, scalpels and forceps, and these usually appear in all of the provinces and unit types. However, it is the legionary fortresses of Germania Superior, mainly at Vindonissa, that have the highest number of probes, as does Carnuntum, possibly because they are common instruments. Scalpels are also common, but more seem to have been found in the two Germanias.

TABLE 5.3: INSTRUMENT TYPES PER UNIT TYPE AND PROVINCE

Lg = Legion and Ax = Auxiliary

INSTRUMENT TYPE	GI Lg	GI Ax	GS Lg	GS Ax	R Lg	R Ax	N Lg	PS Lg	PS Ax	PI Lg	PI Ax	B Lg	B Ax
Spoon Probe	20	8	68	15	1	21	8	28	1	2	8	11	10
Spatula Probe	20	5	49	13	0	13	6	25	0	0	0	3	5
Double Simple Probe	0	1	0	0	0	1	0	0	0	0	0	0	1
Ear Probe	23	6	192	10	0	18	7	113	0	2	4	17	29
Button Probe	0	0	0	1	0	0	0	0	0	0	0	0	0
Olivary End Probe	9	2	3	8	0	11	3	10	0	0	0	9	3
Shears	0	1	0	0	0	0	0	0	0	0	0	0	1
Ointment Pallet	6	2	0	4	0	0	1	0	0	0	0	0	6
Medical Box	2	0	0	1	0	1	0	0	0	1	1	0	0
Instrument Case	0	0	0	0	0	0	0	1	0	0	0	0	0
Spoon Scoop	1	0	0	4	0	0	0	0	0	0	0	0	2
Scratcher	1	0	0	0	0	0	0	0	0	0	0	0	0
Scale	0	0	0	0	0	0	0	0	0	1	0	0	0
Scalpel	12	4	9	19	1	1	1	7	0	1	2	1	4
Bifurcated Hook	1	0	1	1	0	0	0	0	0	1	0	0	0
Hook	1	0	0	7	0	2	0	6	0	0	0	0	2
Needle	0	0	10	3	0	1	0	2	0	3	0	2	0
Cataract Needle	0	0	0	0	0	0	0	0	0	0	0	0	1
Dental Tool	0	0	0	0	0	0	0	0	0	0	0	1	0
Uvula Forceps	1	0	0	0	0	0	0	0	0	0	0	0	0
Rectal Speculum	0	1	0	0	0	0	0	0	0	0	0	0	0
Bone Knife	0	2	0	0	0	0	0	1	0	0	0	0	0
Bone Scraper	0	0	0	1	0	0	0	0	0	0	0	0	0
Cupping Vessel	0	0	0	3	0	0	0	0	0	1	0	0	0
Blade	0	0	0	0	0	0	0	0	0	1	0	0	0
Bone Lever	0	0	0	5	0	0	0	0	0	0	0	0	0
Trepanning Saw	0	0	0	1	0	0	0	0	0	0	0	0	0
Bone Borer	0	0	0	2	0	0	0	0	0	0	0	0	0
Cautery	0	0	0	1	0	0	0	0	0	0	0	0	0

The table also indicates that certain areas not only have a higher number of common instruments, but a greater variety (as would be expected with a higher sample size). Germania Inferior's legionary fortresses, both unit types in Germania Superior and Pannonia Superior's legions (although this is mainly Carnuntum) have the greatest range of instrument types. This suggests that either certain areas were adopting more Roman style medical tools than other areas, or that it might be a product of a greater sample size. One medical object that has a specific regional distribution is the oculist stamp, found mainly throughout civilian settlements in the northwestern provinces; although there are exceptions as examples have also been found in Africa, and even on the remains of a Roman shipwreck off the coast of Italy (Feugère *et al.* 1985). The same pattern appears on Table 5.3, as the majority of stamps were found in Germania Superior and they do not appear in Pannonia

Inferior. Curiously, this pattern also applies for the spatula probes. On the other hand, some instruments were found in most provinces. For example, the majority of sharp hooks were found in the auxiliary units of Germania Superior and in the legion of Carnuntum, but they also appear in Germania Inferior, Raetia and Britannia.

For more specific examples of instrument adoption, one can see that certain instruments are only found in fortifications linked to a single unit. Caerleon, for example, has a possible dental tool (Appendix 10, Table A10.2, number 4; Lee 1862: 67). Whilst engaged in fieldwork I did not see any other instrument of this type, conceivably because similar instruments have not been identified as medical tools by archaeologists, that the identification by Lee (1862: 67) was incorrect, or that it was a tool local to that site or area only.

Other single or unusual instruments were found in other fortifications as well. For example a cataract needle was found at Carlisle (Appendix 10, Table A10.11, number 3) and a rectal speculum was found at the auxiliary fort at Vechten, in Germania Inferior (Appendix 4, Table A4.4, number 1). The speculum might have been used in the removal of missiles, perhaps being the type of instrument

Fig. 13. Possible foetal hook from Mainz. After Lindenschmitt 1889: Tab. 22:13.

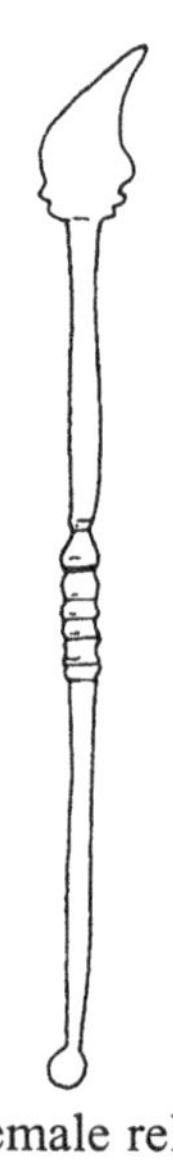

Fig. 14. Possible pterygotum. After Deringer 1954: Fig. 81:1.

described in Celsus (Appendix 3) that appeared to be similar to a Greek letter. Something called a 'scratcher', again without a depiction or description, is noted for Neuss (Appendix 4, Table A4.1, number 70). Although its identification is insecure, it has been retained within this sample. There is also a possible foetal hook that was found at Mainz (Appendix 5, Table A5.1, number 5); though it is mentioned in an older publication without a size being given for the item. If its identification is correct this is a rare instance of a female related instrument being found in a military context (Fig. 13). Dental forceps were found at Vindonissa, and might also have been used in bone surgery (Appendix 5, Table A5.2, numbers 1 & 2).

The auxiliary forts from Germania Superior also have a number of more unusual instruments in comparison with other provinces. Ladenburg had scalpels, hooks and an implement for scraping bone (Appendix 5, Table A5.3). Bingen has a collection of mainly bone-working instruments (Como 1925). The instruments included in the set were cupping vessels, a trepanning saw with circular blades, along with tools used for lifting bones and scalpels (Appendix 5, Table A5.25). Lauriacum (Appendix 7, Table A7.1, number 4) and Neuss (Appendix 4, Table A4.1, number 8) have an instrument called a pterygotum or ear speculum (Fig. 14). Both a female and male catheter are published in the medical findings from Carnuntum (Appendix 8, Table A8.1, numbers 17 and 18).

This closer inspection of the instruments indicates that in most cases only certain areas, or even fortifications, were adopting the use of specific Roman style medical tools, providing greater support for the argument that there were provincial differences in medical care between the frontiers. It is not only medical tools that show this distinction, but other finds as well. Military belt-plates appear more in Germania Superior than any other province; Bishop and Coulston argue that this is because of a greater amount of excavation (1993: 197). However, this is not an entirely secure argument because it should be noted that there has been a substantial amount of excavation in Britain, Germania Inferior and Raetia.

5.6 Testing Distribution

Since not all of the excavated fortifications appear to have any medical care provision, as evident through the epigraphic and instrument remains, perhaps there was a procedure whereby certain fortifications were designated to act as central areas that offered more advanced health care. This idea is considered by Wilmanns (1995a: 108-116) who looked at the distribution of inscriptions and buildings that have been identified as *valetudinaria*. She concluded that there did not seem to be a structural pattern of distribution, but believed that the sick were transported to a place with a doctor or a hospital. However, because the identification of *valetudinaria* is tenuous (Chapter 6) it is important to look at the distribution of instruments and inscriptions from fortifications on the frontiers to see if there is an equidistant spread of fortifications with evidence for Roman style health care. Essentially, the reason for studying the distributions is to see if there might have been certain fortifications that acted as designated areas for medical treatment. Although moving an ill soldier to another fortification does not seem to be a convenient practice it is still worth consideration because it may lead to new conclusions about the arrangement of medical treatment in the army. To test this theory, distribution maps have been prepared to see if the locations of fortifications containing epigraphic and medical implement evidence were equidistantly spaced (Figs. 15-19).

To begin with, Noricum and Pannonia Superior (Fig. 15) only have evidence for Roman style little evidence is recorded for the legionary fortresses of Vindobona and Brigettio. Inscriptions for doctors come from Carnuntum (Appendix 2, Table A2.5, numbers 20-21) and a cemetery outside Brigetio (Appendix 2, Table A2.5, number 22). The majority of the instruments were found at the site of Carnuntum, though the other sites also had them (Appendix 8, Tables A8.1-8.3; Fig. 15).

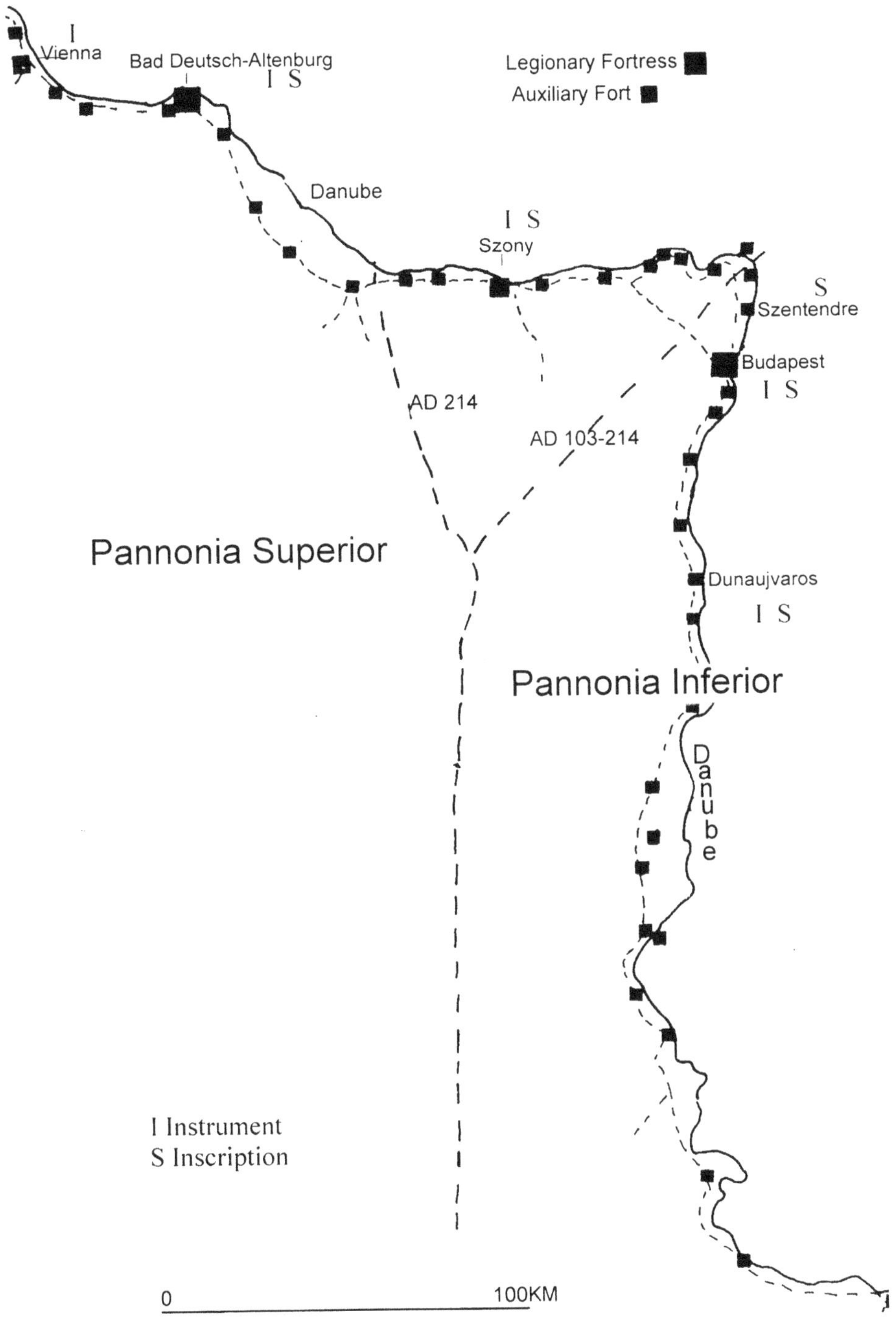

Fig. 15. Distribution map of instruments and inscriptions from fortifications in Pannonia Inferior and Superior. After Mócsy 1974.

medical care from the legionary fortresses. Three legionary fortresses were constructed in the province of Pannonia Superior, with very few auxiliary forts. There is no evidence to suggest Roman style health care in the auxiliary forts, and

Pannonia Inferior has some evidence for health care being offered outside the legionary unit. Not only were the inscriptions found at Aquincum, the only legionary fortress in the province (Appendix 2, Table A2.6, numbers 24-33), but one inscription was found at Intercisa (Appendix 2, Table A2.6, number 35) and another at Ulcisa Castra (Appendix 2, Table A2.6, number 34). There were instruments found at Aquincum and Intercisa (Appendix 9, Tables A9.1-9.2). The units that have evidence for Roman health care are all located within close proximity to each other (Fig. 15).

Raetia, unlike Noricum, does have evidence for medical treatment in the auxiliary forts. The only identifiable inscription was found in the legionary fortress (Appendix 2, Table A2.3, number 18). When looking at the distribution map (Fig. 16) there does not seem to be an even pattern in the distribution of fortifications that have instruments and inscriptions. For the auxiliary forts there appear to be clusters of units with instruments, rather than an even dispersal. The map also shows an unusual pattern of instrument numbers, as some forts with one or two instruments, such as Gnotzheim, are in an area with forts with more medical tools, such as Ellingen.

The clusters of fortifications with evidence for medical care continue to appear in Germania Superior (Fig. 17). Many of the auxiliary forts constructed in the Taunus-Wetterau region have evidence for medical tools, while those with inscriptions are not concentrated in a single area. There is also a noticeable cluster of forts on the Antonine frontier, but few on the Neckar line of fortifications located behind it. The legionary fortresses all have evidence for inscriptions (Appendix 2, Table A2.2, numbers 5-6, 11-13), but only Mainz and Vindonissa have evidence for instruments (Appendix 5, Tables A5.1-5.2).

Germania Inferior seems to have more of an equal distribution of auxiliary units with instruments in the northern section of the province (Fig. 18), whilst the legionary fortresses of Nijmegen, Neuss, Bonn and possibly Xanten have evidence for Roman style instruments and are fairly equidistantly placed in relation to each other. The inscriptions for the fortresses were only found in Bonn (Appendix 2, Table A2.1, numbers 1-2) and possibly Vetera (Appendix 2, Table A2.1, number 4). The evidence found at Vetera is specific to the civilian settlement, but there is always a possibility that soldiers could have opted to be treated by a Roman style doctor in a nearby area.

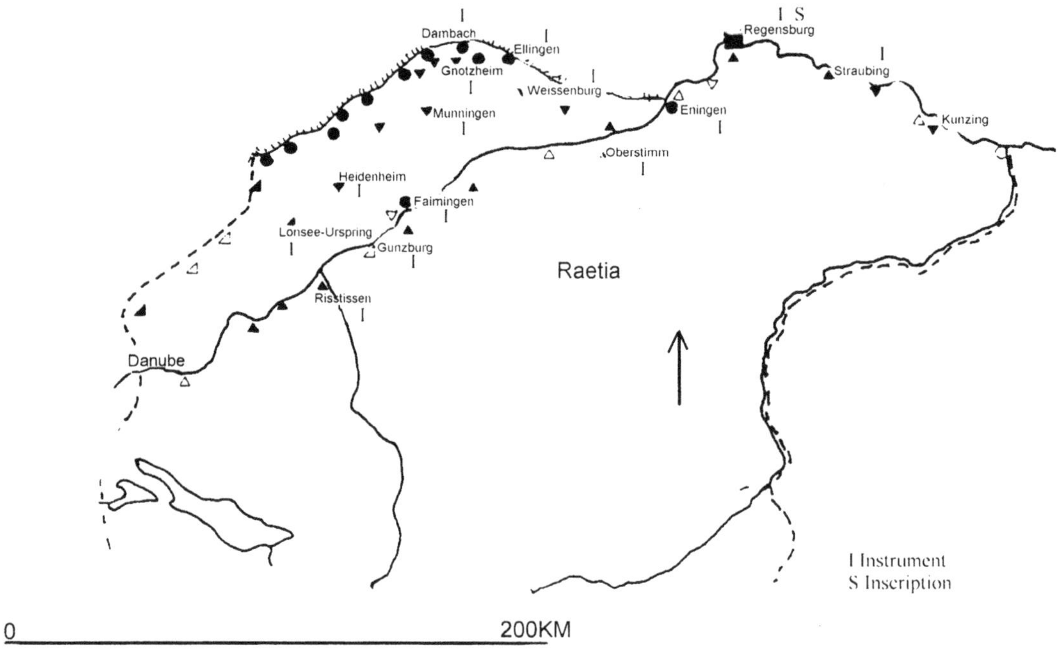

Fig. 16. Distribution map of instruments and inscriptions from fortifications in Raetia. After Schönberger 1969: Fig. 20.

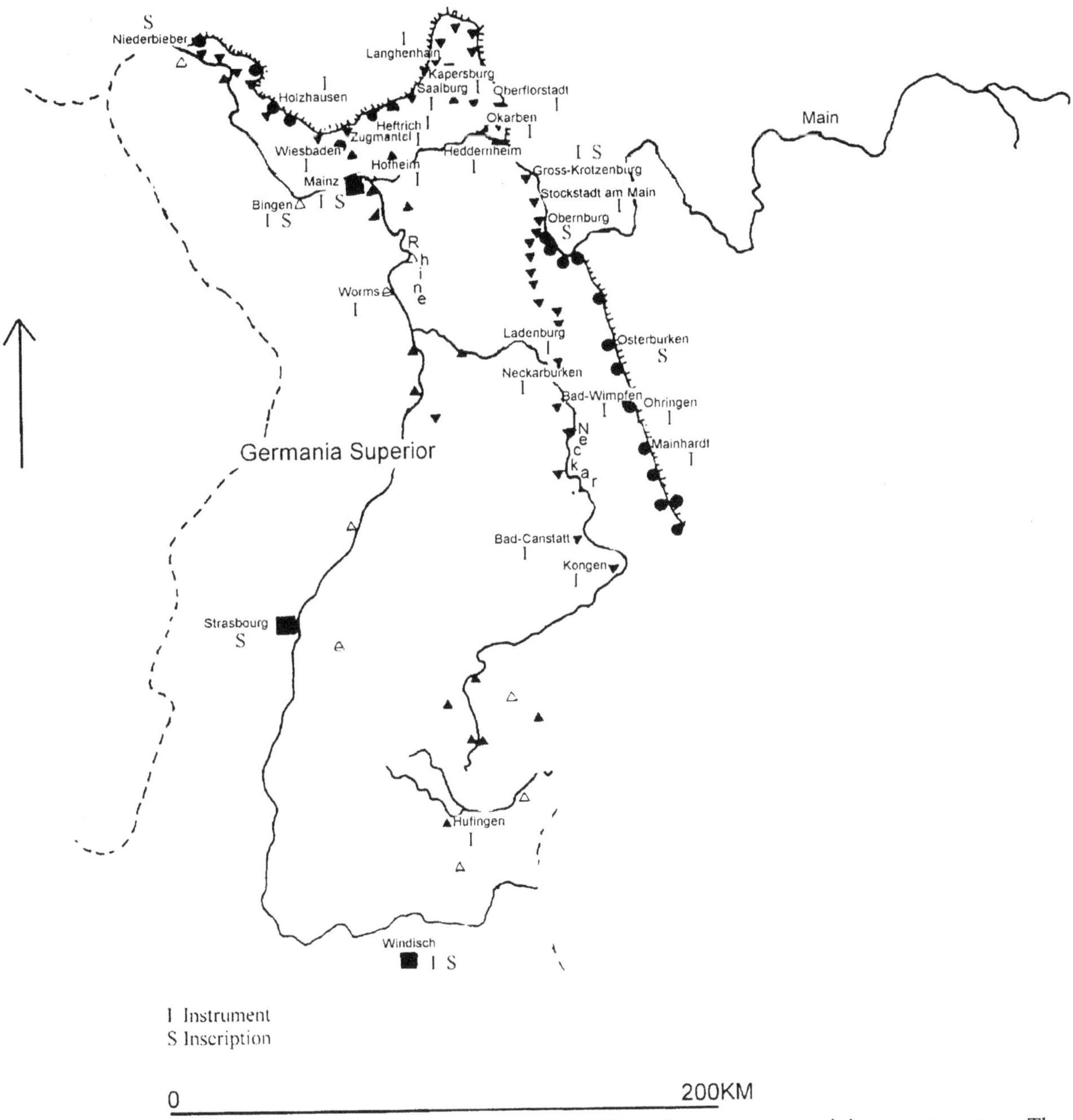

Fig. 17. Distribution map of instruments and inscription from fortifications in Germania Superior. After Schonberger 1969: Fig. 20.

For Britannia (Figs. 19 and 19a) the concentration of units with evidence for medical care was found on the frontier of Hadrian's Wall. Evidence from both inscriptions and instruments was found at the legionary fortress of Chester (Appendix 2, Table A2.7, numbers 36-37; Appendix 10, Table A10.3) and instruments from Caerleon (Appendix 10, Table A10.2). The auxiliary forts in Wales have a very low yield of medical instruments, basically only one or two probes (National Museum of Wales, unknown site). Since most museums and site records for Wales have no instruments or inscriptions, one should question where, or how the soldiers here were receiving treatment. The northern frontier of Hadrian's Wall, however, seems to have a noticeable distribution of instruments and inscriptions. Two auxiliary forts with instruments, Corbridge and Carlisle, were located on main roads leading to Hadrian's Wall from the north and south, whilst in the central area of the frontier there is an inscription for a *medicus ordinarius* at Housesteads (Appendix 2, Table A2.7, number 39). The forts with instruments appear to be located in the central and eastern area of the Wall (Fig. 18), with only a small number of instruments being found in units in the western area of of the frontier (Appendix 10, tables A10.10-10.12).

Having presented basic descriptions of the distribution of units with evidence for medical care per province, models can now be put forward to offer an explanation of how medical treatment might have been arranged in the Roman army. It is clear from the maps that each province varied in arrangement of fortifications with medical tools and inscriptions. Three patterns appear on the distribution maps. Certain provinces have equidistantly spaced fortifications with finds relating to medical activities. These fortifications also seem to be equidistantly placed from one another within the province, in comparison to other provinces. The second pattern that appears has groups of fortifications with evidence of Roman medical tools clustered together on the frontiers. Whilst the final seems to have no pattern at all, and the fortifications with evidence for medical care appear to be randomly spaced.

Britannia, the northern section of Germania Inferior and possibly Pannonia Superior (Figs. 15, 18, 19a) belong to the first pattern mentioned and have the most evidence for central fortifications dedicated to medical treatment. In Britannia, it is possible that Caerleon and Chester acted as medical centres for some auxiliary forts on the Welsh frontier. Yet, they are a far distance from the auxiliary forts on the west coast of Wales, so one would expect that there was some other form of medical treatment made available to these soldiers. Otherwise a sick or wounded soldier or a doctor would have to travel a long way to and from the legionary fortresses. For the frontiers of Hadrian's Wall and northern Germania Inferior the auxiliary forts, along with the legionary fortresses on the Rhine, all seem to be spaced fairly equidistantly apart from one another. The location of the legionary fortresses in Pannonia Superior look to have been better suited to act as centralised medical centres. Here the fortresses are placed fairly equal in distance from one another and each has five to six auxiliary forts located between them. It is therefore possible that medical treatment was offered through these central fortifications, or a doctor was able to travel from these places. Thus, these provinces might have arranged the provision of health care from certain fortifications, rather than at all of the forts.

Noricum and Pannonia Superior (Fig. 15) are interesting because they are the two provinces that only have remains of medical tools and inscriptions from legionary units. It may be that in these places the legions were designated places for soldiers from auxiliary forts to receive treatment, as already described for Pannonia Superior. However, the legionary fortress for Noricum was not based in the centre of the frontier line of the province and many of the auxiliary forts were a long distance from the site, so it would mean that soldiers or a doctor from Lauriacum would have had to travel an unreasonably long distance for treatment. As of yet there is little evidence for Roman style medical treatment in Noricum's auxiliary units that were occupying the sites a century earlier than Lauriacum was constructed. There are a number of

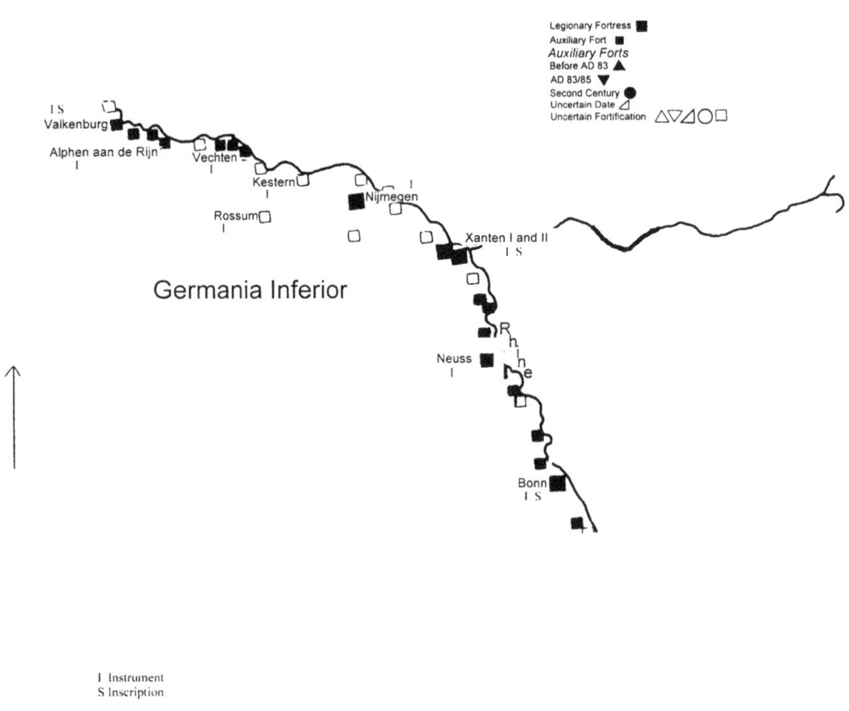

Fig. 18. Distribution map of instruments and inscriptions from fortifications in Germania Inferior. After Schönberger 1969: Fig. 20.

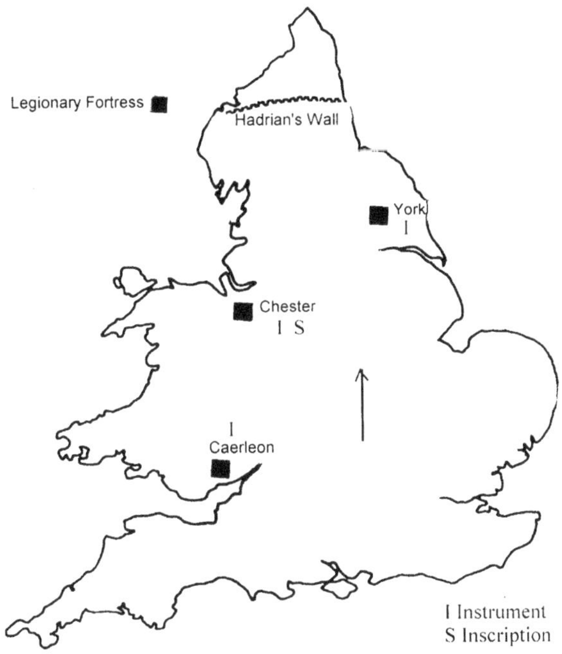

Fig. 19. Distribution map of instruments and inscriptions from legionary fortresses in Britain.

possibilities for this. It may be that the auxiliary units in Noricum, in spite of the lack of evidence, were provided with treatment, or that there might have been some treatment made available by a doctor who travelled from fortification to fortification. Finally, there might not have been any medical treatment, or at least Roman style medical treatment offered in particular units, which may be an indication that each unit was permitted to organise medical care in their own manner.

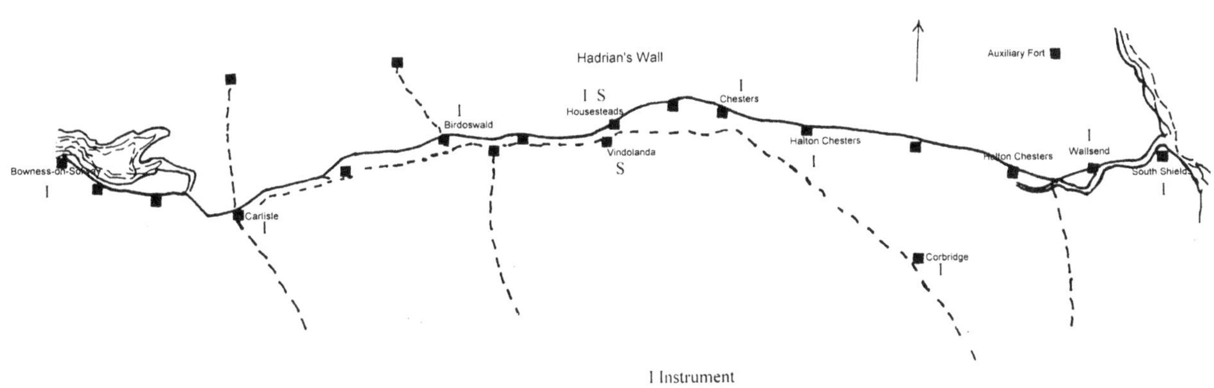

Fig. 19a. Distribution map of instruments and inscriptions from fortifications on Hadrian's Wall. After Breeze and Dobson 1991: Fig. 9.

Pannonia Inferior (Fig 15), like Noricum, has only a little evidence for health care in the province, most of it in the legionary fortress. However, two auxiliary units also have evidence for treatment, but they were constructed in close proximity to Aquincum, so on this basis the theory of a centralised fortification designated for medical treatment does not appear to be plausible. It may be that the fortress of Aquincum was the main medical centre for the frontier because the inscriptions from the auxiliary forts in this province only mention capsarii, who might possibly have provided basic first aid. Intercisca is the only fort with instruments. Overall the evidence from this province is similar to Noricum because Aquincum is a far distance from auxiliary forts in the south of the province.

Raetia (Fig. 16) and Germania Superior (Fig. 17) show evidence for health care in both the legionary and auxiliary fortifications. However, the distribution of the units appears to be in clusters. It might suggest that certain areas of these frontiers were designated as places for medical treatment, or that the units with Roman style medical care might have influenced others close by. In Germania Superior one of the groups of units appears in the Taunus-Wetterau region because many were constructed during the reign of Domitian, when there was a military campaign (Chapter 3). The same might be true for the Antonine frontier beyond the River Neckar in Germania Superior. Since Raetia saw little military action, perhaps the groups of units with evidence for medical care were influenced by neighbouring troops. Thus, looking at the distribution of instruments on a regional scale presents further evidence that there were variations between the frontiers in the way medical care was provided.

TABLE 5.4: LIST OF AUXILIARY FORTS WITH NAMED UNITS WHERE MEDICAL TOOLS HAVE BEEN RECOVERED

MI Number of Medical Instruments, Belgica refers to Gallia Belgica

FORT	PROVINCE	UNIT TYPE	UNIT NAME	PROVINCE	MI
Vechten	GI	Cohors millaria equitata Ala Cohors quingenaria equitatae	Brittonum Thracum Hispanorum	Britain Thrace Spain	17
Valkenburg	GI	Cohors quingenaria equitata. Cohors quingenaria equitatae	Gallorum Thracum	Gaul Thrace	4
Heftrich	GS	Numerus	Catherensium	Noricum	2
Zugmantel	GS	Cohors quingenaria	Treverorum	Belgica	19
Holzhausen	GS	Cohors quingenaria	Treverorum	Belgica	2
Saalburg	GS	Cohors quingenaria	Raetorum	Raetia	9
Groß-Krotzenburg	GS	Cohors quingenaria	Vindelicorum	Noricum	1
Wiesbaden	GS	Cohors quingenaria Cohors quingenaria Cohors quingenaria Cohors quingenaria Cohors quingenaria	Dalmatiarum Pannoniorum Thracum Delmatarum Raetorum	Dalmatia Pannonia Thrace Dalmatia Raetia	4
Neckarburken	GS	Cohors quingenaria equitata	Aquitanorum	Gaul	1
Bad Wimpfen	GS	Cohors quingenaria Cohors quingenaria Cohors quingenaria equitata	Aquitanorum Hispanorum Germanorum	Gaul Spain Germany	2
Stockstadt	GS	Cohors quingenaria Cohors quingenaria. Cohors quingenaria	Hispanorum Gallorum Gallorum	Spain Gaul Gaul	1
Langenhain	GS	Cohors quingenaria equitata	Aquitanorum	Gaul	1
Öhringen	GS	Cohors quingenaria Cohors quingenaria	Helvetiorum Belgarum	Helvatia Belgica	1
Mainhardt	GS	Cohors quingenaria equitata	Asturum	Spain	1
Straubing	R	Cohors quingenaria	Raetorum	Raetia	21
Weißenburg	R	Ala	Hispanorum	Spain	6
Gnotzheim	R	Cohors quingenaria Cohors quingenaria equitata	Bracaraugustorum Thracum	Spain Thrace	1
Dambach	R	Cohors quingenaria equitata	Aquitanorum	Gaul	1
Dunaújváros	PI	Ala Cohors milliaria sagatorum	Tungrorum Hemesenorum	Belgica Syria	15
South Shields	B	Cohors quingenaria equitata.	Gallorum	Gaul	10
Wallsend	B	Cohors quingenaria Cohors quingenaria equitata	Nerviorum Civium Romanorum Lingonorum	Belgica Gaul	3
Halton Chesters	B	Ala	Pannoniorum	Pannonia	2
Chesters	B	Ala	Asturum	Spain	13
Housesteads	B	Cohors milliaria Numerus Numerus	Tungrorum Frisiavonum Hnaudfridi	Belgica Frisia Germany	6
Birdoswald	B	Cohors milliaria. Cohors quingenaria	Tungrorum Dacorum	Belgica Dacia	5
Corbridge	B	Cohors milliaria equitata	Vardullorum	Spain	23
Carlisle	B	Cohors quingenaria	Gallorum	Gaul	3

5.7 Comparison of Material Culture

Military events and/or provincial organisation might have had some effect on the way that medical care was organised in the army. Yet, if one considers actions to be the main reason for regional variation one must ask why so few medical tools exist in certain areas that saw military operations, such as Pannonia Inferior? Illness and injuries would have been common in daily activities including the large scale building projects and training, so evidence of medical care is also to be expected in areas that were not as militarily active, such as Noricum.

Here I would like to develop the idea that variation within medical practice in the Roman army extended not just as a result of regional systems of organisation, but because units and soldiers from different ethnic groups retained something of their that Roman medical care was offered. Whilst both types of units were clearly offered treatment there is, however, very little evidence for widespread care being offered to all the units. own traditions of healing. It may be that on occasion they were influenced by the people occupying the region in which they were stationed. It could also be that they were influenced by Roman style medicine, but rather than adopting it outright they changed aspects to suit their own understandings of medical treatment.

In the previous chapter an examination was made to see if there was any evidence of certain groups adopting the use of Roman style doctors, or at least calling their doctors by Roman titles. It seemed that groups from Gaul had the most evidence for inscriptions that referred to Roman style medical personnel; however the numbers were too small to make the study wholly valid. To continue with this line of investigation the auxiliary forts with known units that contained medical implements were compared. This was done to see if only certain units were adopting Roman style medical tools, or if there is a random pattern of units utilising medical tools. Of course this does not necessarily imply that they were using such instruments for the same purposes.

Table 5.4 contains data from 27 auxiliary forts with known units and the number of medical tools that had been found within them. One initial problem with this study is that certain forts had a number of units stationed at them, and without good contextual information it is impossible to know to which unit the instruments belonged. Out of the 27 entries, 16 forts (59%) on the list have single units, or at least are only known to have had one unit stationed at the site. Statistically one may argue it is not a very sound comparison; however, the examination is still worth considering in order to establish whether or not certain patterns begin to emerge, as with the epigraphical comparison. In fact from the 16 forts with instruments a pattern does begin to appear. First of all there are seven units from Gaul, equalling 39% of the total number of forts with instruments. The Treverii and Galliae have two forts each, and there are three forts with instruments for the Aquitanii. Units from Spain (Asturum, Hispania and Vardullorum) occur four times or 31% of the time. Also included are two groups from Noricum, two from Raetia and one from Pannonia. When comparing this with the inscriptions (Table 2, Chapter 4) it is very interesting to note that in general the emerging patterns in both studies match. The units from Gaul have both inscriptions and Roman style instruments. One Norican unit of the *Vindelici* has both an inscription of a doctor and an instrument (at Groß-Krotzenburg). This is the only fort that has both types of evidence.

As mentioned, the difficulty with the data presented in Table 5.4 is that some forts had a number of units of different origin stationed at them. When looking at those associated with a number of units the same pattern begins to appear: groups from different areas of Gaul appear ten times, groups from Spain three times, whilst Raetia and Pannonia appear once. There are also potential linkages between finds of inscriptions and instruments for these units that might tell us which groups were using the instruments. The Syrian unit at Dunaújváros, the unit from Gaul at Valkenburg and Tungria at Housesteads all had inscriptions and instruments, so it is possible that the tools might have belonged to the troops with inscriptions. Although one can argue that the sample is too small, there is a recurrence of units from Gaul and Spain, suggesting that certain ethnic units were more open to adopting aspects of Roman style medicine.

The next stage of the analysis was to investigate whether any similarities existed between units from certain regions and specific types of medical instruments (Table 5.5). This was undertaken in order to investigate whether certain forms of surgery or medical practice were more openly adopted or performed by certain ethnic groups. The table shows the home of the unit and the instruments. There were of course units throughout the empire with the same name, and on this table where there was an instance when two different units with the same name from different forts had the same type of instrument found in it they are designated with a '+' with them.

TABLE 5.5: MEDICAL INSTRUMENTS PER SOCIAL GROUP

C= Catharensum; V = Vindelici; A= Aquitani; G = Gallorum; T = Treveri; R= Raeti; Var=Vardulli; Ast=Asturum; H = Hispani; P = Pannoni

INSTRUMENTS	C	V	A	G	T	R	VAR	AST	H	P
Spoon Probe	1	1	1+1	2	6	2+6	2	3	3	2
Spatula Probe	0	0	0	0	2	1+5	3	1	1	0
Ear Probe	0	0	0	8	5+1	7	8	7	2	0
Scalpel	0	0	0	1	3	1	3	0	0	0
Surgical Knife	0	0	0	0	0	0	2	0	0	0
Hook	0	0	0	1	0	0	0	0	0	0
Cataract Needle	0	0	0	1	0	0	0	0	0	0
Olivary End	1	0	0	0	1+1	2	2	0	0	0
Spoon Scoop	0	0	0	0	1	0	1	0	0	0
Double Ended Olivary	0	0	1	0	1	0	0	0	0	0
Double Simple Probe	0	0	0	0	0	0	1	0	0	0
Forceps	0	0	0	0	0	1	1	0	0	0
Ointment Pallet	0	0	0	0	0	1	1	2	0	0
Oculist Stamp	0	0	0	0	0	2+2	0	0	0	0
Button Probe	0	0	0	0	0	1	0	0	0	0
Shears	0	0	0	0	0	0	0	1	0	0

Unfortunately Table 5.5 shows relatively little, but it is worth discussing because some items are more common to certain groups than others. There are two instruments that appear to be common to all, or most, of the groups: the spoon probe and the ear probe. One instrument that seems more common to a single group is the spatula probe from the Spanish units. There are three groups that share more instruments in common than other units, those from Raetia, Belgica (Treveri) and Spain (Vardulli). It seems that Raetia and Belgica have more than one unit sharing the same instrument types, possibly implying that certain units had adopted specific Roman instruments, or surgical procedures. In support of this, one can look at oculist stamps that appear more frequently in the northwest, mainly Gaul (Feugère, Künzl and Weisser 1985). Here they appear to be common for the units from Raetia and examples are not associated with other known units.

Other support for these observations comes from another source of evidence, graves containing Roman style medical tools from civilian sites. Patterns appear in Künzl's (1983) study of surgical instruments from tombs. Gaul and Spain have more burials, whilst Britain and Noricum have very few with 3 each. Britain now has four burials with instruments (Jackson 1997, Crummy 2002). Gallia Aquitania has four burials and Gallia Belgica has 15 burials. Gallia Lugdunensis and Narbonensis have one each. In Germania Inferior 16 graves with medical instruments were found in and around legionary fortresses and large civilian settlements. Eleven of these were from Cologne. Germania Superior had seven. Hispania does not have many tombs with instruments, but a few exist in each of the three Spanish provinces. One tomb is known of in Baetica, four in Lusitania and two in Tarraconensis. Thus, it appears that the areas with more so-called doctors' burials are the same regions from which military units with strong evidence of Roman style medical practice came.

The virtual absence of epigraphic and artefactual remains from other regions, such as Britannia, Dalmatia and Dacia (shown on Table 5.4), suggests that not every unit coming into contact with Roman ways of life were automatically adopting new ways. These patterns appear in the so-called doctors' burials as well: Britannia has only two burials and Dacia and Dalmatia have one each (Künzl 1983). Interestingly, a number of Spanish groups are not connected with evidence for inscriptions or instruments (Appendix 1, Part 2). This may be because of the limited scale of the excavation at the sites they are known to have occupied, or that only certain Spanish units adopted aspects of Roman medicine. The argument taken here is that medical treatments more familiar to those in Italy were made available to the different auxiliary units, but were rejected or changed by units with different ideas about health care and treatments of the body. Such a scenario would hardly be unique for the Roman world. For example, with Roman Britain Hingley argues for the continued use of roundhouses by indigenous groups as part of a rejection of Roman concepts of lifestyle (1999: 146-7). There is also evidence of auxiliary soldiers buried at Kempten in Bavaria, who combined both German and military identities through their grave goods (Wells 1999: 135-6). Interaction is not a simple process of diffusion between an active donor and a passive recipient (Deitler 1995: 90). Deitler describes how, in studies of Greek contact with groups in what are now France and Bavaria, Hellenocentric readings of interaction between the different societies have been created because modern European cultures tend to place the classical world at the zenith of civilisation (Dietler 1995: 90). Romanocentric readings of the past are also created on account of this belief, and they assume that any culture coming into contact with Rome would have wished, after seeing the Roman way of life, to adopt a similar lifestyle because of its supposed superiority. For example Roman technology is often seen to be better than that of provincial population (Hingley 1999: 147).

Such attitudes do not escape Roman medicine. It is assumed that those who did not have classical medical care would have wanted it because modern scholars have regarded it as superior to the less understood forms of provincial medicine. It seems to be an underlying assumption that is demonstrated in arguments about Romanisation, such as with Wilmanns, who states that Roman style medicine would have been openly adopted in the army by the 2nd century (1995b: 121).

Künzl does discuss evidence for native and Roman interaction in regard to medicines by showing that Romans did adopt some 'Celtic' medicinal plants; plants being described by their indigenous name and not a Greek or Latin one (1991: 189). Although Künzl suggests possibilities for interaction, the army is still seen as a homogeneous group, employing similar medical practices. Moreover, this underlying supposition of the superiority of Roman medicine, as it seems to the author, is demonstrated by a lack of study into provincial practices of medicine; again Künzl does so to an extent, but it is almost always viewed in the context of Greek influence on 'Celtic' and Germanic medicine before a Roman influence (1991: 185). One reason for this is that archaeologists only concentrate on the understood aspects of Roman medicine from the Latin and Greek medical literature and rarely look for other forms of medical practice through archaeological remains – this is a 'text restrained' archaeology. Künzl states there was a collision of the Roman republic with the 'Celts' in the 1st century BC leading to a confrontation between a technologically superior *Hochkultur* and a developing one (1991: 185). Yet there were many problems in classical medicine: there was no anaesthesia, no guaranteed cure, and no standardisation, which could cause confusion in other culture's interpretations of the subject. It is possible, as demonstrated by the lack of Roman style medical instruments and inscriptions from some military contexts, that certain auxiliary units may have rejected Roman medical practice; or if tools were found, adapted them to their own understanding of how to use them.

Since Gallic and Iberian societies have the most evidence for Roman style medical treatment, an examination was made to see if there were more 'Roman' aspects in their culture present than in others. The understandings of native groups within the empire have traditionally lain in the scope of prehistory, and there is little interaction between those who study Roman archaeology and those who study the native except at the very point of transition. Furthermore, Romanists tend to use the classical historical sources to try and understand the life-styles of native groups, but when comparing the archaeology there are often obvious exaggerations made in the sources along with many misunderstandings. Along with the use of classical sources, scholars also rely on 19th century linguistic designations of the terms 'Celtic' and Germanic, yet by looking at the material culture of these groups it is clear that even if they were in the same linguistic group socially there were many variations (Wells 1995: 173-4). The Treveri for example, although they lived in Gallia Belgica thought of themselves as German through their ancestry, but in their religion had adopted Gallic traits (King 1990: 153-5). By looking at more general aspects of both cultures it is clear that they adopted aspects of a Roman lifestyle to different degrees. For those who lived in Gaul it is obvious that some things Roman were adopted, such as attitudes towards cleanliness, as more baths and toilet instruments appear, but perhaps this says something about their attitudes towards their bodies before the Romans arrived (Woolf 1998: 242). In terms of association it seems that groups in Gaul did have more contact with the Romans, and it is possible that they were more willing to accept Roman medical treatment, or at least have doctors with Roman titles in their units and to use instruments. With the exception of Baetica, which seems to have been more accepting of a Roman lifestyle, the rest of the Iberian Peninsula still retained its language, art, religion and oppositional attitudes to Rome (Curchin 1991: 178; 181-6). It could be that certain aspects of Roman life-style were adopted, or adapted by different Iberian groups as is evident through the inscriptions and remains of medical instruments.

5.8 Deposition of Finds

It has been mentioned throughout this chapter and in Chapter 1 that an understanding of the deposition of Roman instruments could tell us much about the way they were intended to be used, and about attitudes towards disease and medicine. It is argued that this interpretative approach can inform us about medical practice between the different units' specific attitudes towards medicine and the body. From the outset it should be made clear that the uses and meanings of objects (medical tools included) extend beyond the obviously functional. Because of the way in which they are made and used, all objects carry meanings (Hodder 1989; Shanks and Tilley 1987), and their significance in turn affects the manner in which they are employed in practice and deposition (Hodder 1982). Deposition of all classes of material culture can include casual dumping and "more directed, intentionally structured incorporations that are consciously bound up in specific symbolic values" (Whittle *et al.*: 1999: 355). Because of the varied, contextual importance of material culture, rubbish is not a universal category as indicated by Moore's study of the Marakwet (1982). She demonstrates how items are discarded according to their gender association. Deposition is a reproduction of the symbolic categories that constitute their culture. Every culture perceives refuse in a different manner, and objects can carry complex symbolic associations that condition how they are discarded. By looking at depositional patterning in the archaeological record, attitudes towards objects can be presented as well as more general attitudes intrinsic in a specific society.

Studies of deposition in relation to the Roman army rarely consider complex questions about how and, more importantly, why objects are deposited in specific places. In general deposition tends to be understood in the functional terms of recycling, refuse disposal and deliberate clearance (Bishop and Coulston 1993: 34). According to Bishop and Coulston there are not as many metal finds as one might expect from Roman military sites because metal objects were frequently recycled (1993: 34). Their argument is convincing for some aspects; however, not all metal objects were recycled, and some objects are found in some very strange deposits indeed. It has been argued that a box of equipment from Corbridge, buried beneath the floor of the building identified as the *fabrica,* or store building (Bishop and Dore 1988: 128) was intended for recycling (Bishop and Coulston 1993: 35). However, it is questionable why something meant for recycling was carefully packed in a chest with the armour wrapped in cloth and placed under a floor. Whilst Bishop and Coulston suggest (1993: 37) the hoard was awaiting repair, one must question why it was left there for centuries and why it was buried? Other possibilities for its deposition suggest themselves, including it being some form of votive deposit. This is not the only box of equipment to be found buried. A hoard was found at Ribchester, which contained intact pieces of armour, some that had been de-silvered and some that were damaged. It is suggested that it was either put away for future use, or awaiting recycling (Jackson and Craddock 1998: 100). Again it is questionable why such a mix of objects would have been buried? One thing that they have in common is that both might have belonged to Spanish units. The Ribchester hoard may have belonged to the Ala II Asturum, and the Corbridge hoard might have belonged to the Cohors Vardullorum. Perhaps, although only a suggestion, the practice of burying objects had a ritual, rather than practical function in Iberian culture, and this might indicate that there were different ideas about deposition amongst different groups within the Roman empire. It might also have been considered practical to bury objects awaiting recycling because there were magical practices associated with the work of blacksmiths in Iron Age and even Roman times.

Another argument is that objects were buried during deliberate episodes of clearance. Again, this line of reasoning is often taken as 'fact' without discussion of other suggestions. In the case of the unusual deposition within the Newstead pits, argued by Bishop and Coulston to be related to clearance (1993: 34), it is possible to see this material as being deliberately and ritually deposited (Clarke and Jones 1994). In some instances human skeletons were buried in these pits, suggesting that the action of burial was more than simple clearance, but perhaps comprised votive boundary offerings (Clarke and Jones 1994: 120). In civilian contexts, infants and body parts were buried in villa sites in Roman Britain (Scott 1991: 117) and appear to have had a ritual significance, as some were laid in foundations and on the axis of the house. Other possible examples of ritual deposition can be seen in the burial of cavalry helmets in the environs of the legionary fortress of Nijmegen (van Enckevort and Willems 1994: 127-134). Although they were not all in perfect condition, similar to the objects at Corbridge and Ribchester, such objects would probably have been purposefully deposited because of their symbolic, rather than economic, value (Clarke and Jones 1994: 119).

The cultural or 'identity' value of an object will often determine the way it is deposited. Bird-headed winged pendants, for example, are mainly found in areas where Thracian cavalry units occupied sites. These objects might have been the unit's (Bishop and Coulston 1993: 197). Since they have not been recycled perhaps the Thracian soldiers had a specific practice or belief about how the objects were to be discarded. Another example of possible ritual deposition is seen at the site of Velsen, where along a ridge near the site a mixed set of objects was discovered (Bosman 1995: 89). Bosman notes that there were 59 military items found along with bone and indigenous pottery. The majority of the bone is horse, and 90% of the pottery is indigenous. Deposits like this seem to have been a Frisian rather than a Roman practice, and Bosman questions whether the Romans recognised the ritual importance of the site and used it along with the local Frisians, or perhaps whether it belonged to Frisian soldiers (1995: 94). These examples are certainly suggestive of cultural variations in deposition with Roman military sites.

The body is a prime source of symbolism, and it is not surprising that the placement of objects closely associated with it should incorporate complex rules. Shoes were ritually deposited in wells and house foundations (van Driel-Murray 1999: 135-7). Objects associated with clothes and hair have also been found in wells (Allason-Jones and McKay 1985). It is conceivable that other items associated with the body, such as medical instruments, could carry a ritual significance as well (Baker 2004). An object that had been used in medical practice might have had its significance increased because of its association with a specific person or the sick body. It is interesting in this context to note the occurrence of two Roman medical instruments at Stonehenge (Cleal *et al.* 1995: 433, nos. 32, 35), along with a large group of coins, pins and brooches (Cleal *et al.* 1995: 431) – practical evidence that is suggestive of cult activity.

Medical tools might also have been considered to be polluted if they had been used in an unsuccessful operation, or belonged to a dead or rather unsuccessful doctor. In such cases they may have been deposited in specific areas because they were considered somehow harmful, or taboo, so they were disposed of in order to keep them from 'infecting' people or places (Baker 2004).

The difficulty with assessing the detail of depositional practices is that many of the fortifications were examined in the late 19th or early 20th century, and records of their find spots were not kept. It would have been interesting to continue with the theme of known auxiliary units to see if there might have been more information on cultural variation in depositional practices. Nonetheless, the record keeping does, as yet, not allow for such questions to be considered. However, those sites where recording was clear will be discussed to see if there are any provincial differences in deposition.

In a few instances there is sufficient contextual detail to study intra-site patterning. We can start with the fortress of Chester (Fig. 20). Only 13 tools were found in the fortress. They came from a few specific areas of the site. Three instruments

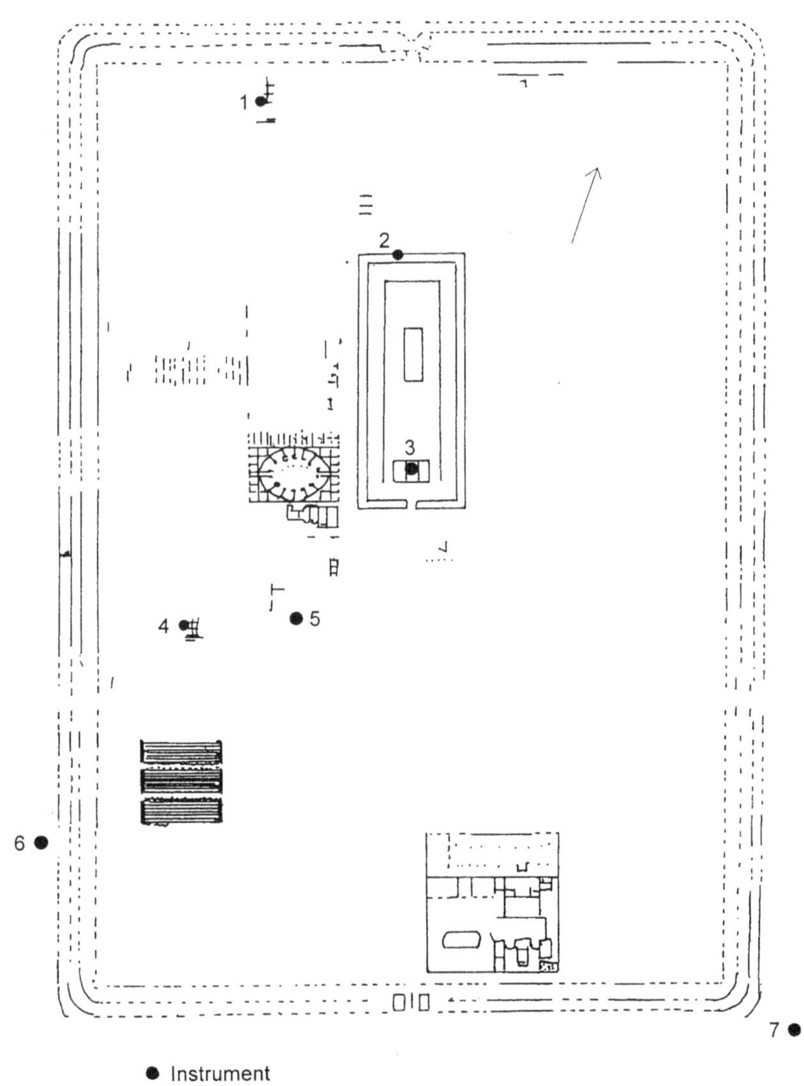

Fig. 20. Distribution of medical instruments in the fortress of Chester. After Mason 2000: 410.

were found in the courtyard building (Nrs. 2 & 3), two of which were broken. Three were found in what has been identified as the first cohort's barracks (Nrs. 4 & 5), one in a northeast barrack (Nr. 1), four in the *vicus* (Nrs. 6 & 7) and one pair of forceps was found in the amphitheatre, located outside the fortress. The reason for a small number of instruments might be because of the amount of excavation at the site, or perhaps indicating that instruments were only used or deposited in specific places.

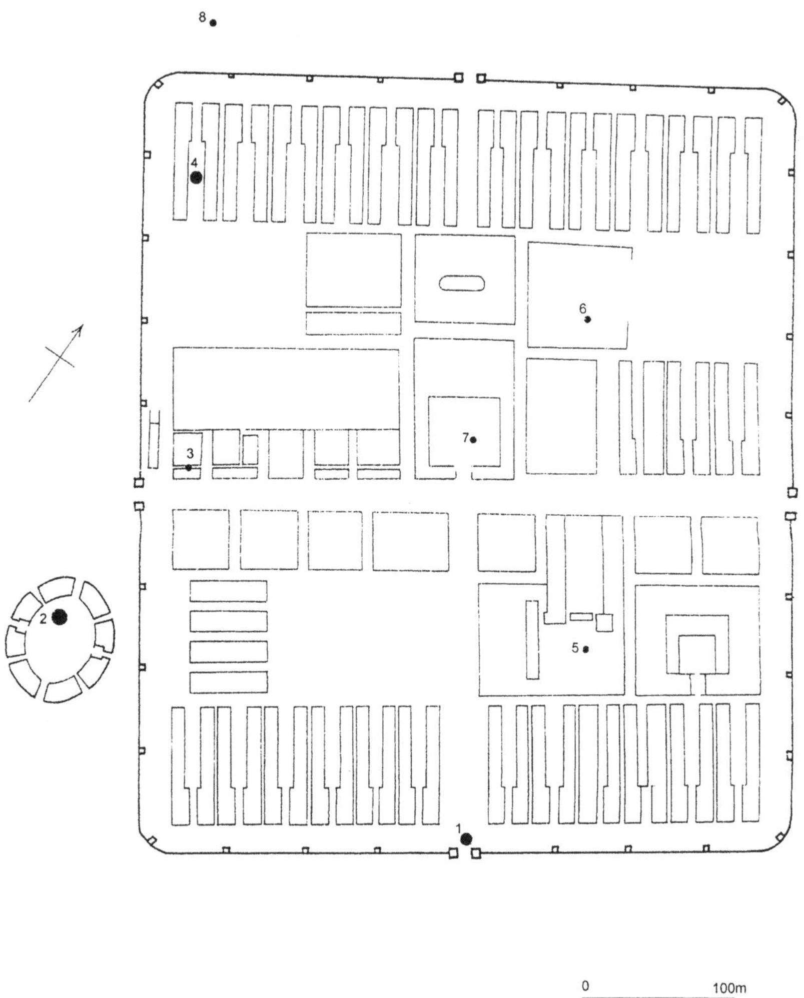

Number on Fortress	Number of Instruments
1	5
2	5
3	1
4	4
5	2
6	2
7	1
8	1

Fig. 21.Distribution of medical instruments at Caerleon. After Boon and Williams 1967.

The site of Caerleon, located in southeast Wales, has yielded 38 medical instruments. When examining their distribution (Fig. 21), it becomes immediately apparent that the instruments seem to appear in clusters, albeit in small numbers. The areas they are concentrated in are mainly in the tower/rampart area (1), the amphitheatre (2), the barracks (buildings 3 & 4), the baths (5) and a possible workshop (6). The rampart area had five probes of varying sorts, two of these instruments are broken, one bent, but the other two were in good condition. Five instruments were found in the amphitheatre: three were broken and two in good condition. The barracks of the first cohort had a spatula probe in good condition buried in a post-hole, itself a rather unusual context (3). The barracks in Prysg field (4) has one probe with inscribed lettering on it and three ear probes in good condition. A surgical needle and a few probes were found in the so-called workshop (6). The baths and the vicus drains also have a higher number of instruments, and with the baths it seems that this might be one place where surgery was performed because children's teeth showing signs of surgical extraction were found in the drains (Zienkiewicz 1986: 223). One broken spoon probe was found in the headquarters building (7). One scalpel was found outside the fortress in a so-called rubbish pit (8). From the patterning it is clear that there is some form of clustering of instruments, which might indicate specific places where they were made, used, or permitted to be deposited. Most interesting are the ones found in the rampart area of the fortress and in the post-hole of the barrack. In the case of the scalpel found in the rubbish pit, since it was in good condition one can ask if it had been deliberately deposited because of pollution taboos? It might also be asked if the pit was for rubbish or whether it really served another purpose?

The fortress of Neuss in Germania Inferior has three areas where instruments seem to be clustered (Fig. 22). One of these is described as the hospital (1), and it has 10 instruments, mainly probes, and four scalpels. The other area is a group of barracks (2), where seven instruments were found. Seven

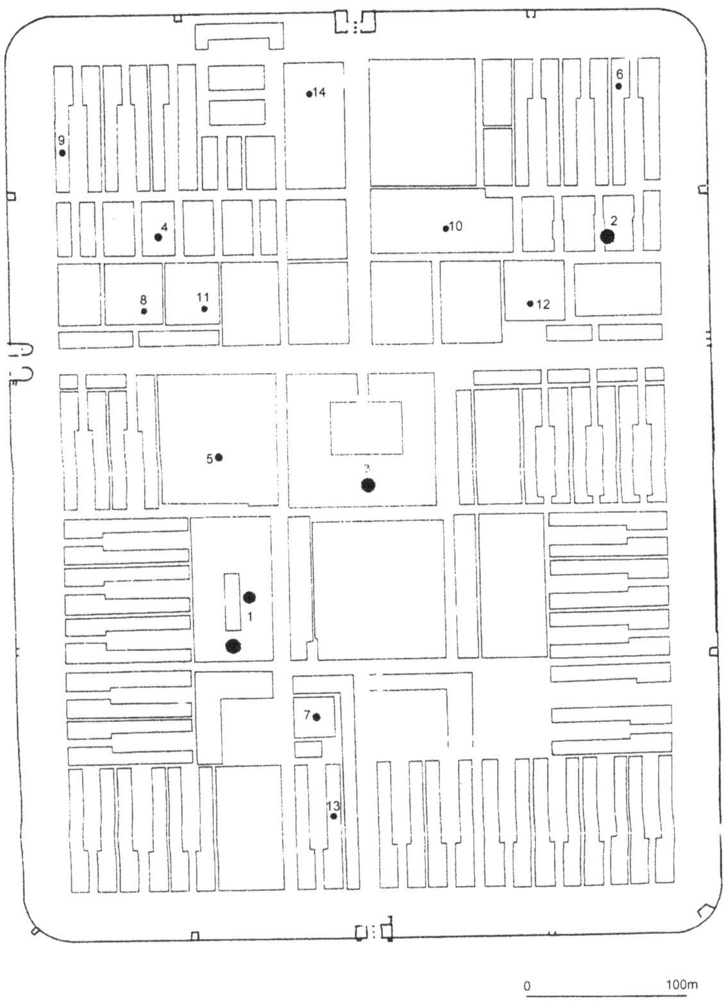

Number on Fortress	Number of Instruments
1	15
2	6
3	7
4	2
5	2
6	1
7	2
8	1
9	1
10	1
11	1
12	1
13	1
14	1

Fig. 22. Distribution of medical instruments from Neuss. After Johnson 198: Fig. 17b.

instruments, mainly ear probes, and all in good condition, were found in the headquarters building (3). Two instruments were possibly found on the corner tower, but they might have come from building four. The bath had a few instruments (5) and one or two were scattered around other areas of the fortress. Three probes and one scalpel were found in the south section of the fortress, but the exact location of the instruments is not known (Lehner 1904 and Watermann 1970). As with Caerleon, it is noticeable that the instruments appear in clusters, but in Neuss they appear in different areas of the fortress. There is the possibility of instruments being deliberately deposited in the ramparts, but this is not completely certain.

The auxiliary fort at Oberstimm (Fig. 23) in Raetia has nine instruments with details of their find spots recorded (Schönberger 1975). The buildings they seem to appear in are the possible workshop (Nrs. 1 & 2), which has four instruments and a courtyard structure (Nrs. 3, 4 & 5). Neither one is identified as the hospital building. Again the clustering appears to be a common aspect to instrument finds.

The auxiliary forts of Birdoswald and Housesteads in Britain (Figs. 24 and 25 respectively) also have the find spots of instruments recoded. Yet, the numbers are too small to note whether patterns appear in their deposition.

Vindonissa, has the highest number of instruments (325), and again they were found in clusters (Fig. 26). Sixty instruments were found in an area called the Schutthügel, a rubbish deposit located outside the fortress (1). Sixty instruments were found in this deposit and a number of them were in good condition. The fact that many are in good condition suggests that the instruments were ritually deposited and might have been placed in this region because they were considered unclean and associated with disease. It is also possible that they were thrown over the side of the fortress as a boundary offering (See Baker 2004 for further discussion on this topic). The barracks do not have many instruments with seven in total (2 & 3), but the central area of the fortress has a cluster of 57 instruments (6-17). The so-called hospital has 13 instruments as well (5). One instrument was found in the south gate tower (13), something seen at Caerleon. There were also a few other instruments scattered around the fortress, but it is noticeable that they were generally deposited in groups.

In order to 'test' the validity of these distributions, the location of surgical instruments was compared to that of another common artefact type - horse-

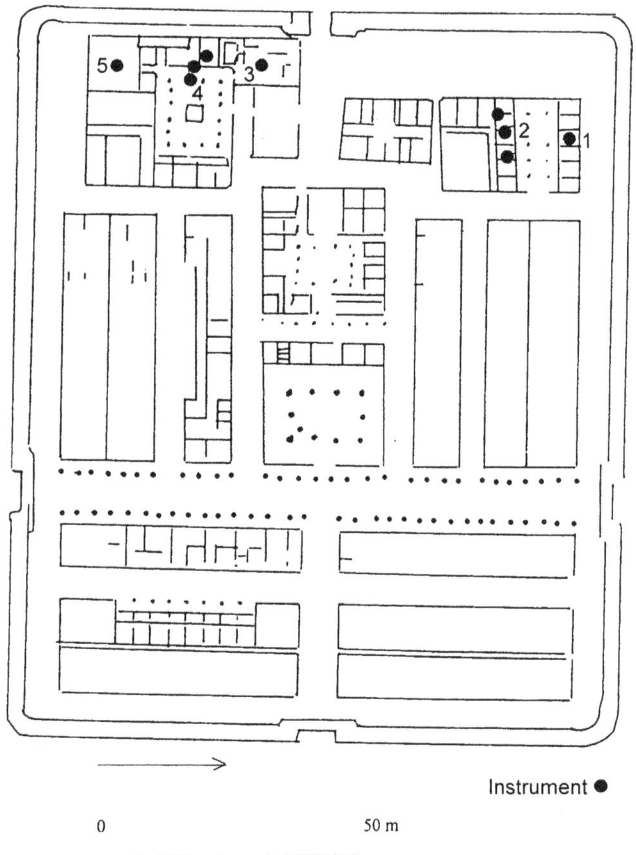

Fig. 23. Distribution of medical instruments from Oberstimm. After Johnson 1983: Fig. 180.

trappings (Fig. 27). Ninety-one were found in the Schutthügel (1), 13 in the so-called hospital (5), 13 in area (4), 34 from the area of the *principia* (6-20), 18 from the barracks (3, 4, 22, 24, 25), 18 from the amphitheatre (28), whilst there were more found in other areas around the fortress. This seems to suggest that different types of objects were found in different areas of the fortress, perhaps because each had specific places of deposition, storage or manufacture. Thus, there does seem to have been a difference in the places metal objects were discarded within Vindonissa, suggesting disposal practices may have varied according to item.

Other forms of ritual deposits are those found in tombs. In the context of Roman burials with medical tools Künzl states that tombs are the best way to see ancient reality (1986a: 130), because they offer a closed context from which to observe the past. What should be said is that they offer a very selective view of reality, since burial practices frequently present a distorted view or idealised image of a dead

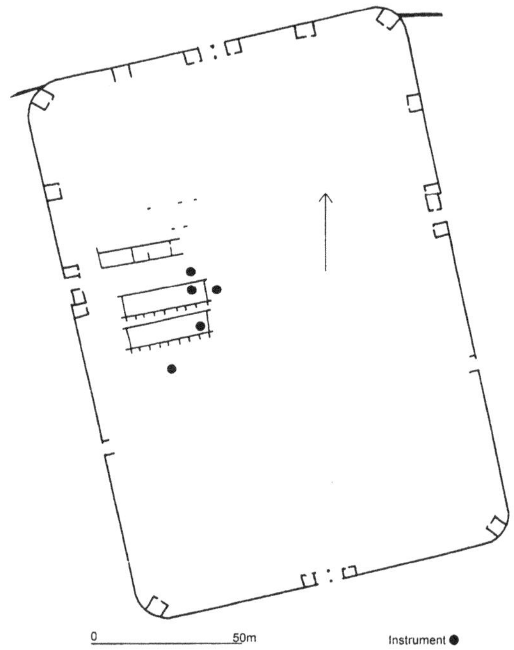

Fig. 24. Distribution of medical instruments from Birdoswald. After Wilmott 1997. Fig. 24.

person and social relationships (Parker Pearson 1999). An example of this comes from beaker burials from the British late Neolithic where arthritic skeletons were often buried with the remains of hunting equipment. This assemblage probably displays how the deceased, or his family wished to be remembered, rather than showing a realistic view of the dead person's true role in life (Thomas 1991). It is likely that Roman burials with medical tools tell us more about the selection of instruments that were permitted to be placed within the tombs and had a symbolic importance for their deposition than any kind of clear reality.

Fig. 25. Distribution of medical instruments from Housesteads. After Johnson 1983: Fig. 199.

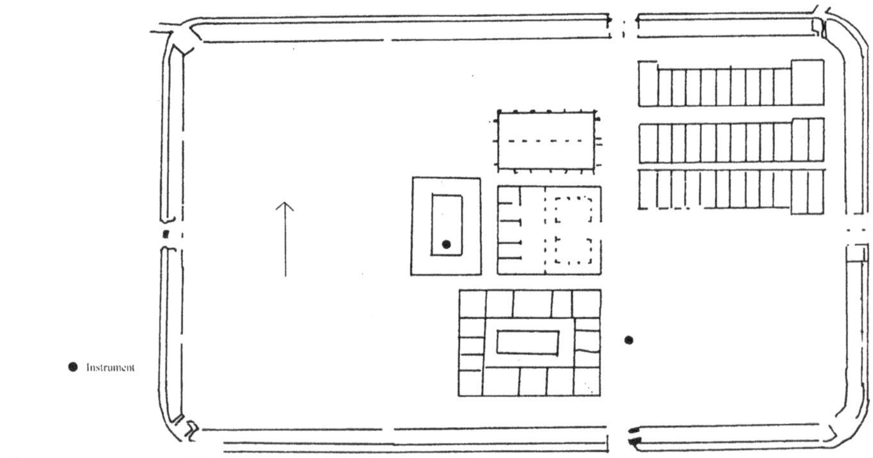

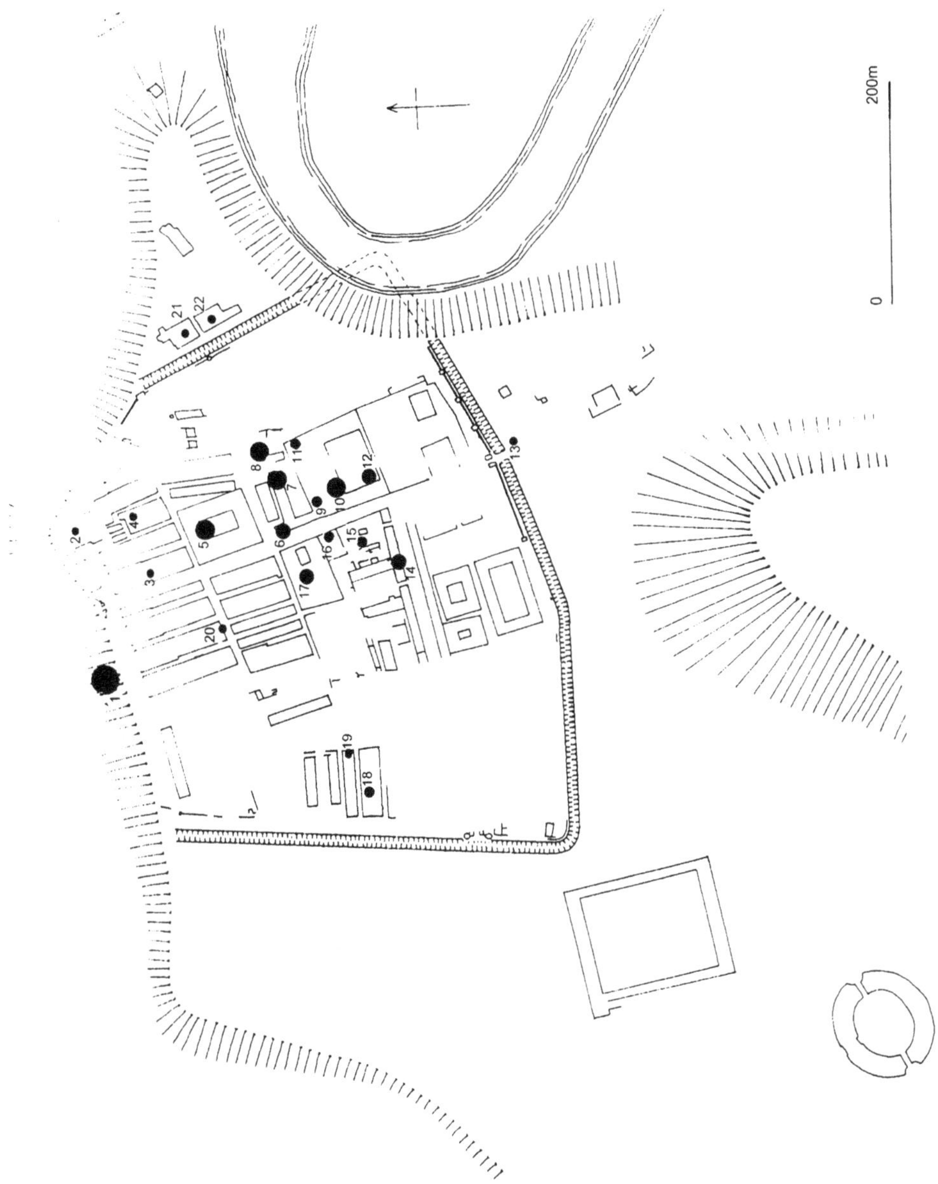

Number on fortress	Number of Instruments
1	60
2	1
3	1
4	1
5	13
6	3
7	7
8	13
9	2
10	10
11	2
12	5
13	1
14	4
15	4
16	2
17	6
18	3
19	1
20	1
21	1
22	1

Fig. 26. Distribution of medical instruments from Vindonissa. After Unz and Deschler-Erb 1997: Fig. 2.

Usually instruments were found in small quantities, probably as token offerings, rather than the entire medical kit. Where it seems that complete kits have been found in graves, for example those at Colophon (Caton 1914) and Bingen (Como 1925), instruments might be considered as personal objects, part of the doctors' identity, and therefore buried with them. It might also be perceived that the doctor was so horrible that his or her instruments were buried as a means of ridding them

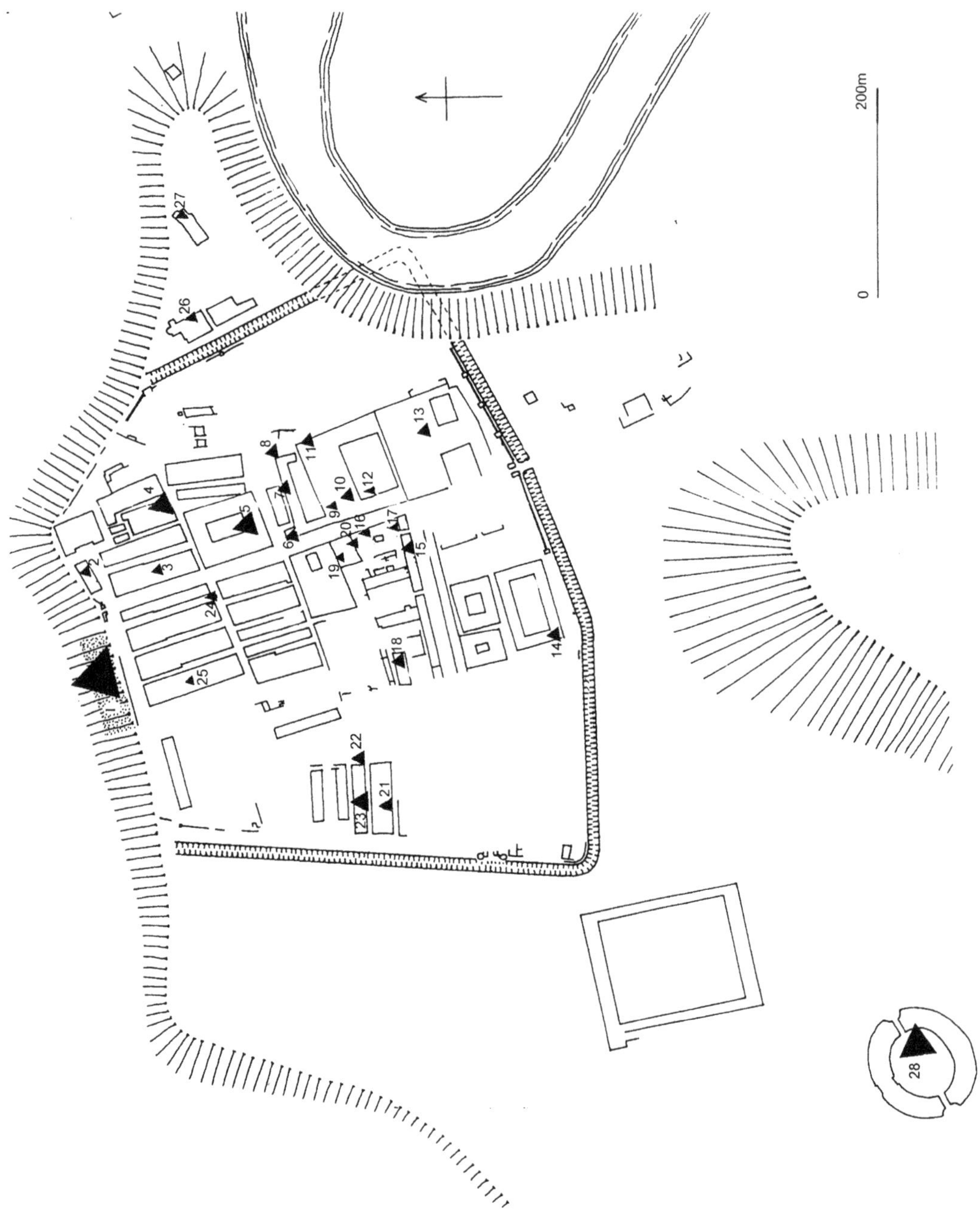

Number on Fortress	Number of Instruments
1	91
2	2
3	2
4	13
5	13
6	6
7	5
8	6
9	3
10	7
11	4
12	3
13	4
14	5
15	2
16	3
17	2
18	7
19	1
20	3
21	4
22	6
23	9
24	2
25	1
26	3
27	2
28	18

Fig. 27. Distribution of horse-trappings from Vindonissa. After Unz and Deschler-Erb 1997: Fig. 2.

from society. The deposition of instruments in tombs would have almost certainly had a symbolic value different to those found within fortifications. Perhaps they were not even part of the person they belonged to, but belonged to a family member, as might be the case with the instrument found in the child's tomb in Worms, Germany (Künzl 1983: 78). Thus, the tombs only show a single view of a complex reality.

Overall it is noticeable that each fortress has different areas where the instruments were deposited and each contained different numbers of instruments. The majority do not seem to appear in a random pattern, but in clusters. Some instruments seem to have been deposited as part of ritual practices, especially those in the rampart areas of the fortresses and the one found in the post-hole at Caerleon. Those instruments that were most likely deposited as rubbish were sometimes found in good condition, begging one to ask if they were thought to have been polluted, or if they belonged to a dead soldier or doctor and were thus considered 'unlucky'. Furthermore, it is suggested that the different patterns of deposition within each fortification may be the manifestation of different cultural attitudes. Thus with these differences one can think back to the anthropological examples of medical practices to understand that medicine is culturally specific, and that even if one cannot say anything with certainty this exercise has hopefully made us think more about attitudes towards small finds and cultural variations in the military.

5.9 Civilian Treatment

A question that was raised in the previous chapter was whether there might be evidence for military doctors treating civilians living in the area of fortifications. There was one inscription from Drobetae that seemed to suggest this did occur. The only other evidence of medical interaction comes from the literature of Soranus and Celsus who described other practices. Nonetheless, these do not answer the question about who was caring for whom. To look at this in closer detail the medical tools can be used to see if there is any evidence for more gender specific instruments, particularly ones that relate to female care. The majority of instruments are not gender specific and can be used on all ages and genders. Yet, gynaecological tools and catheters were intended to be gender specific, so they can be used in this study to try and determine whether care was provided for others who were not in the army. Scott has pointed out that women and children are often not looked for in the archaeological record (1997: 5), and this is the case with the Roman army, where it is assumed that it is a male dominated society with few women, so they are rarely considered. Yet, soldiers had wives, indigenous women would have lived near fortifications and there would have been interaction, so by looking for gynaecological instruments, one might be able to say whether the military doctors cared for non-soldiers. The provision of care probably depended on the beliefs and the rules and regulations, extent and nature of relations between the military and civilian populations of those living in the fortifications, rather than their gender.

Fig. 28. Possible screw-bolt of a vaginal speculum from Niederbieber. After Gaitzsch 1983: Fig. 1.

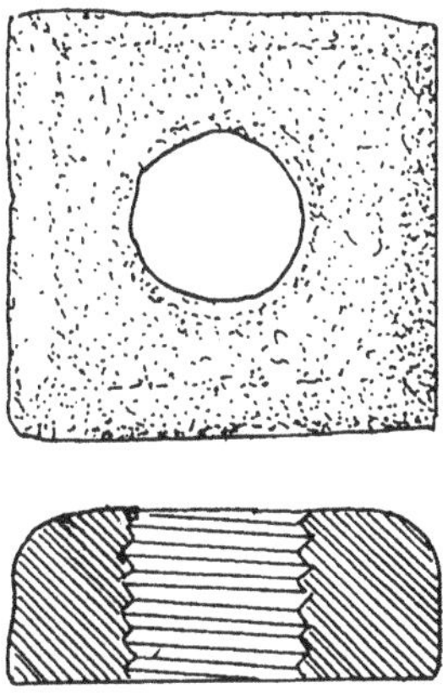

The female catheter from Carnuntum (Appendix 8, Table A8.1, number 19) and the foetal hook from Mainz (Appendix 5, Table A5.1, number 5) suggest that care was available to women on the frontiers. No provenance was noted for either instrument, so it is not clear if they were found in the fortresses or in the extra mural settlements. Yet, since the instruments tend to be Roman in design, it at least suggests that Roman style medical practices might have been made available to the civilians or the soldiers' wives. There is also argued to have been a possible bolt for a screw piece to a vaginal speculum (Fig. 28) from the site of Niederbieber (Gaitzsch 1983: 596). This piece was not included in the appendices because it cannot be attributed with absolute certainty to a speculum and perhaps belonged to another object, related to carpentry for example. Milk-teeth from the fortress baths at Caerleon suggest that health care was available for people other than soldiers; in this case children (Zeinkiewicz 1986: 223). Baths outside the fortress at Vetera and an inscription of a doctor from the site indicate that there might have been Roman health care available to the civilians in the area. From some evidence, the teeth in the bath and instruments from the bath, medical treatment definitely seems to have been offered to civilians, but the instruments can only be used to suggest this possibility, as none are truly gender specific.

5.10 Conclusion

The archaeological remains of instruments have demonstrated that the medical care system varied between provinces. Although one cannot say much about the specific details of differences in medical care and traditions in the Roman army, it can be said that there are variations in the frequency and use of Roman medical inscriptions, Roman style instruments and depositional practices amongst different units. These may be based on different reasons: military and political events, provincial organisation, and there may be a link to different cultural perceptions of body and medicine. With a closer look at the deposition of instruments, and with a better awareness of how various societies defined medical tools and their use, one could make more informed comparisons of the sites and units to see if there are differences in military medical care. However, from our current understanding of the information available and reliance upon earlier archaeological reports, one is limited in the interpretations that can be made, but it is hoped that future investigations will consider these problems with more care. Thus, under the facade of the Roman army lay a mixture of different cultural traditions - a complex milieu of indigenous and Roman.

CHAPTER SIX

QUESTIONING THE IDENTIFICATION OF *VALETUDINARIA*

6.1 INTRODUCTION

The next step to understanding medicine in the Roman army would logically be to compare the remains of buildings identified as hospitals in order to see if they too are specific to certain units or frontiers. In spite of the fact that many people use these buildings to support their interpretations of Roman medical care (e.g. Breitwieser 1998: 61-7; Davies 1989 (1970): 221-4; Jackson 1988: 134-6; Künzl 2002: 28-9; Majno 1975: 382; Nutton 2004: 178-9; Penn 1964: 257; Richmond 1952: 3; Salazar 2000: 81; Wilmanns 1995b: 103-16) there is a need to assess whether there is sufficient archaeological evidence to sustain the interpretation of these structures as *valetudinaria*. This issue is raised because the identification of the Roman military hospital was made at the beginning of the 20th century and has been accepted without question since that time. Over the last century or so there have been numerous archaeological excavations of so-called hospitals in Roman fortifications, but the interpretation of these structures continues to be made in the same manner, regardless of new archaeological methods and theoretical means of interpretation.

There is no question that *valetudinaria* did exist in some legionary and auxiliary fortifications; they are sometimes, though rarely, mentioned on inscriptions and in other literary sources, discussed below. Archaeologically the first Roman military *valetudinarium* to be identified was that at the legionary fortress of Neuss, located on the lower Rhine (Koenen 1904: 180-2). Koenen identified the building as a *valetudinarium* because it contained a room with ten probes (Appendix 4, table A4.1) and four scalpels were found in other rooms of the structure (Appendix 4, table A4.1). Besides the instruments, the layout - a building with a number of small rooms, or wards, divided by small hallways that would aid in keeping the rooms quiet - was similar to the plan of German civilian and military hospitals (Figs. 29-32) of the 17th, 18th and 19th centuries (Brat 1966; Jettner 1966: 82, 144-5), and this would have influenced his understanding of how a hospital should be arranged. Following his naming of the building, others with a similar design were accepted as *valetudinaria* without question, which they still tend to be. As Bidwell says "courtyard buildings in or behind the central range have long been identified as hospitals; conclusive evidence of their function has never been forthcoming from auxiliary forts, but much larger courtyard buildings in fortresses have been satisfactorily identified as hospitals" (1997: 71). Yet, Bidwell does not explain what the evidence is for this satisfactory identification, as 'hospitals' are not the only buildings to have had instruments found within them as can be seen in the previous chapter. Press also shows a willingness to accept Koenen's identification as she said, "the discovery of the building at Neuss brought an answer to the question concerning the layout of the legionary hospital's design and plan" (1988: 69). Press goes on to say, "some archaeologists had doubts as to the correctness of the identification of the building, but the discovery of other buildings with a similar plan confirmed Koenen's opinion" (1988: 69). Unfortunately, she does not explain who the archaeologists were that had doubts, nor does she say what the doubts were, nor why they had them. Yet, how could a building with a similar plan confirm the identification of the *valetudinaria*, especially since many do not have any archaeological material to support this; it merely shows that other structures of this layout were constructed in other fortresses, but it should not be taken for granted that they were intended to be hospitals. Moreover, these are not the only structures to have a courtyard plan. *Principia* (Johnson 1983: 104-132), *praetoria* (Johnson 1983: 132-9), some *fabricae* (Johnson 1983: 163-4, 183-8) and some storage buildings (Johnson 1983: 164) also have courtyard plans. Some of these buildings' identities are fairly secure, as *principia* were to be found in the centre of fortifications and certain *fabricae* have definite evidence for metalworking, such as at Oberstimm (Johnson 1983: 185). Yet not all of these buildings appear to have assured identities, as there have been arguments over whether the building at Corbridge was a *valetudinarium*, *fabrica* or storage buildings (Hanson *et al.* 1979; Johnson 1983: 163, note 152). There are also granaries, or storage buildings from Italy constructed in a corridor plan that are similar in plan to some auxiliary 'hospitals' (Johnson 1983: 164). Thus, the inclination to accept the identification of a building as a *valetudinarium* on the basis of four scalpels and one room with medical instruments (all of which can serve non-medical functions), and a possible anachronistic preconception of how a hospital should be arranged, indicates that there is a need to re-examine the evidence to see if the identification of this building type is secure, or if it was and is based on a tenuous argument.

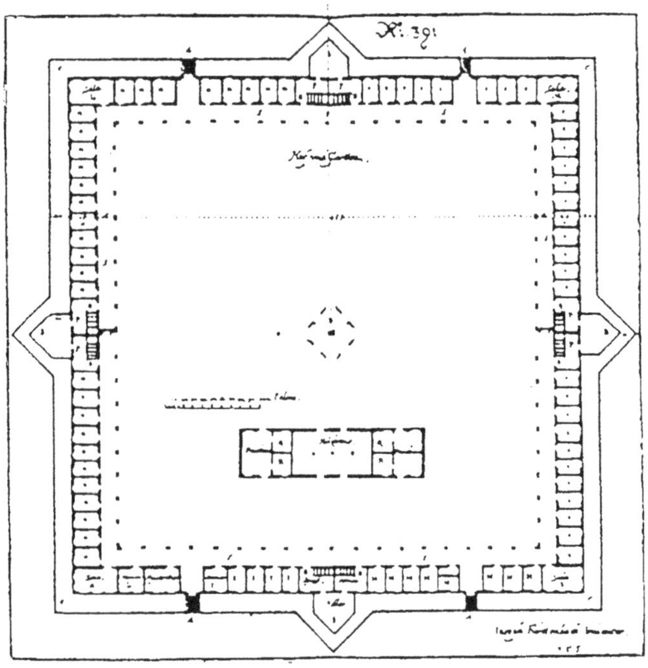

Fig. 29. Plan of a 17th century hospital or poor-house from Germany. After Jettner 1966: Fig. 37.

The main issue of this chapter is to ask whether one can securely define the structures that have been identified as hospitals, as *valetudinaria*. The second point is to see if the buildings identified as hospitals share the exact plan or if they are different. This comparison can be used to continue questioning the hypothesis that there were variations within the Roman army and this could be related to medical practice. To do so the literary sources, architectural remains and remains of artefacts from within the structures will be studied.

6.2 Literary Evidence

The literary evidence unfortunately provides us with little explanation about how *valetudinaria* were expected to appear. Hyginus is the only writer from the Roman period who provides us with information that *valetudinaria* were to be a part of every marching camp at least at the time he was writing in the late 1st century, and this expectation is carried over by scholars for the construction of *valetudinaria* in permanent fortifications (e.g. Bidwell 1997; Johnson 1983; Press 1988). Questions are raised about the

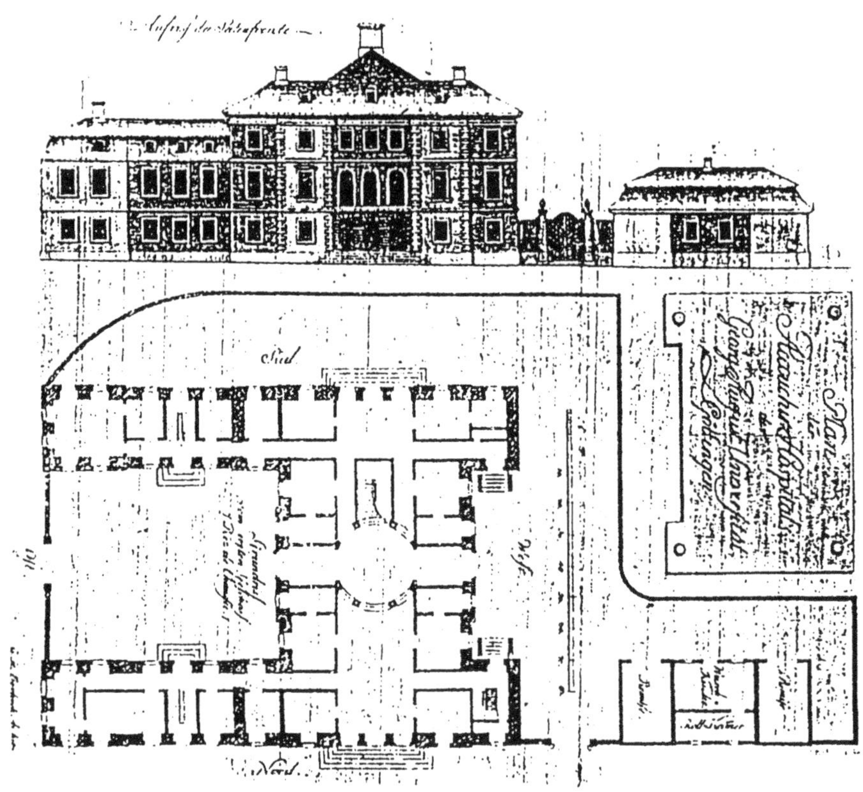

Fig. 30. Plan of an 18th century hospital from Göttingen. After Jettner 1966: Fig. 75.

identification of *valetudinaria* in auxiliary forts, but never in legionary fortifications (e.g. Bidwell 1997: 71; Johnson 1983: 163-4), because there is a strict expectation that the *valetudinaria* should be of a similar and easily recognisable plan. Buildings of comparable plan appear in all fortifications, but perhaps there is too much of an expectation that they were to all serve the same function. Since the buildings identified as *valetudinaria* in auxiliary forts are not of the same plan, more questions are raised about their existence than in legionary fortifications. The only two definite epigraphical sources that mention *valetudinaria* for a specific fortification come from auxiliary forts. An inscription from an auxiliary fort, Mantissa Addendorum, occupied by a second cohort of *equites*, at Stojnik in Serbia (Appendix 2, number 42), has the word *valetudinarium* inscribed on it. Sadly the provenance of the inscription is not noted. Had the inscription been associated with a particular building, perhaps the structure could have provided an understanding about the possible layout of hospital buildings. A tablet from the fort of Vindolanda also mentions the word *valetudinarium*. The tablet contains a fragmentary list that mentions 343 men who were associated with the workshop. It states that of the 343 men, 12 were shoemakers, then it lists builders for the bath house, the word *valetudinarium* and the fragment continues with other references to positions associated with the *fabrica* (Bowman and Thomas 1994: 155). Since the text is damaged there is no indication as to whether the word *valetudinarium* is associated with those who built it, worked in it, or made tools, such as instruments, for it, but what it seems to do is provide a link with the *fabrica*.

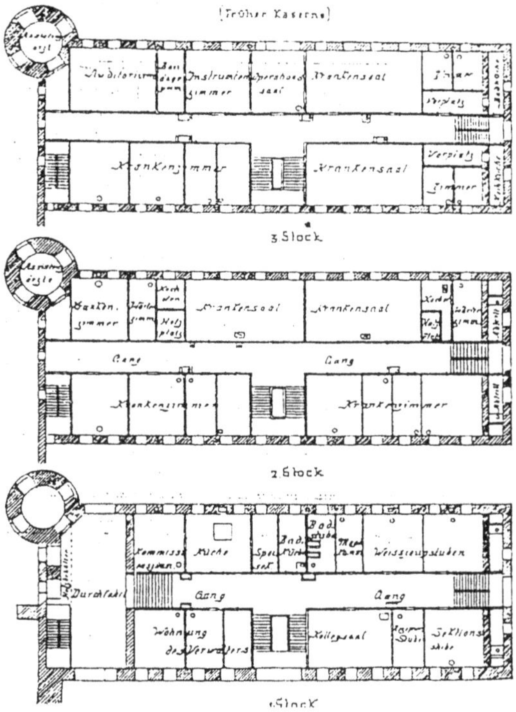

Fig. 31. Plan of a 19th century hospital from Heidelberg. After Jettner 1966: Fig. 83.

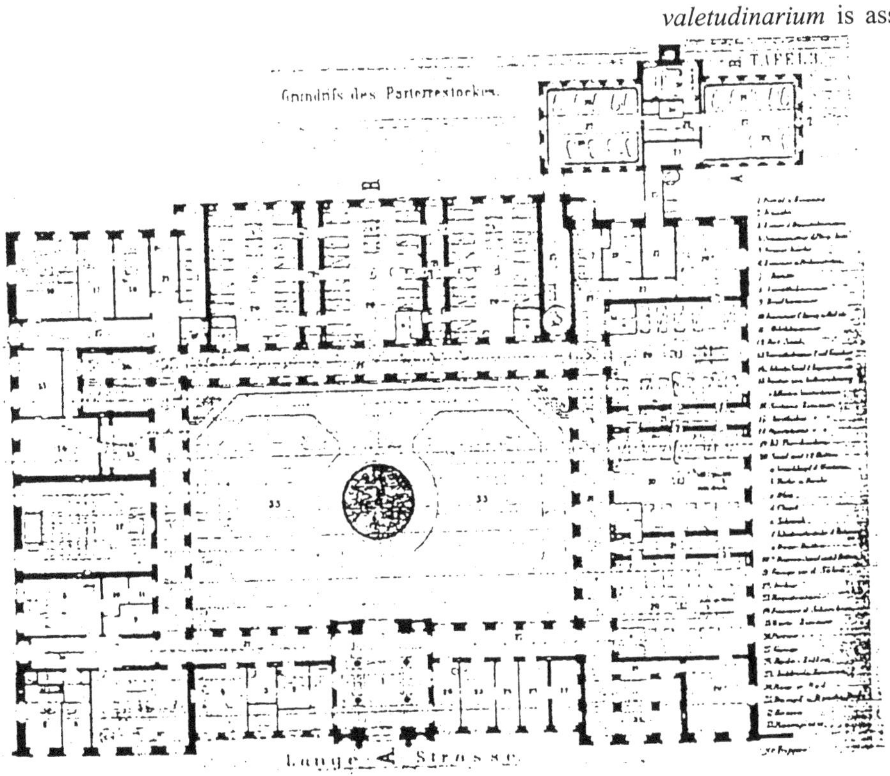

Fig. 32. Plan of a 19th century hospital from Frankfurt. After Jettner 1966: Fig. 92.

As mentioned earlier, Hyginus provides us with a slightly better description of the location of the *valetudinarium* in the fortification in his *Liber de Munitionibus Castrorum*. According to Hyginus (4), the *valetudinarium* was to be constructed beyond the *praetorium*, or the commanding officer's private quarters. As a means of keeping the building quiet, he suggested that the *veterinarium* and the *fabrica* be constructed about 70 Roman feet away from the *valetudinarium* to prevent noise from entering the building. It is often assumed that his suggestion for the location of the building is followed (e.g. von Petrikovitz 1975: 98), but when comparing fortifications of both the legionary and auxiliary units it becomes immediately apparent that each has a different arrangement of buildings, and the buildings that have been identified as *valetudinaria* are not always located in the area that Hyginus suggests. Sometimes they are located closer to the *fabrica* and the barracks, which might have been rather loud places at certain times during the day or night with soldiers' movements. Of course Hyginus was discussing the location of areas in temporary camps mainly made of tents so the distances could have varied from those made of wood or stone, and things might have been different depending upon the materials used in the construction of buildings in permanent fortifications.

The closest epigraphic evidence for the existence of *valetudinaria* in legionary fortresses comes from inscriptions of the *optio valetudinarii*. Two inscriptions were found in Lambaesis in Africa (CIL VIII 2553; CIL VIII 2563) and one was from an unknown unit in Italy (CIL VI 175). From the area of study one was found in Bonn (Appendix 2, number 1) and two from Aquincum (Appendix 2, numbers 25 and 26). All of these are definitely from legionary fortresses, with the exception of the inscription from Italy, which is thought to have come from either a *cohors urbana* (Wilmanns 1995b: 152-3). The only inscription that has a find spot recorded is one from Aquincum (Appendix 2, number 25), and it is assumed that where it was found was the location of the *valetudinarium* (Wilmanns 1995b: 214); however there is very little structural evidence to support the statement. Even if it were from the *valetudinarium* the lack of architectural remains fails to provide information about the layout of the building. The inscription from the so-called hospital at Aquincum was found with another one that mentions a *medicus* (Appendix 2, number 24). Both were erected as altars dedicated to healing deities, so it might relate to an area of a temple rather than a *valetudinarium*. There are other inscriptions that are thought to be associated with *valetudinaria*, but these mention doctors rather than a person associated with a specific structure. Two were found together at Chester (Appendix 2, numbers 36 & 37), but the area where they were found that Wilmanns identifies as a *valetudinarium* (1995b: 207 & 214) has very little structural evidence and has not been thoroughly explored or understood (Mason 2000: 410). A piece of *spolia* from Carnuntum that mentions the word *capsarius* was found built into a wall of the so-called hospital building (Appendix 2, number 20). Given that this is a piece of *spolia,* built into a wall, it is most likely not in its primary context, making it almost impossible to use as support for the identification of the *valetudinarium*, if that is what the structure was. It may have been incorporated within a later building phase of the *valetudinarium*, but one cannot say whether the inscription defines the building as such.

Another indirect indication of hospitals existing in fortifications is provided by a papyrus fragment found in Egypt (BGU 1564=Sp 395, papyrus Egypt 138; Campbell 1994: 239). The fragment, which has been mentioned previously, is an order form from a military *valetudinarium* in Cappadocia requesting a white blanket to be sent to the fortification. The order requested that the blanket should be plain and white, eight feet, eight inches (6 cubits) long, five feet, eight inches (4 cubits) wide and weighing three pounds nine ounces (4 minae). It was also asked in the order that the blanket be of good, soft pure white wool without any stain and that is to be well woven, firm, with finished hems, satisfactory without damage. It was ordered in the second year of Antoninus Pius' reign. Since the inscription mentions the blanket being of pure white wool and with no stain, this gives an impression that hospitals, or at least items associated with the body, were kept clean. One is inclined to ask whether such standards were made of all *valetudinaria*, or only in certain units or provinces, as the importance of cleanliness of items might not have been an universal phenomena in Roman health care. Perhaps it is only the items associated with the body rather than the structure that were expected to be clean. Unfortunately, Hyginus and other writers do not mention anything about this aspect of the *valetudinaria*, and one is only left with the suggested possibility that some *valetudinaria*, at least, might have been maintained as clean buildings.

An interesting point that can be made about Hyginus' suggestion for *valetudinaria* is that they were to be located along with the *fabrica* and the *veterinarium*. These three buildings were used for a form of repair and craftsmanship, be it of the body or something else, an association that was noted from the Vindolanda tablet mentioned above (Bowman and Thomas 1994: 155). Thus perhaps the *valetudinarium* was expected to be in the area of these buildings by means of metaphorical and functional association.

Other primary historical sources that discuss the placement of wounded and ill soldiers on Roman military campaigns have been used by modern medical historians to support the existence of *valetudinaria* (e.g. Davies 1989: 221-2; Johnson 1983: 159-65; Nutton 1969: 262-3; 1995b: 49-51; Scarborough 1976: 78-9). Nutton believes that the *valetudinarium* was based on a group of tents (1995: 49). When the Latin or Greek is examined carefully it becomes clear that the meanings of some historical statements might have been over-interpreted, as the sources relate to soldiers on campaign, not in permanent fortifications. One example of a historical source that is interpreted by Davies to be evidence of a *valetudinarium* is from Hadrian's biography, where a statement is made about how he would visit the sick in their quarters, which is a demonstration of his being a concerned emperor whilst on campaign: "*Aegros milites in hospitiis suis videret*" (SHA *Hadr.* 10. 3). It is important to point out from this passage that Hadrian visited the sick in the *hospitium,* rather than in a *valetudinarium*. *Hospitium* is similar in meaning to the Greek word *ξενοδοχεῖον* and can be translated to mean a place for foreigners to stay, or a place to receive hospitality. Thus the Latin indicates that the sick and wounded were not necessarily placed in a *valetudinarium* for treatment or recuperation, but perhaps in another part of a building, or in a separate area of the campaign fortification.

The biography of Severus Alexander (SHA *Severus Alexander* 47. 2) also describes him visiting the sick in their tents: "*aegrotantes ipse visitavit per tentoria milites*", again implying that this was probably a common practice, or at least expected of emperors and generals. Since the writer uses the word for tent, rather than *valetudinarium*, the suggestion is that the soldiers were placed in their tents, but whether this is meant to be specific tents for the sick is not certain. Simply because he visits the sick and wounded in their tents does not automatically indicate a separate area, or set of tents. It is possible that the sick were placed with others, healthy or wounded, in their ranks. As the plural for tents is used it might imply a single group of tents used as a *valetudinarium*. There is a further suggestion that the soldiers were placed in their regular tents from Tacitus. Tacitus says that in the same tents some nursed the wounds of brothers, others of relatives: "*Isdem tentoriis alii fratrum, alii propinquorum volnera fovebant*" (*Hist.* 2. 45). From these three statements it is difficult to say if *valetudinaria* were set up during all military campaigns, only a few, or if they were set up at all.

According to Majno (1975: 382) a quotation by Livy (10. 35. 7) provides the reason why *valetudinaria* were created. Livy states that during the Samnite Wars in 294 BC soldiers sharing quarters with the casualties were dispirited because they were kept awake by the groans of the wounded and the dying:

> "*sed militum iacere animos; tota nocte inter volnera et gemitus morientium vigilatum esse*".

The statements from Tacitus and that about Severus Alexander expressed the idea that even after Livy wrote the wounded might still have been placed with the healthy soldiers on campaign. At the same time there is no evidence to say they were not placed somewhere separately. Moreover, none of the statements mentions the term *valetudinarium*, so it is impossible to say when, or why *valetudinaria* might have been established. Majno's statement can only be taken as a suggestion, but it does display the fact that soldiers, at least during the time Livy was writing (as his statement might have been made on situations with which he was familiar rather than what actually happened), were most likely living with the wounded. Yet, all of these comments refer to soldiers on campaign and provide no strong evidence to suggest how *valetudinaria* might have developed in permanent fortifications. None of the writers tells us who was supposed to be in the tents. Perhaps only those who were suffering from certain ailments or types of wounds were admitted.

In support of the fact that *valetudinaria* might not have been made available to soldiers on campaign is the literature mentioning wounded soldiers being left behind in friendly villages if they were unable to continue with the march. Obviously, if a troop had to continue with marching there might not have been time to set up a *valetudinarium* and the soldiers could have been left behind in a friendly settlement. The idea of leaving soldiers in this situation is also mentioned well after the time Hyginus was writing. Julius Caesar did this during his campaigns in Africa. He halted for the evening to care for the sick and the wounded and if they became too much of a burden he sent them to stay behind in the local village:

> "*Labienus saucios suos, quorum numerus maximus fuit, iubet in plaustris deligatos Hadrumetum*" (*BA* 21. 2).

He also mentions halting to care for the wounded during the Gallic Wars for three days in order to tend to the wounds and to bury the dead:

> "*cum et propter vulnera militum et propter sepulturam occisorum nostri triduum morati eos sequi non potuissent*" (*BG* 1. 26. 5).

The biography of Severus Alexander continues by saying that if the soldiers did not regain their health the emperor would have them sent to the most upright house-holders or highly esteemed matrons in the cities and country districts near to the campaigns:

> "*per civitates et aegros patribus familias honestioribus et sanctioribus matrionis eos*

distribuebat", (SHA *Severus Alexander* 47. 3).

It appears that if there had been *valetudinaria* on campaign, as Nutton argues there were (1969: 266, note 1) on account of the shape of the so-called *valetudinarium* at Haltern appearing to be like a group of tents, then soldiers would not have been placed in their tents or left behind in friendly villages. Furthermore, the conditions of being on campaign, with frequent movement, may have made it impractical to construct such specialised buildings as *valetudinaria*.

For soldiers not on campaign there is the possibility that perhaps only patients suffering from certain diseases or wounds were expected to be placed in the *valetudinarium* for recuperation. The daily report from Vindolanda, mentioned above, lists the number of soldiers who were available for their daily duties and the numbers and whereabouts of those who were absent (Chapter 4; Bowman and Thomas 1991: 62, 66; Bowman and Thomas 1994: 93-4, 98). Ten percent of the soldiers who were absent were missing because of illness. Again those who were ill were divided into three categories: those suffering from eye problems, injury and illness. One suggestion for this division is that the three groups were divided because they had different places to convalesce. For example, those who were absent because of illness might have been left to recuperate in their barracks. It was mentioned in Chapter 4 when discussing the possible interpretations of the Vindolanda tablet of a daily strength report that this division might have been an indication of a specific doctor being provided for these treatments, but then one must ask where the treatments were being offered, suggesting the possibility that there might have been different ideas about how a *valetudinarium* should be constituted according to the different military units' understandings. Supporting this is a papyrus fragment from Egypt that comprises the remains of a soldier's letter to his parents. The soldier, stationed in Egypt, was ill because of food poisoning caused by rancid fish. In his letter he mentions being fed by members of his troop (P. Mich 478 in Davies 1974: 130). This could imply that he was cared for by fellow soldiers - had he been in a *valetudinarium* he would probably have mentioned a doctor or someone else associated with the medical field feeding him. At the same time it might also be an indication that soldiers sometimes helped their ill comrades, either in their barracks, or in the *valetudinarium*. This could indicate that the soldiers in some units, when ill, may have stayed in their barracks depending upon the nature of the disease. It might also be an indication of specific troops using different care that was not standardised across the empire. Again more questions are raised about the nature of the *valetudinarium* from this statement.

A comparison of descriptions of civilian *valetudinaria* could be useful; unfortunately, however, descriptions of civilian *valetudinaria* are even more vague. Xenophon speaks of a man suffering from an eye disease leaving a doctor:

> "*καὶ ἐντυχὼν τινι ὀφθαλμιῶντι ἀνθρώπῳ ἀπιόντι ἐξ ἰατρείου*" (Hellenica II. 1. 3).

From this it seems that in some instances, people were able to visit the doctors' home. Celsus is the only Roman writer who mentions *valetudinaria* outside a military context and comments that the larger the building the less treatment there was made available to the people by the person in charge of running the structure: "*et qui ampla valetudinaria nutriunt, quia singulis summa cura consulere non sustinent*" (Proemium 65). This statement in itself indicates that such structures did exist. There is another suggestion by Harig that there might have been *Tabernae Medicae* (1971: 185-7; Jackson 1988: 65), or basically a shop where one could receive treatment. Galen also mentions visiting patients in their own homes; though it has been argued by Horstmannshoff that he did this mainly for the wealthy. It is also known from Galen that doctors would have patients visit their homes (1995: 84-5, 91). It is possible that poorer patients might not have received visiting doctors, but had to visit the doctor's themselves, if many doctors held the same attitudes as Galen about whom they preferred to treat. Another suggestion is that civilians were treated with folk-remedies by those whom they deemed wise enough to understand their problems; perhaps both visited each other, yet this is not mentioned in the medical literature. The civilian evidence points to a number of possibilities for people to receive treatment, suggesting that there may not have been one specific place for civilians to have health care offered to them and this should be kept in mind when the archaeological material is considered for the Roman military.

6.3. STRUCTURAL EVIDENCE

To add to our understanding of *valetudinaria*, the archaeological evidence for the structures needs to be considered in detail to see if there is enough support for their current identification. The first Roman military *valetudinaria* were identified early in the 20th century, though curiously such attributions have rarely been questioned. A re-examination of the evidence will help by either presenting stronger evidence for such existing identifications, or it will demonstrate that there is insufficient data to state what such buildings are, and that one must be more cautious when accepting archaeological interpretation as fact, or truth, without question.

However, before discussing the architectural features of the buildings identified as *valetudinaria*, an issue that must be discussed centres around the arguments over the development of *valetudinaria* in the Roman world. Debates exist in scholarship about how Roman military *valetudinaria* came to be. Some scholars feel that they should have developed out of pre-existing structures, whilst others feel they represent an innovation specific to the Roman army.

According to Haberling (1909: 442) civilian settlements functioned as *valetudinaria* first and he believed that the sick and wounded soldiers were cared for by the local population, just as they were during the military campaigns. This could be correct in some cases; however, no broad archaeological study has been made to see if there is supporting evidence for this. Some medical tools were found in civilian settlements, such as at Caerleon and Chester, for example (Appendix 10, Tables A10.2 and A10.3), but the context of the finds is only recorded for an area in general, rather than a specific structure. Moreover, these civilian settlements are contemporary with the fortresses and not the pre-existing structures. This theory remains possible given the fact that there are reports of soldiers being left behind in friendly villages whilst on campaign. However, it cannot be said with any certainty whether a *valetudinarium* developed from places in the *vici*, as there is no structural evidence on which to base a comparison, and even if there were, the structures of *valetudinaria* in the fortifications might not have been based on those in *vici*.

Krug believes that the *valetudinarium* developed from accommodation provided in religious sanctuaries, such as that for Aesculapius at Epidaurus, (1984: 207-8). From the archaeological remains it seems very likely that sanctuaries had rooms provided for those who visited to rest, and possibly to receive medical treatment in cases of sanctuaries relating to healing. These rooms are thought to have had space for a number of separate beds, rather than private accommodation (Krug 1984: 207-8). It is debatable whether the doctors treated patients in these rooms or if they were treated elsewhere. Perhaps treatment in certain places depended on the type of disease. It is known that doctors resided at the sites as well as 'spiritual healers', such as priests and priestesses. It may be that both worked with one another, but without better evidence one is unable to make any specific statements about what actually occurred at the healing sanctuaries. One way to be healed was by a visitation from or vision of a god, probably Aesculapius, in a dream or hallucination. Whether these buildings were the inspiration for *valetudinaria* is also difficult to determine because they had a religious function. On the other hand, we assume that Roman *valetudinaria* would have been fairly rational (i.e. conforming to our notion of being a purely functional structure), with the exception of possible cult rooms, but it may be that some troops, depending upon their beliefs, placed their unhealthy soldiers in buildings that were associated with religious functions, rather than the identified *valetudinarium*. Or perhaps the *valetudinarium* was religious in nature.

Harig feels that the *valetudinaria* were developed in the military (1971: 84). The site of Haltern is argued to have the first *valetudinarium*, because it was a fortification constructed during the reign of Augustus on the Lippe frontier. Harig argues that they were part of the emperor's development of the health care system. Again this cannot be determined, especially when there is a question about whether *valetudinaria* have been identified correctly. Since all of the arguments regarding the development of *valetudinaria* are conceivable, but have very little supporting evidence, one cannot say with certainty what the origins of *valetudinaria* were.

After the structure at Neuss had been acknowledged as a *valetudinarium*, buildings with similar designs were also recognised as such. The general layout of the structures identified were similar; however even these vary from one fortification to another in terms of their size and the detail of their plan. Generally, the structures are based on a rectangular plan constructed around a central courtyard (i.e. Baatz 1970: 8-10; Jackson 1988: 136-7; Kunzl 2002: 28-9; Majno 1975: 382-96; Nutton 1969: 262-3, 2004: 178-9; von Petrikovitz 1975: 88; Salazar 2000: 81; Scarborough 1976: 68 Wilmanns 1995b: 104-5). The buildings in legionary fortresses had a courtyard that was surrounded on three sides by an inner row of small rooms, or 'wards'. The inner ring of rooms faced onto a hallway that was surrounded on three sides by an outer ring of wards. Each ward consisted of two rooms divided by a small hall, each of the two rooms opened onto the small hall, rather than onto the larger central hall. The rectangular plan described is more commonly found in the legionary fortresses; smaller versions of the rectangular plan surrounding a courtyard are seen in some auxiliary forts, but with only one ring of rooms surrounding the courtyard. Another plan that has been identified as a *valetudinarium* for auxiliary forts is a rectangular structure with a central hall surrounded on four sides by a single row of small rooms. The front of the structure is understood to be the area where the reception room, operating theatres, kitchens and rooms with a religious function were placed. These rooms were identified on understandings of rooms incorporated into hospitals in the 19th century. Salazar also notes that there is not enough evidence for operating theatres within *valetudinaria*; although she assumes that this would make more sense than a situation where the doctors moved from room to room; yet she rightly points out that the Greeks and Romans might have had different ideas about 'common sense' arrangements (2000: 70, 81-2).

Legionary buildings that have been identified as *valetudinaria* occur at Inchtuthil, Caerleon, Vetera I and II, Haltern, Neuss, Bonn, Vindonissa, Carnuntum and Lotschitz in inner Pannonia Superior, and Novae on the lower Danube in Moesia Inferior. There are also some argued to be in the fortresses at Chester, Vindobona, Lauriacum, Regensburg and Aquincum, but these have even fewer structural remains for their identification to be relied upon with any certainty. In auxiliary forts so-called *valetudinaria* have been identified at Housesteads, Benwell, Pen Llystyn, Wallsend, Valkenburg, Oberstimm, Wiesbaden, and Künzing. Presented below is a detailed discussion of each so-called *valetudinarium*.

6.3.1 Legionary Structures

Haltern (Fig. 33). The structure identified as a *valetudinarium* was built in the praetentura and was oriented on a north-south axis. It dates to the late 1st century BC, and was probably built for the campaigns of Drusus. The structure was built in the courtyard style, but was not entirely excavated so there is some question about the actual size of the building. Stieren (1928; 1930: 197) believes that it was roughly 43.0 x 80.0 metres and that the inner courtyard measured 33.0 x 63.0 metres. The north half of the building was studied, and what was excavated measured 50.5 x 76.5 metres, equal to 3,863 sq. metres. The inner hall of the building measured 26.5 x 40.0 metres equalling 1,060 sq. metres. Twenty-five wards were found, but there is an estimated number of 50. They each measure 3.5 x 4.0 metres and are thought to have had enough room to hold two or three beds (Schultze 1934: 59). The little hallways between the sets of wards measured one metre in width. There were no characteristic finds from the building that would indicate it was intended to be used for health care purposes (von Schnurbein 1974: 67-8; Jettner 1966: 1-2). The one medical find from the site was a lead stopper from a medicinal jar that had the words *radix Britannica* inscribed on it, which was a medicine for scurvy. The inscription was found in the *principia* not the *valetudinarium* (Johnson 1983: 161; Stieren 1928: 70).

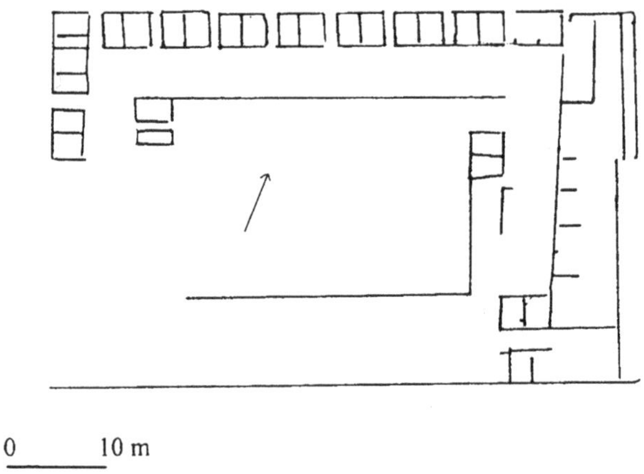

Fig. 33. Plan of the valetudinarium *at Haltern. After Jettner 1966: Fig. 1.*

Vetera I. (Fig. 34) This structure was constructed between 47-54 AD for the two legions, V and XXI, stationed at the fortress. It was built in the courtyard style on the west side of the fort south of the *via principalis* in the *praetentura*. It measured 73.0 x 58.4 metres or 4,320 metres square. The main hallway that runs around the interior of the building is 5.0 metres wide. The entrance is located on the north side of the building. Vetera I's valetudinarium was fully excavated. The entrance had a number of rooms constructed on the outer porticoes that are claimed to be shops. These are thought to be a means of keeping the building quiet, though the degree of silence would depend on the types of shops that were constructed onto the front of the building. The first room is described as an entrance hallway and measured 9.3 x 14.0 metres. The connection to the *via principalis* is through a large corridor hall, measuring 8.4 square metres. Following the entrance was a large hall that was divided into three parts by two rows of Corinthian columns (Oelmann 1931: 225). There are two small rooms located to the side of the large colonnaded room that were suggested to have been used for an admissions' office and possibly doctor's accommodation. At the side of one of these rooms was a niche claimed to hold the figure of a healing god, but there are no archaeological remains of such a figure, or any object found within the niche. Sixty small rooms were found surrounding the central courtyard and each measured roughly 3.4 x 3.0 metres. Moreover, they were thought to have held two beds, equalling 120 in total. This would not seem to be many beds for two legions, given that the average estimated number of beds is 6 to 10 per cent for an entire legion. A possible operating theatre was suggested for the room that jutted out into the courtyard. This measured 8.0 x 12.6 metres. A kitchen was suggested for the large room to the left of the so-called operating theatre (Jettner 1966: 3-4). A bathing complex was found near the entrance of the building (Lehner 1929: 126-32). The presence of drains found running beneath

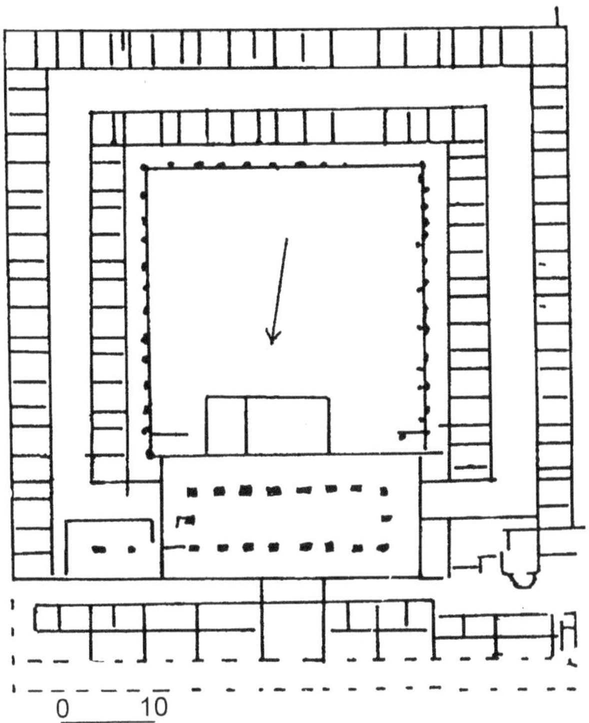

Fig. 34. Plan of the valetudinarium *at Vetera I. After Johnson 1983: Fig. 117.*126-32).

the building suggests that there might have been toilets in the structure (Böcking 1987: 137; Pitts and St. Joseph 1985: 30, 95; Schultze 1934: 58; Watermann 1980: 30).

Vetera II (Fig. 35). The second legionary fortress at Vetera also had a building that has been

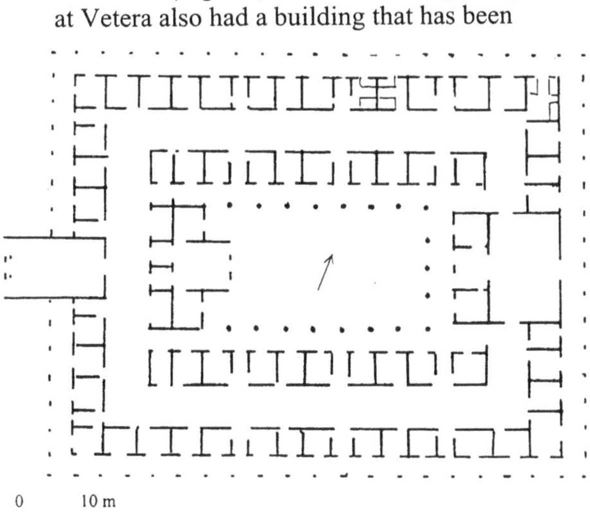

Fig. 35. Plan of the valetudinarium *at Vetera II. After Majno 1975: Fig. 9.36.*

identified as a *valetudinarium,* believed to have been built during the reign of Nero. It was erected around a large courtyard surrounded on three sides with sets of two rooms. One of the larger rooms in the structure was argued to have been an operating theatre (Böcking 1987: 137). It is a square building 83.5 metres on the outside with an interior circuit of rooms of similar form measuring 40.2 metres. The building is 1,616 metres square (Böcking 1987: 137; Pitts and St. Joseph 1985: 30; Watermann 1980: 30).

Neuss (Fig. 36) This so-called *valetudinarium* has an uncertain date and may have been constructed in the Claudian or Neronian periods. The building was excavated between 1887 and 1901, and was found to be of a standard courtyard plan, but a little more than half the building has been revealed. It was built in the *latera praetorii* on the south side of the *via principalis* and opposite the *praetorium* or the commanding officer's quarters. Measuring 89.0 x 49.0 metres, it had a colonnaded portico on its front. From the portico its interior was reached by a long entrance hall. There was a group of smaller rooms in the area of the entrance and these might have been cult rooms. One of these rooms had a hearth that could have been used for religious purposes, but may also have served another function. The remaining three sides of the

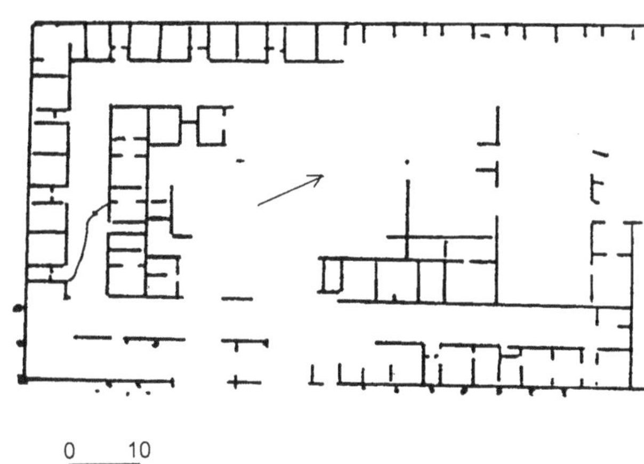

Fig. 36. Plan of the valetudinarium *at Neuss. After Johnson 1983: Fig. 160*

rectangular hallway were divided into wards (Jettner 1966: 4-5). A courtyard measuring 11.4 x 8.6 metres was discovered and it had a peristyle, possibly covered, surrounding the four sides of the area (Haberling 1909: 448-50). The room claimed to be an operating theatre jutted into the courtyard and it also had a hearth. The building had about 60 wards that measured 5.13 x 3.6 metres. Based on evidence of a drain, a toilet is believed to have been in the building (Schultze 1934: 59-61); however, no remains of a latrine have been uncovered. It was the south-east corner of room 51 where ten medical implements were found, and along with them were pottery vessel fragments, pieces of bone, oyster shell and egg shell (Koenen 1904: 180-2).

Herbs were found in the *valetudinarium* during excavations in the 1960s, and argued to have been used for medicinal purposes (Knorzer 1963; Watermann 1978: 1-2). Whether they were used here or stored in the structure cannot be said with any certainty.

Bonn. The so-called *valetudinarium* was excavated in 1954 and found to have been of the courtyard style. It is thought to have been built somewhere between AD 180 and the third century. It was constructed in the *praetentura* on the west of the *via principalis*. It has not been fully excavated so it is estimated to have measured 110.0 x 90.0 metres, and argued to have been able to hold 180 sick or wounded soldiers (Jettner 1966: 6; Watermann 1980: 30). Yet, the structural evidence does not reveal enough information to support these statements with any certainty.

Vindonissa (Fig. 37). Located in the *praetentura*, the building identified as a *valetudinarium* was constructed of stone and measures 70.0 x 60.0 metres or 4,410 metres square (Anonymous 1970-71: 33; Pitts and St. Joseph 1985: 30; Tabanelli 1958: 41; Watermann 1974b: 353; Watermann 1980: 30). It was built in a similar courtyard style as the other legionary structures thought to be *valetudinaria*. The courtyard was surrounded on three sides with small wards and measured 37.8 x 26.6 metres, with a large entrance room in the front of the building. The structure was located on the *via principalis* next to the *principia* (Simonett 1937: 202-3).

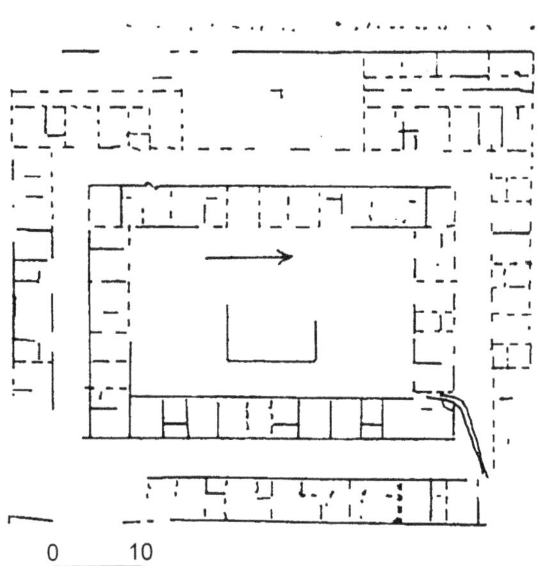

Fig. 37. Plan of the valetudinarium *at Vindonissa. After Johnson 1983: Fig. 117.*

Lauriacum. This structure argued to be a *valetudinarium* was not fully excavated. The remains measure 90.0 x 50.0 metres and it was built in stone (Breitwieser 1998: 57; Watermann 1980: 30). It lies in the *praetentura*. The fortress was constructed after the Marcomannic Wars, so the structure dates to the late-2nd century and it had three building phases. The third phase is dated by coin evidence to at least the reign of Valentinian I. It has a six metre wide corridor and a 58.5 x 22.5 metre courtyard. The last third of the building has water channels, which might represent a latrine (Swoboda 1937: 265). Twenty-three wards have been found, measuring 5.6 metres wide and estimated to have had places for six beds in each room (Swoboda 1937: 270).

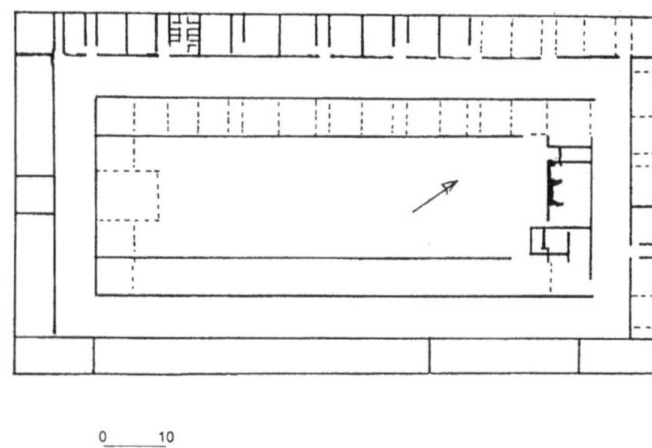

Fig. 38. Plan of the valetudinarium *at Lotschitz. After Majno 1975: Fig. 9.36.*

Lotschitz (Fig. 38). Although this is not located on the front line of the frontiers the fortification has a building identified as a military *valetudinarium* and will be taken into consideration here. The structure was constructed in the typical courtyard style and measures 123.0 x 68.0 metres. It dates to the 2nd century (Tabanelli 1958: 45). It had two larger rooms that are argued to have been an operating theatre or an entrance hall (Lorgar 1919: 117-8). Estimations have been made that there was enough room to hold 420 beds (Swoboda 1937: 270).

Regensburg The stone building claimed to have been a *valetudinarium* has seen very little excavation (Watermann 1980: 30). Thus there is little structural evidence on which to base its claimed existence.

Vindobona. This building, too, has hardly any structural remains, making its identification as a *valetudinarium* questionable. It is thought to be a *valetudinarium* because it is located in the *praetentura* and because one of two altars found in the building had the name Aesculapius inscribed on it. Furthermore one probe was found within the structure, along with other non-medical finds of green and brown glass, tile fragments, part of a sieve and a knee fibula (Neumann 1965; Watermann 1980: 30). Most of the finds date to the 2nd and 3rd centuries (Breitwieser 1998: 55-6; Neumann 1965: 99-113). Since there was an altar found *in situ*, a suggestion was made that the room probably had a cult purpose associated with healing gods, yet this does not necessarily indicate that it was intended to be the cult room of a *valetudinarium*. The first altar reads

[I(ovi)] O(ptimo) M(aximo)/ Apollini/et Sirona[e/Ae]sculap(io) Ae]sculap[io]/P(ublius) V(otum) S(olvit)/l(ibens) l(aetus) m(erito).

The second altar found in the structure reads

Ap(ollini) So(li) et Sir[o/n]ae (Neumann 1965: 103; Neumann 1980: 28).

Since other gods are mentioned as well, there is no reason why this altar was particularly associated with the cult room of a *valetudinarium*.

Carnuntum (Fig. 39). The stone building claimed to be a *valetudinarium* measures 82.0 x 73.0 metres or 5,890 metres square. It was built in the latera praetorii located on the corner of the via Quintana and the via praetoria. (Breitwieser 1998: 51-2; Haberling 1909: 441; Pitts and St. Joseph 1985: 30; Watermann 1980: 30). The structure was excavated in 1904 and found to have been constructed in two periods. The building of the second period is an example of the so-called courtyard *valetudinarium* structure (Haberling 1909: 452 and 454). The main entrance is located on the eastern side of the building. Unlike other structures there is not always a division of wards into two rooms, but sometimes they are grouped into three and four rooms together. The outer circle of rooms had one room with a hearth, which is argued to have been used for the kitchen. One of the rooms was decorated with *opus spicatum*. Two other rooms had clay floors. Rooms 10 and 11 were heated by a hypocaust. Room 15 was constructed with flue tiles from a hypocaust on its southern wall. Room 16, two rooms away from room 15, has a T-shaped hypocaust beneath its floor. The inner ring of rooms is little like those in other *valetudinaria*, as one room had a hypocaust and another a small stone trough (Groller 1906: 53-5). The courtyard had a landing with steps on its west side, something that does not seem to appear in the other buildings identified as *valetudinaria*, with the exception of Novae. There were some architectural remains found in the courtyard - part of a column shaft, part of a column foot and a Corinthian capital. In the middle of the courtyard was a possible well or a hole for the column. The south front of the main room 37 had a hypocaust. A drain was constructed on the west part of the main building on the 48.0 metre *cloaca maxima* of the camp. It was 70.0 cm high and 50.0 cm wide (Groller 1906: 57-62).

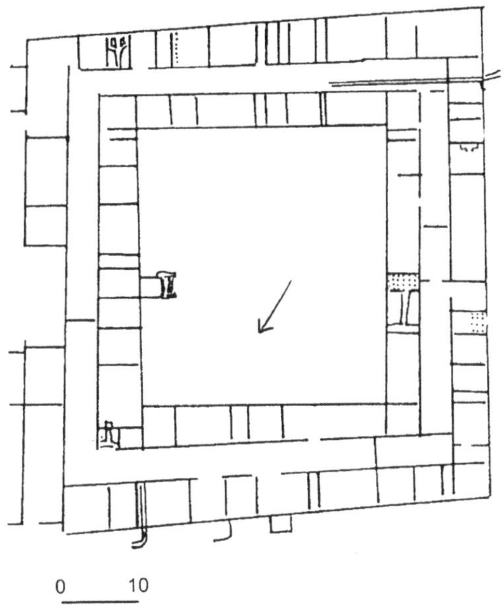

Fig. 39. Plan of the valetudinarium *at Carnuntum. After Haberling 1909: Fig. 4.*

Novae (Fig. 40) Although this fortress is not in the area of study, being in the lower Danube, it is mentioned to demonstrate that buildings of similar plan were found in other parts of the empire as well. The structure was situated in the *praetentura* and measures 5,970 square metres. The average size of the wards measured 5.35 x 4.70 metres and is estimated to have enough space for two to six beds. There was a latrine found in the western wing and a storeroom of lamps (Press 1988: 77).

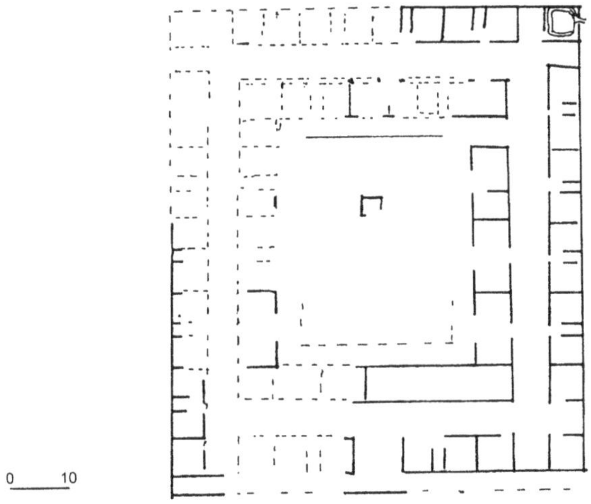

Fig. 40. Plan of the valetudinarium *at Novae. After Dyzcek 1988: Fig. 1.*

One room did have a few instruments, but they are said to have been broken, and could have been placed in the *valetudinarium* for another reason. Novae is one of the few buildings to have had a contextual study of artefacts (Dyzcek 1995), and it displayed some interesting patterning in the distribution of objects (discussed below) that make one question the identification of such structures even more. It also appears to have had a small temple in its courtyard.

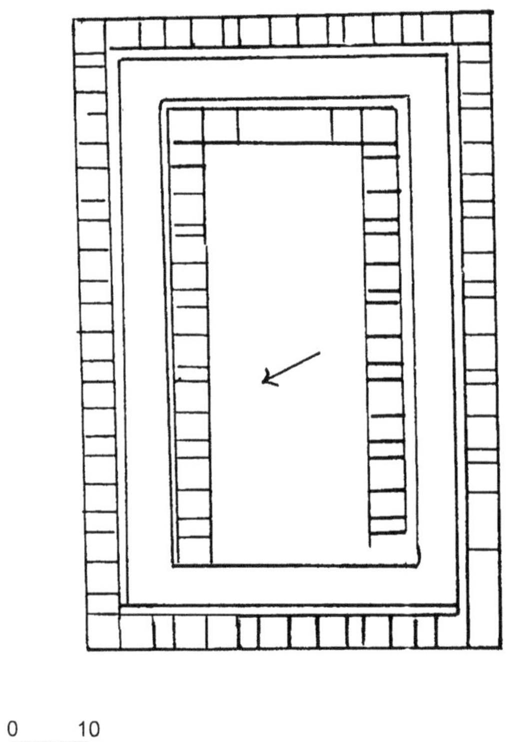

Fig. 41. Plan of the valetudinarium *at Inchtuthil. After Johnson 1983: Fig. 117.*

Inchtuthil (Fig. 41). The *valetudinarium* in this fortress was excavated in the summer of 1957 and found to have 60 wards located around a central courtyard. The building was constructed on the left side of the *latera praetorii*, corresponding with the *fabrica* on the right side, and adjacent to some barracks. The building measures 91.44 x 58.52 metres equal to 5,351 metres square (Pitts and St. Joseph 1985: 95). The courtyard measured 21.33 x 59.74 metres or 1,274 metres square. The main entrance was located on the south-east facing the granary. There was no forehall or large reception room, and the main entrance gave access to the main circulatory corridor through a small vestibule. At the south-east end of the inner range of rooms was a hall, room A, that measured 13.41 x 4.88 metres flanked by two smaller rooms, measuring 3.66 x 4.88 metres, and is suggested to have been the operating theatre. The reason for this definition is that one of the small rooms was equipped with numerous hearths argued to have been used to sterilise instruments. Since the Romans were unaware of sterilisation, and furthermore probably would not have needed a number of hearths even had they been used for this purpose, another function for the room must be sought (perhaps a workshop or kitchen). The wards measured 3.96 x 4.27 metres in size. It has been suggested that there were four beds in the *valetudinarium* for each *contubernium,* or 40 beds for each century, which is quite a large amount of space for ill and wounded soldiers. Few material remains were found to suggest the purpose of the structure (Pitts and St. Joseph 1985: 91-101).

Caerleon. The fortress is Flavian in date, but was rebuilt in the early 2nd century and partially demolished at the end of the 3rd century. Since little excavation has taken place the building claimed to be a *valetudinarium* has very little structural evidence. The main argument for its identification is based on its similar position to that of other buildings identified as *valetudinaria* at the fortresses at Haltern, Lauriacum, Xanten and Lotschitz that are in the *praetentura*. This building took the typical form of a double range of rooms separated by a wide longitudinal corridor, flanking three sides of a courtyard. A large hall, 25.0 metres in length, projected into the courtyard. The central corridor was 6.7 metres wide. It is difficult to give an estimate of the number of rooms. In the outer range they measured some 3.6 by 4.6 metres. Internally they appear to have been divided into sets of three with a small hall dividing them. There were no latrines found, but a possible drain for one was uncovered. Tanks were found in the courtyard that may have been used to collect rain from the roofs of the building (Murray-Threipland 1964: 86-123). It is believed that the rainwater would have been used for medical purposes, but since many Roman houses had *impluvia* to catch rainwater for the purpose of drinking, it seems unlikely that the water would have had a special medical purpose. The numerous remains of amphorae suggests a concentration of imported commodities in this building, perhaps storage. A handle from one suggests that it was Amirian wine, a white wine from Italy that had medicinal purposes. No surgical instruments were found in the building (Boon 1972: 75-7). At the end of the 3rd century the tanks in the courtyard were filled in (Wilson 1965: 199).

Chester. The so-called *valetudinarium*, located behind the *principia*, has little in the way of structural remains. It was excavated in 1980 and measured roughly 65 x 150 metres. It was first identified as the commanding officer's quarters (Frere 1983: 297-8), but the true purpose of the structure is not understood (Mason 2000: 410).

6.3.2 Auxiliary Structures

Valkenburg (Fig. 42). This auxiliary fort was thought to have had a wooden *valetudinarium* constructed in the 1st century. Built as a smaller

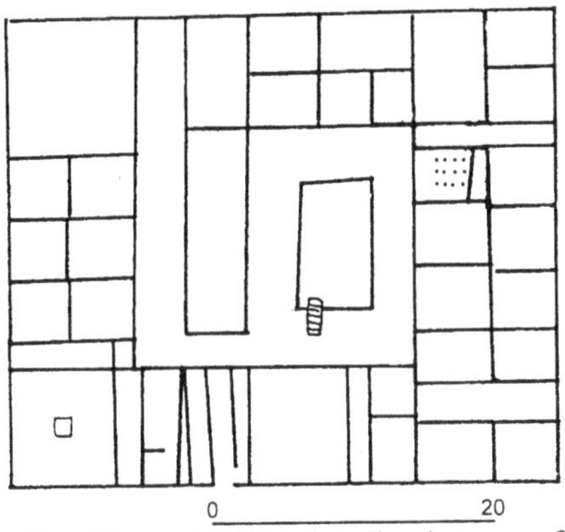

Fig. 42. Plan of the valetudinarium *or* fabrica *at Valkenburg. After Johnson 1983: Fig. 140.*

version of the courtyard style, the structure measures 35.0 x 12.0 metres. It is located in the *praetentura* (Watermann 1980: 30). However, it has also been argued to have been a *fabrica* (Schönberger 1979: 135-41), demonstrating the difficulty in defining the building on its structural evidence alone.

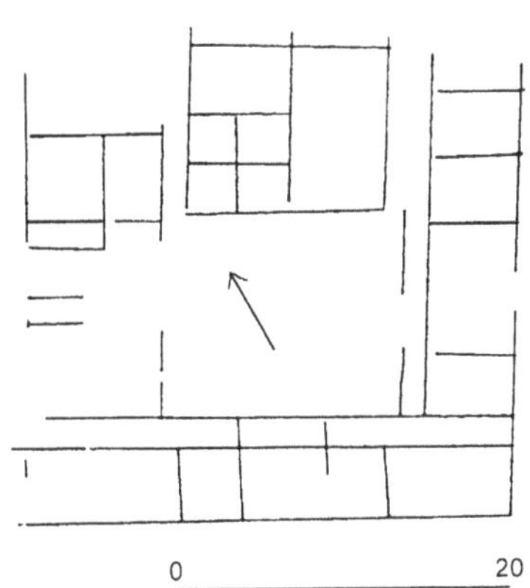

Fig. 43. Plan of the valetudinarium *or* fabrica *at Wiesbaden. After Johnson 1983: Fig. 140.*

Wiesbaden (Fig. 43). This so-called stone *valetudinarium* was erected in the *praetentura* of the fort. It measured 15.0 x 22.0 metres (Watermann 1980: 30). It was built on a long rectangular plan with a central hallway (Schönberger 1972: 54).

Fig. 44. Plan of the valetudinarium *at Oberstimm. After Johnson 1983: Fig. 121.*

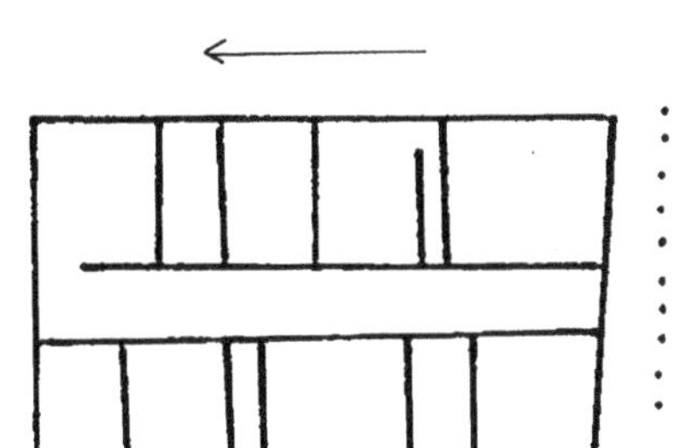

Oberstimm (Fig. 44). The building claimed to be a *valetudinarium* was constructed in a rectangular plan around a central hall in the *latera praetorii*. It measures 18.0 x 13.0 metres (Watermann 1980: 30). The *valetudinarium* dates to roughly AD 40 to 69. There were small corridors between the double rooms. There may have been a latrine in the northeast corner (Hassall 1983: 115; Schönberger 1972: 57-62). It was built next to the *fabrica* and behind the *praetorium* (Johnson 1983: 238)

Künzing (Fig. 45). This building identified as a *valetudinarium* was erected during the 1st century in the *praetentura* of the fort. The wooden

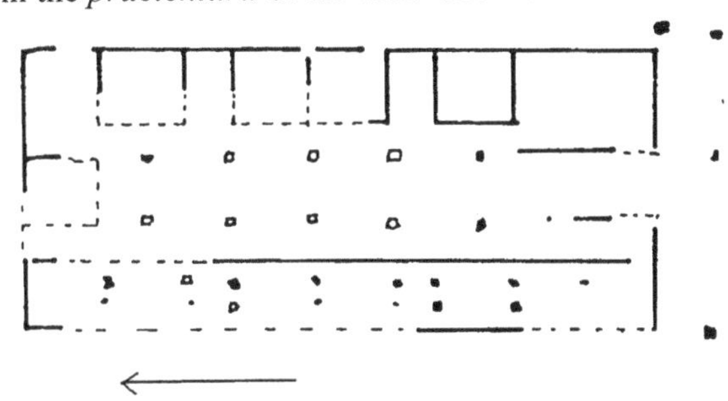

Fig. 45. Plan of the valetudinarium *at Künzing. After Johnson 1983: Fig. 121.*

structure measured 30.0 x 15.0 metres (Watermann 1980: 30). It was a rectangular structure running around a central corridor. The entrance was located on the north wall and measured 3.2 metres wide. The first room, room one, was especially large measuring 7.5 by 5.3 metres (Hassall 1983: 107; Schönberger 1975: 53-4).

Corbridge (Fig. 46) The building at Corbridge originally identified as a *valetudinarium* has since been argued to be a *fabrica*. Building 5 inside the large forum at the site was first identified as a *valetudinarium* because of its similarity to the buildings at Künzing and Oberstimm, having a series of rooms laid out on both sides of a central corridor. It measured 28.0 x 13.0 metres and was

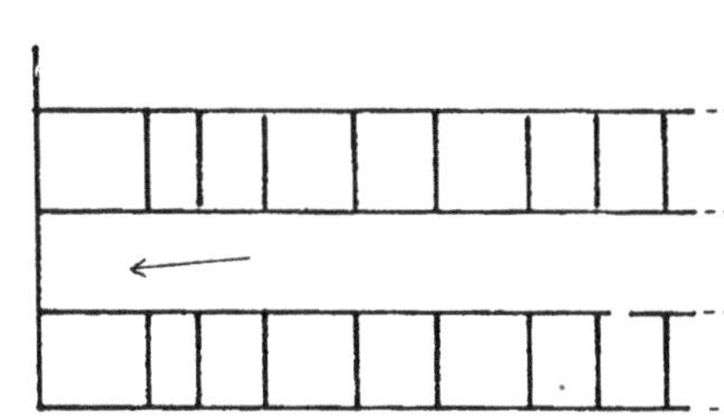

Fig. 46. Plan of the valetudinarium *at Corbridge. After Johnson 1983: Fig. 121.*

made of stone (Daniels 1969: 97-101; Gillam and Tate 1971: 8; Richmond and McIntyre 1938-39: 132-4; Watermann 1980: 30). An iron bound chest was located under the floorboards of the structure, and contained the remains of armour, weapons and tools. Davies argued that these were put away to rust, so that the rust could be used for medicinal purposes (Davies 1969/70: 177). Nevertheless, it should be asked why someone would have placed the metal objects in a chest if they wished them to rust quickly and why these objects were not retrieved. The plan of the building also resembles workshops, as pointed out by Daniels (1969: 126). However, another suggestion is that its proximity to the granary that makes it more likely to be a store building. The building at Corbridge was similar to store houses in Rome (Bishop and Dore 1988: 128). Again the building at Corbridge is a good demonstration of how a single structure could have a variety of purposes.

Housesteads (Fig. 47). The stone building identified as a *valetudinarium* has been much discussed (Bosanquet 1904; Charlesworth 1976; Crow 1995: 50-1; Wilson 1972: 306-8), and comparison has been made with other auxiliary structures identified as *valetudinaria*. Measuring 30.0 x 22.0 metres it was built in the courtyard style (Watermann 1980: 30). The building was located in the *latera praetorii* behind the

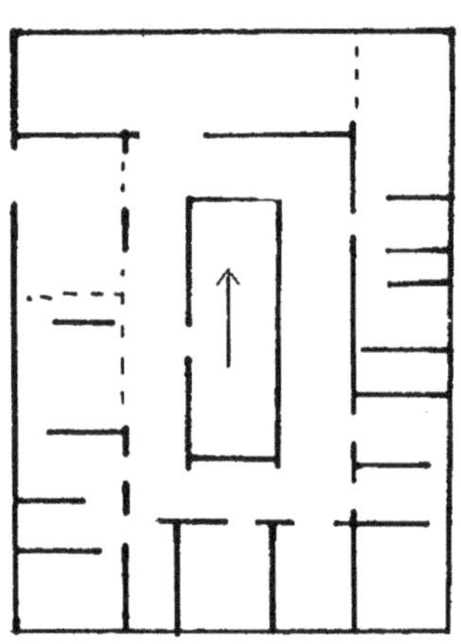

Fig. 47. Plan of the valetudinarium *at Housesteads. After Johnson 1983: Fig. 121.*

headquarters building. It had a west entrance that led onto the *via decumana*. The central courtyard was surrounded by a low wall that supported a colonnade. On the north side of the structure close to the western entrance, a large room was constructed that has been claimed to have been the operating theatre. Around the other three sides of the courtyard were smaller rooms. There was a latrine in the lower southwest corner. It was first excavated in 1904 (Bosanquet 1904: 239) and re-examined in 1970 and 1971. In 1971 most of the Hadrianic plan from the east range of rooms was excavated (Wilson 1971: 250). The structure was found to be different from the plan published by Bosanquet in 1904. Most rooms in the south range had three floor levels, each composed of earth and pebbles and some walls had been altered. There was a series of drains that were not connected with latrines, but have been suggested for the ablutions of the building (Wilson 1972: 306-8). Bosanquet found cross walls in the large room, which tends to suggest that at one point the room was smaller.

There are possible remains of hearths found in the eastern end that show burning so intense that they may have been used for metal working (Charlesworth 1976: 19). There are other suggestions that the structure could have been an armoury or a workshop; however it is generally assumed that it was a *valetudinarium* (Crow 1995: 50-1).

Benwell (Fig. 48). The so-called *valetudinarium* was built immediately behind the commandant's house on the south side of the *via quintana* in the

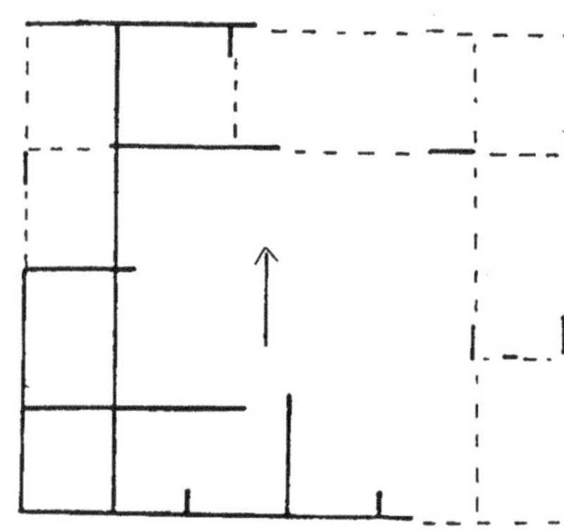

Fig. 48. Plan of the valetudinarium *at Benwell. After Johnson 1983: Fig. 121.*

praetentura. It was another courtyard building similar to that at Housesteads, measuring 24.70 x 22.50 metres. It proved impossible to excavate the building in its entirety, so only the west wing and part of the north-south wing were examined. The wings were divided into a series of small rooms and one larger room was found projecting into the courtyard. The position of the structure within this fort provided the sole indication to archaeologists that this was a *valetudinarium* (Simpson and Richmond 1941: 22).

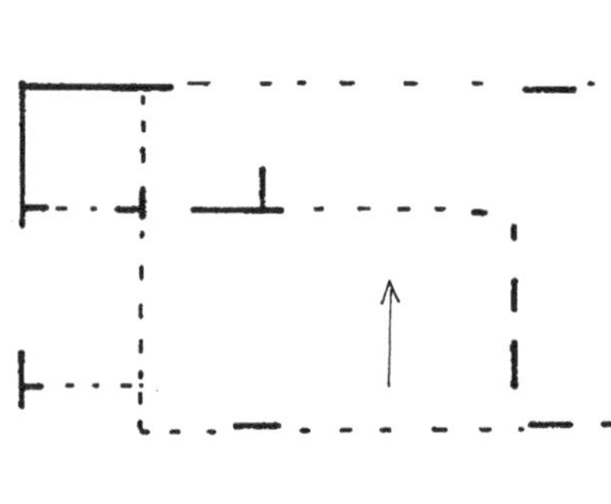

Fig. 49. Plan of the valetudinarium *at Hod Hill. After Johnson 1983: Fig. 121.*

Hod Hill (Fig. 49). A timber building claimed to be a *valetudinarium* located in the *praetentura* south of the *via principalis* was excavated in the 1950s. It measures 24.3 x 18.29 metres with a central courtyard, while the hall measures 18.29 metres long and 7.62 metres wide. The amount of space allotted for the wards is about 48.78 metres, thought to have accommodated roughly 90 beds, or about 12.5 per-cent of the population. This was for a total strength of 718 men (Richmond 1968: 85-6).

Wallsend (Fig. 50). The building identified as a *valetudinarium* was excavated in the early 1980s and was re-examined in the later 1990's and was identified because of its location in the *latera praetorii* (Frere 1983: 289). In 1984 the range in the north was excavated and shown to have had undergone later modifications. Overall the building measured 15.0 by 23.6 metres. A large room excavated in the north was argued to be an operating theatre. A latrine was found in the southern end of the structure (Frere 1984: 277).

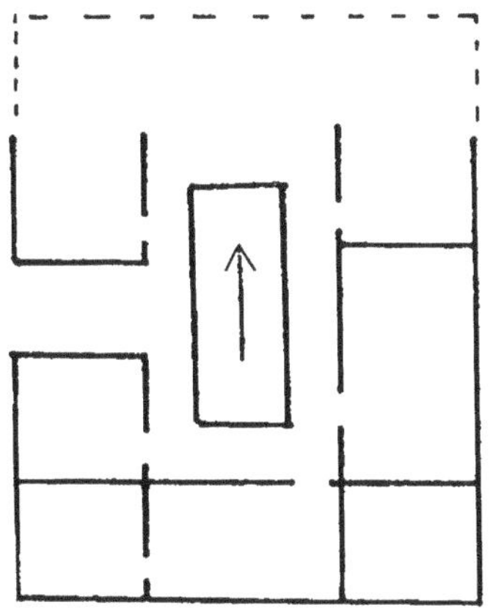

Fig. 50. Plan of the valetudinarium *at Wallsend. After Johnson 1983: Fig. 121.*

Fendoch (Fig. 51). The so-called *valetudinarium* was in a position of relative seclusion north of the commandant's house in the *latera praetorii*. It was 12.19 x 32.3 metres long. The building had a long central corridor. There were eight wards in the east and another room identified as a reception hall found in the west (Richmond and McIntyre 1938-9: 132-4).

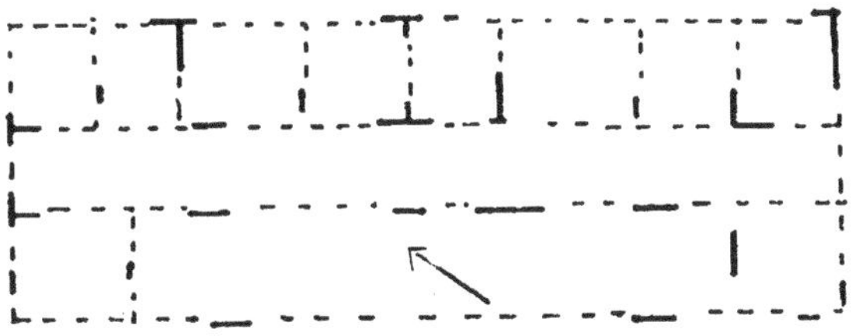

Fig. 51. Plan of the valetudinarium *at Fendoch. After Johnson 1983: Fig. 121.*

Pen Llystyn. The central section of the fort had the commandant's house, the *principia*, two granaries and a long building with 11 rooms identified as the *valetudinarium*. For the most part the so-called *valetudinarium* was clearly exposed. Its identification was made on the grounds that it is analogous to the structure at Fendoch. It was 45.73 metres long by 7.62 metres wide. A row of ten wards was found. Burnt patches almost certainly representing hearths were found in the two main rooms located at the end of the structure (Hogg 1968: 133-4).

6.4 Discussion of the Structures

The descriptions and figures of the *valetudinaria* demonstrate notable variations between each structure in terms of plan and location. To begin with, the buildings are usually compared according to their size and structural layout, so this will be discussed first, followed by descriptions of room types, summary analysis of their locations within the fortifications and finally other possibilities for the function of these structures.

6.4.1 Size and Structural Layout

The size of the legionary structures ranges from 73.0 x 58.4 metres at Vetera I to 123.0 x 68.0 metres at Lotschitz. The central hall-style buildings identified as *valetudinaria* located in auxiliary forts range from 18.0 x 13.0 metres at Oberstimm to 35.0 x 12.0 metres at Valkenburg, and the courtyard style structures in auxiliary forts range from 30.0 x 22.0 metres at Housesteads to 24.7 x 22.5 metres at Benwell. There is some disagreement amongst the sources that provide information about the sizes of the structures, so the sizes given are sometimes approximations. A reason for this is that many buildings have only been partially excavated, and the extent of the rest of the structure is speculative. By looking at the figures of the structures it is clear that the majority of the buildings' plans are based on conjecture, rather than surviving architectural remains. Despite this problem, there is still a noticeable difference in the scale of the remaining buildings. If the buildings are *valetudinaria* then they were not constructed on a standard scale.

6.4.2 Description and Arrangement of Rooms

Each building has a different arrangement of interior rooms, promoting the idea of variation within the army even further. In the legionary fortresses, those buildings that have been excavated thoroughly all have a courtyard plan with two rows of wards. Yet, the wards are of different sizes. For example, although small, Caerleon's measures roughly 3.6 x 4.6 metres and Neuss' 5.13 x 3.6 metres. The auxiliary fort at Künzing has wards measuring 4.3 x 3.8 metres, even though the sizes of these are not very different they are also similar in size to barrack rooms. The barrack at Valkenburg measures 3.5 x 4.0 metres in the larger of the two rooms and 3.5 x 2.0 metres in the smaller front room. Housesteads, only having a larger single room, measures 3.5 x 8.0 metres (Johnson 1983: 169 fig. 129), which is longer than the two rooms combined at Valkenburg. Since the rooms in both structures are thought to have been intended for sleeping, comparisons were made of rooms in buildings thought to have had different purposes to see if there are noticeable differences in size. The *fabrica* at Wiesbaden, for example (Fig. 43), has rooms of many different sizes and shapes, but the smaller ones measure in the range of 4.5 x 3.5 metres and 3.0 by 3.0 metres (Johnson 1983: 186). The tribune's house at Inchtuthil again has rooms of various size but some are similar in size to the *valetudinaria* rooms, measuring 3.5 x 5.0 metres, 4.0 x 4.0 metres and 4.5 x 6.0 metres (Johnson 1983: 138, fig. 104). If one looks at the fortress of Inchtuthil (Fig. 54) and the fort of Oberstimm (Fig. 55) as visual examples of room comparisons within fortifications, it begins to become apparent that many of the room sizes within different structures of the same fortification are of similar size. Finally a comparison of room sizes in the *principia* shows that the size of the bedrooms in *valetudinaria* cannot be used to

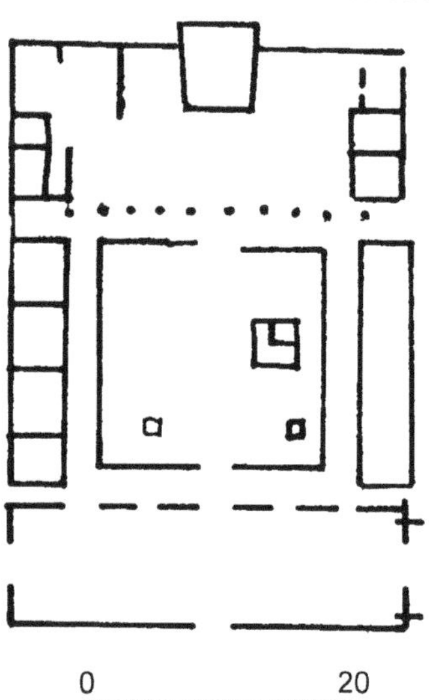

Fig. 52. Plan of the principia *at Saalburg. After Johnson 1983: Fig. 95.*

determine the function of the structure, as the rooms measure 3.5 x 4.0 at Valkenburg, 4.0 x 4.0 at Saalburg (Fig. 52) and 4.0 x 3.5 at Künzing (Fig. 53), for example (Johnson 1983: 124, fig. 95, 129 fig. 98). The bedroom size of the *valetudinarium* and the *principia* room size at Künzing are very similar.

The different kinds of room within a structure are also used to determine the purpose of the building. Von Petrikovitz (1975) and Press (1988) believe that all *valetudinaria* had baths, but there is certainly not enough evidence from the structural remains to support this assumption. The so-called *valetudinarium* in Vetera I had a bath and some rooms in Neuss and Carnuntum had a hypocaust system, which are often associated with bathing, but can also have been used to heat rooms. Warm rooms would certainly have been sensible for the sick and wounded soldiers, as well as the provision of their own baths, preventing the need for them to leave the comfort and warmth of the *valetudinarium*. Bathing was a means of treatment in Roman times and some soldiers were even sent to baths for recovery, such as at Baden Baden in

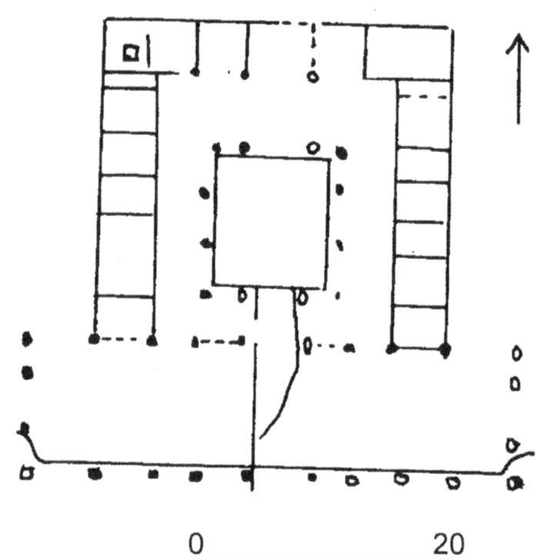

Fig. 53. Plan of the principia *at Künzing. After Johnson 1983: Fig. 95.*

Germania Superior, Baden in Switzerland and Aquae Sulis (Bath) in Britannia (Doppler 1970/71: 26). It is possible that some *valetudinaria* did have private baths for the sick, but it is also possible that if baths were not provided in the structure then the sick were either sponge bathed, sent to the camp bath, or might not have been bathed, depending on the beliefs of the unit towards the care of the ill and the disease's association with cleanliness. Moreover, heating might only have been provided depending on the environmental understandings of the illness and its cure, as discussed previously with building constructions.

It is also expected that latrines were placed in all of the so-called fortification *valetudinaria* (e.g. von Petrikovitz 1975: 101). Again this assumption is not fully supported by the archaeological remains. There was a possible latrine found at Housesteads and one at Wallsend. Neuss, Vindonissa and Lauriacum had drains running out of the structures, but their intended purpose has only been assumed to be for latrines. There are no archaeological remains of toilets in these structures and not all drains were intended for the purpose of sewage removal. The placement of a latrine in *valetudinaria* would make common sense; however the sick soldiers might have been encouraged to use the camp latrines, as a means of obtaining fresh air when they walked to the structure, or if they could not, perhaps 'bed-pans' were used. Latrines might not have been the nicest smelling places, and Hippocrates (Decorum 15) warns against the sick being placed in an area that reeked of foul odours, so perhaps latrines were not placed within the structures, assuming they are *valetudinaria*.

Operating theatres are integral to any modern hospital, and so there is another expectation the Roman *valetudinaria* were to have such rooms as well (Schultz 1934). Salazar notes that there is nothing in the literature to support the rooms' existence (2000: 81). The only indication we have about the rooms in which doctors had to work is from Celsus, who recommends a well-lit area to perform a cataract operation:

> "*Post haec in advorso collocandus est, luco lucido, lumine adverso, sic ut contra medicus paulo altius*" (7. 7. 14C).

The Hippocratic writer of *In the Surgery* (III) stated that the surgeon was to be placed conveniently to the part of the body that needed treatment. Quite often it is suggested that the patient sat rather than lay down (e.g. Celsus 7. 7. 14C). Archaeologists believe that the physical remains of rooms that protrude into the courtyard such as at Neuss and Vetera I were operating theatres, because it is believed they would have had brighter light and fresher air (von Petrikovitz 1975: 101). This argument complies with the statements of Celsus and the Hippocratic writer, but it does not explain why the larger rooms in other structures such as at Housesteads, Wallsend, Künzing and Oberstimm have been defined as operating theatres on account of the need for space of the equipment and doctor's movement. In comparison, modern operating theatres need room for an operating table, electronic equipment, a team of surgeons and nurses, large lamps and tanks for anaesthetic gases. No Roman operating theatre, if they existed, would have needed room to accommodate the same number of items that are used in modern surgery. A painting of Aeneas from Pompeii depicts him standing whilst having a spearhead removed from his thigh (Ramage and Ramage 2000: 180, fig.

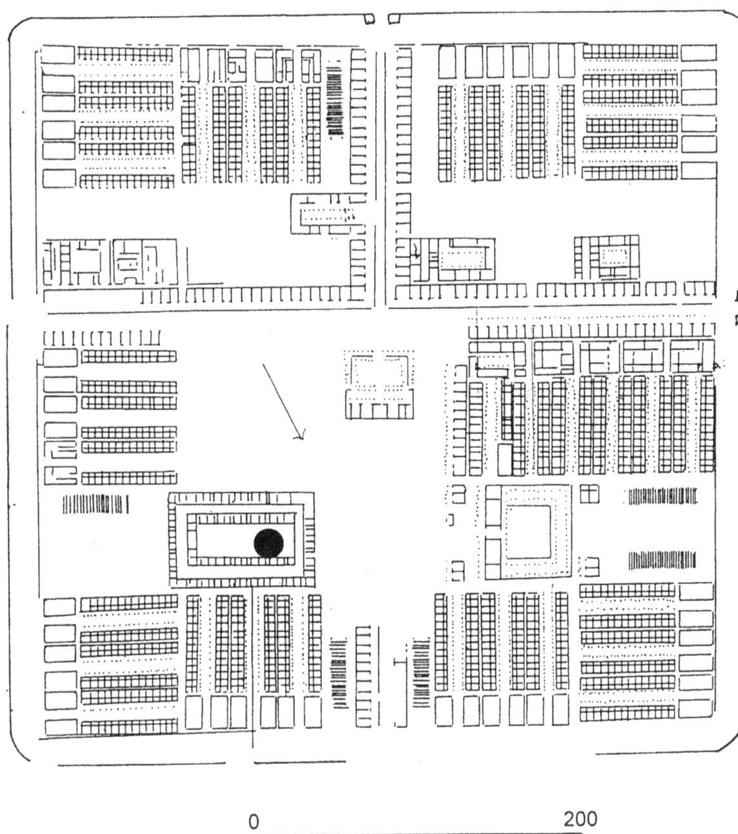

Fig 54. Plan of Inchtuthil marking the valetudinarium. *After Johnson 1983: Fig. 17.*

The final two rooms that are mentioned repeatedly in the descriptions of *valetudinaria* are the possible kitchen and cult room. Some of the structures have hearths within them that were originally suggested to have been used by doctors to sterilise their instruments (Schultz 1934: 55). However, as it became clear that sterilisation was not practised by the Romans the hearths were then argued to have been used as a component in kitchens, again playing upon 'common sense' arguments because modern hospitals always have cooking facilities. Though kitchens in Roman fortifications are not widely known of because it seems that most soldiers were expected to cook their own meals. It may be that the soldiers cooked for their sick comrades in their barracks, rather than there being kitchen staff in the *valetudinaria*. Hearths are often found throughout many buildings and could have had a variety of functions, such as cooking, heating, craft activities and so forth. The hearths in the so-called *valetudinarium* at Housesteads have evidence for high temperature burning (Crow 1995: 50-1), probably an indication of metalworking rather than cooking, making it probable that this particular building might have been a workshop. Without secure contextual records of the archaeological finds from rooms with hearths it is impossible to say what their intended function or functions were.

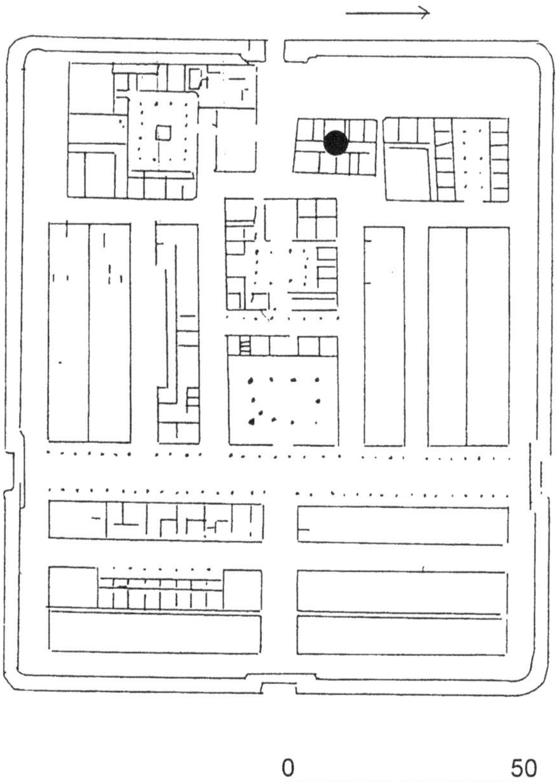

Fig. 55. Plan of Oberstimm marking the valetudinarium. *After Johnson 1983: Fig. 180.*

Rooms claimed to have a sacred or religious function are also thought to have been part of all the *valetudinaria*, but evidence is lacking from most places. The structure at Vindobona had two altars found within one room (Neumann 1965: 103; Neumann 1980: 28). However, one of the altars had been reused as *spolia* in part of the wall of the building, whilst the other was found *in situ*. The altar found *in situ* was dedicated to Aesculapius and Jupiter, whilst the other was dedicated to Apollo. A small shrine dedicated to the healing deities of Aesculapius, Hygia, Jupiter and Minerva was uncovered at Novae (Dyzcek 1995: 201-2). A building that has altars dedicated to gods of health need not necessarily be a *valetudinarium*, it could have had another function, perhaps as places were 'clubs' or religious societies would meet (Johnson 1983: 30, 111). Some forts had buildings used for places for socialising and these were often based around religious activity, making it plausible that the room at Vindobona and the structure at Novae might have been used for a social and/or religious function.

6.4.3 Location of the structures

Every Roman fortification has a different layout of buildings, from this difference it is clear that Hyginus' description of a marching camp was either based loosely on what he saw at the end of the 1st century AD in permanent fortifications, or that marching camps might have followed a stricter plan than was adhered to in the case of permanent fortifications. As mentioned, the building that has been identified as the *valetudinarium* was not always found in the area of the fortification that Hyginus recommends, but was constructed next to different buildings, such as barracks, *fabrica, principia, praetoria* and granaries. If, on the contrary, Hyginus was followed then the plan of the *valetudinarium* varies because not all of the buildings located behind the commanding officers' houses are of the same design.

The legionary fortresses of Haltern (Fig. 56), Vetera I (Fig. 57), Bonn (Fig. 58), Vindonissa (Fig. 59), Vindobona, Lotschitz, Lauriacum (Fig. 60), Caerleon (Fig. 61) and Novae had buildings claimed to be *valetudinaria* in the praetentura, whilst others were constructed in the *latera praetorii*: Neuss, Carnuntum (Fig. 62), Inchtuthil (Fig. 54) and Chester. In the auxiliary forts the so-called *valetudinaria* located in the *praetentura* were at Valkenburg, Wiesbaden, Künzing, Benwell and Hod Hill. Those in the *latera praetorii* were found at Oberstimm (Fig. 55), Housesteads (Fig. 63), Wallsend (Fig. 64) and Fendoch.

Another problem with undue dependency upon Hyginus as a source is that many of the identified *valetudinaria* were found next to *fabrica*, barracks, baths and granaries. Hyginus suggested that the *valetudinarium* be constructed in a quiet place, yet again his advice does not seem to have influenced all who built the structures, because the locations of many of the so-called *valetudinaria* do not appear to have been in quiet areas. Vetera I was located next to a gate with possible shops constructed at its entrance, whilst Künzing's argued *valetudinarium* was built between a gate and a granary and in front of a barrack block. The *fabrica* next to the possible *valetudinarium* at Oberstimm and across the way from Inchtuthil were probably not quiet either. Barracks and a bath building were constructed in the area of the *valetudinarium* in Vindonissa. Caerleon's might have built next to a *schola*, a 'clubhouse' or place for socialising. This brings us back to questioning what the Romans thought of as quiet, as one would not expect shops and the granary during deliveries and daily distributions of grain to be peaceful, especially if the soldiers and workers were talking, moving goods, carts and so forth (Rickman 1971). The same problem might occur in the barracks and baths. Gates could also have been noisy places when carts were brought through them.

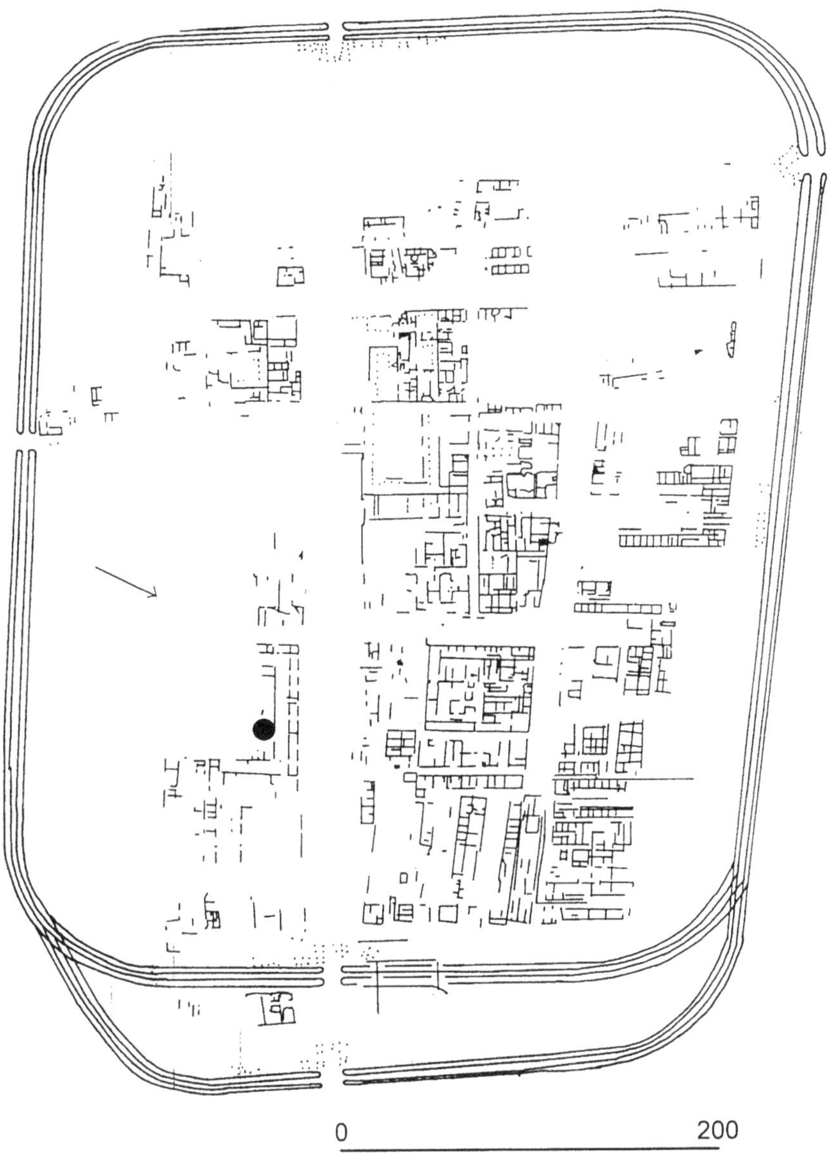

Fig. 56. Plan of Haltern marking the valetudinarium. *After Johnson 1983: Fig. 176.*

It has been made clear by Vegetius that soldiers were expected to live in a healthy area (Chapter 3). This is supported by a statement of Vitruvius (6.1) who says that the human body requires a certain climate to live comfortably and that buildings and rooms should be constructed in a manner to assure this comfort. He argued that rooms ideally should be arranged according to the season in which they were being used. The summer dining room in a villa, for example, should face north because it will be cool and dry. It would seem that if there were recommendations for structures to be constructed in a salubrious manner the architects of the *valetudinaria* would have considered this point, as it is a building associated with the health and well-being of the body. However, when looking at the placement of the so-called *valetudinaria* in their fortifications, evidently the advice of Vitruvius might not have been followed because the *valetudinaria* were not all constructed in the same area of each fortification and their orientations vary as well. Housesteads, for example, faces west, Künzing faces east and Oberstimm faces south. The same discrepancy is found in the legionary fortifications. Caerleon's entrance is thought to have been placed to the east whilst Neuss' faces north. The other difficulty with this is that we are relying on a Roman writer from 1st century AD Italy in order to explain how a healthy building should be constructed, when there is the possibility that units from different areas and different time periods (as attitudes do change through time) would have had other ideas about what constituted a healthy aspect of a building.

6.4.4 Structural comparisons

The *valetudinarium* is not the only building within Roman fortifications to have had a courtyard plan, so it is rather difficult to base its identification on this aspect alone. If one wishes to identify *valetudinaria* on the basis of structures with courtyard plans and rooms surrounding the centre, other buildings such as the commanding officer's quarters in most fortifications and the tribune's houses at Vetera I and Vindonissa could also be identified as *valetudinaria* rather than private residences. Some even had hypocaust systems and baths like the structures identified as *valetudinaria* at Vetera I and Carnuntum. Even though it is the double room arrangement that has been taken as essential for the identification of *valetudinaria* there is not enough recorded evidence from archaeological site reports to support the fact that these were bedrooms. With this in mind, and with very few contextual studies having been made of the artefacts from these structures, one could easily identify many buildings as *valetudinaria* on their plans alone.

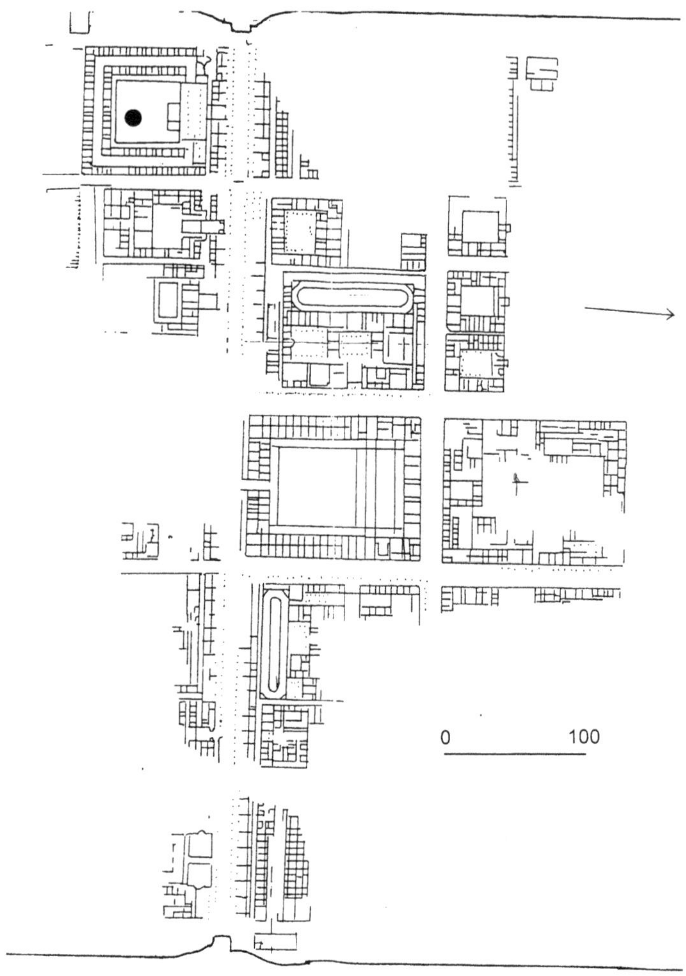

Fig. 57. Plan of Vetera I marking the valetudinarium. *After Johnson 1983: Fig. 186.*

Not only can other buildings be identified as *valetudinaria*, but the so-called *valetudinaria* also show signs of having served different functions, such as storage places or workshops. Courtyard plan buildings have been identified by as workshops because of the remains of slag pits and hearths from metalworking at Inchtuthil, Corbridge, Oberstimm, Wiesbaden and Valkenburg (Johnson 1983: 183). The workshop at Wiesbaden also had the remains of a hypocaust in two of its rooms (Johnson 1983: 185), just like the *valetudinarium* at Carnuntum. Thus, it is important to note that perhaps other buildings besides dwellings had hypocausts and it is not a strong means of identification for a *valetudinarium*. The so-called *valetudinarium* at Valkenburg has not only been identified as a *valetudinarium* (Watermann 1980: 30), but on occasion as the *praetoria* and *fabrica* in the fort (Schönberger 1979: 135-41). The building was identified on its ground plan, but it was not until more studies were made of the hearths and artefacts that a more positive identification as a workshop was made. This should be taken as a word of caution for anyone intending to use the ground plans of a building as proof of its function.

The presence of medical tools has also been taken as supporting the identification of *valetudinaria*. However, simply because instruments were found in structures does not automatically imply that they were used in the building as medical tools. Other objects found with them are rarely recorded, which is unfortunate given that they might help in the identification of the use of the tools. Tools in the *valetudinaria* at Neuss and Novae (Dyzcek 1995: 202) were generally found in a single room, perhaps indicating a place of storage or manufacture. The majority of the tools from Novae were broken, so perhaps they were discarded here or were in storage for recycling. Furthermore, the finds might have been deposited after the building went out of use. Here again the identity of buildings should be based on thorough contextual studies of all the finds. Only then should comparisons be made of similar style buildings to see if the same sorts of finds are appearing in similar types of buildings.

6.5 Cultural Views of Space

The finer details of the *valetudinarium* arrangements are described as if the buildings were modern hospitals. The sleeping arrangements are discussed by Majno (1975: 387) and von Petrikovitz (1975: 101), who state that there was probably space for four or five people, each having their own beds (Fig. 65). To the modern reader, this seems perfectly reasonable; nonetheless we know very little about the sleeping arrangements of the Romans. When looking at other cultures it becomes clear that the one person or couple per bed is not always the norm. The Pennsylvania Dutch or Amish practice bundling (www.Horseshoecc and www.fortklock), whereby they use their beds as places for discussion and courting in the winter months. Since the Amish do not have heating in their houses they find that it is more comfortable and practical to invite a guest to sit under the covers of their beds for warmth. In order to avoid possible 'temptation', a length of wood known as a bundling board is placed down the centre of the bed separating the two occupants. Mention can also be made of the 16th century 'great bed of Ware' (held in the Victoria and Albert Museum) that could have slept about fifteen people. In the Inns of colonial America an overnight visitor paid for a space rather than a room and might have had to sleep in the same bed with a stranger, or even on the floor. These three

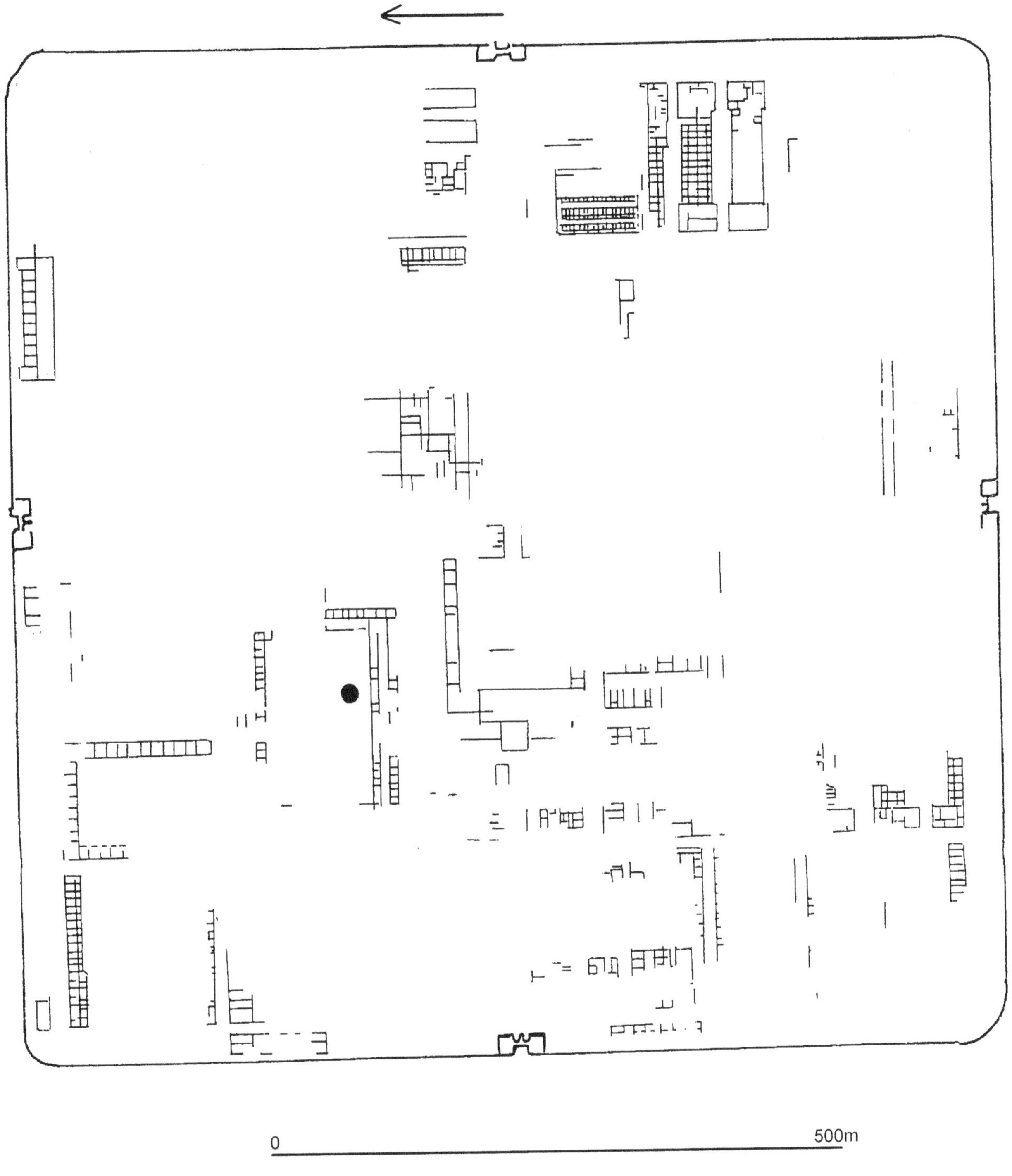

Fig. 58. Plan of Bonn marking the valetudinarium. *After Boon 1967.*

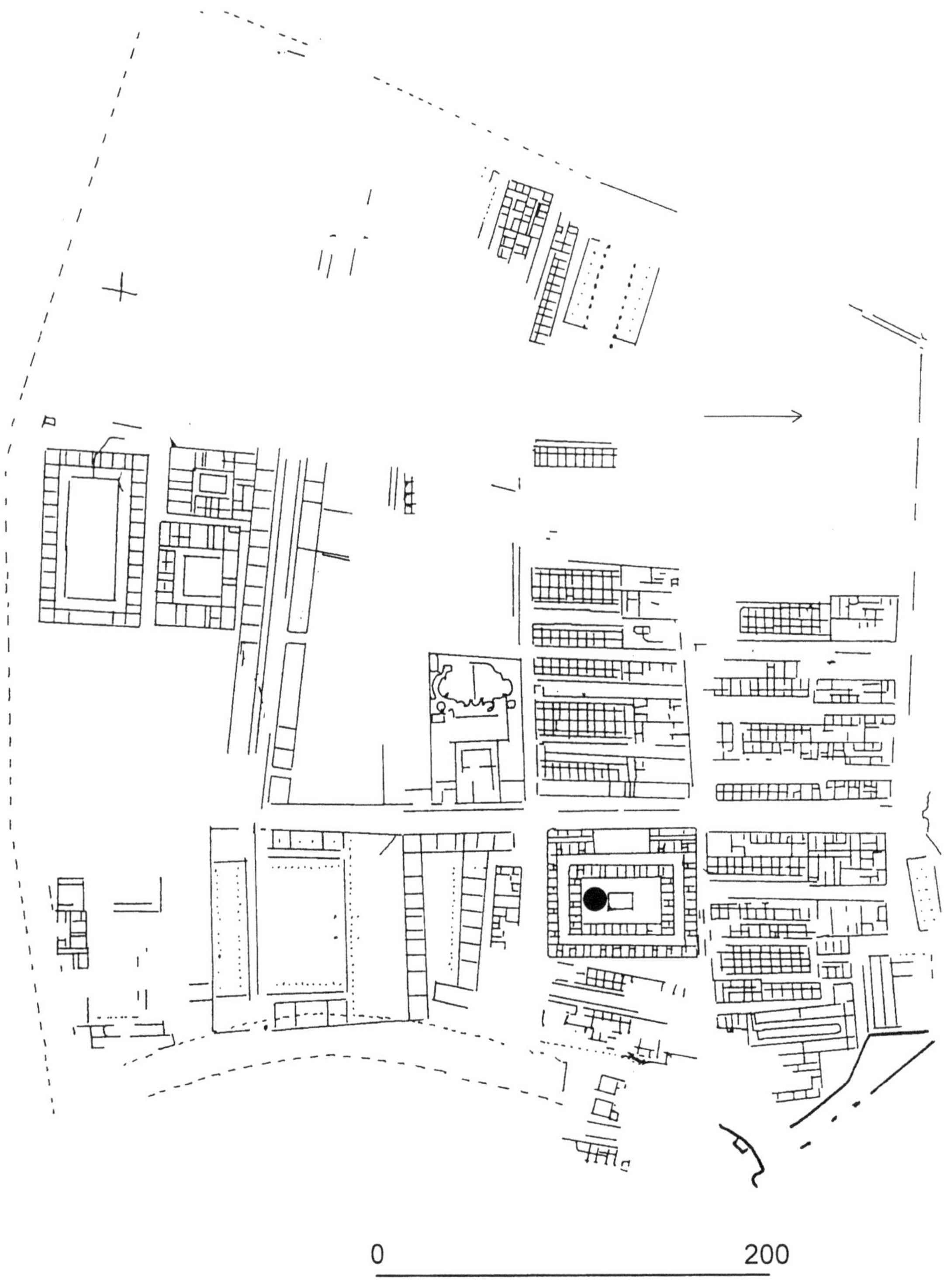

Fig. 59. Plan of Vindonissa marking the valetudinarium.
After Johnson 1983: Fig. 178.

we learn that a patient was placed in rooms according to the environment, but we do not know if the person was at home, in a *valetudinarium*, or in a room or bed alone.

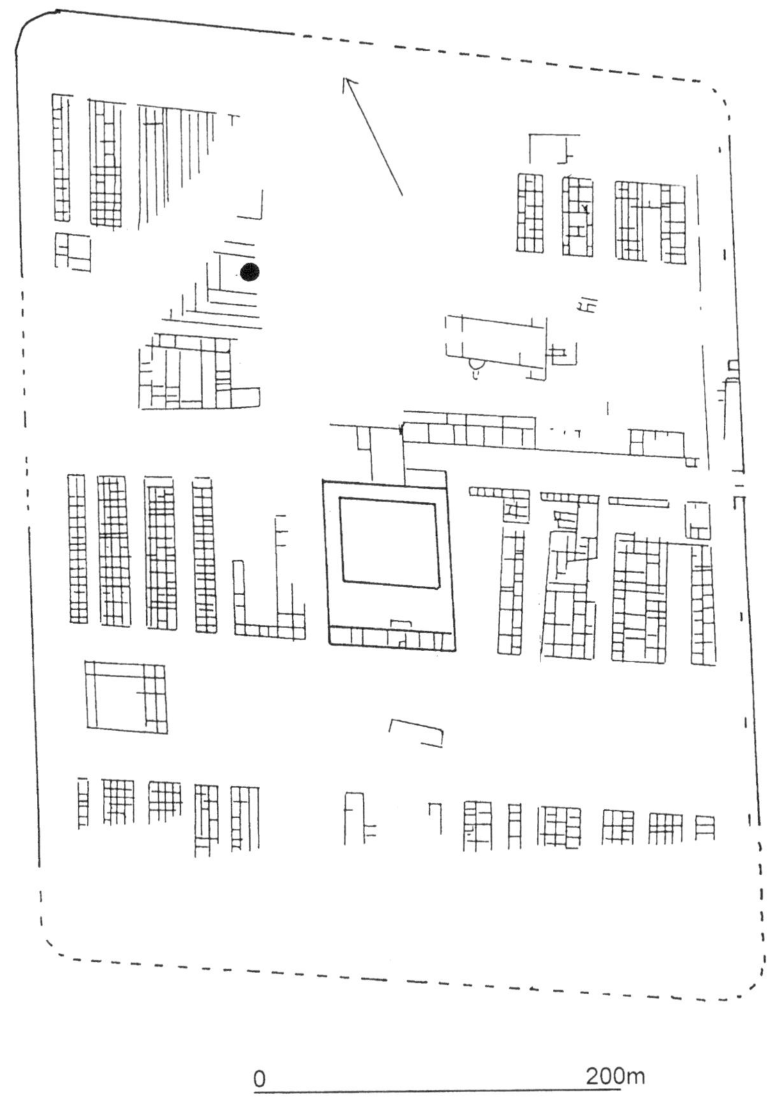

Fig. 60. Plan of Lauriacum marking the valetudinarium. *After Boon 1967.*

The anthropological study of proxemics reveals that people define their space and environmental surroundings according to their cultural norms (Argyle 1988: 184; Deetz 1977: 25). In certain cultures people will stand closer to one another whilst speaking to people than in other cultures. Arabs, for example, will stand closer and face each other more directly than Americans (Argyle 1988: 58). This space does not only affect the manner people use non-verbal communication with their body, but also the way they organise their architectural arrangements as well as their domestic and office furnishings (Argyle 1988: 185-7; Rapaport 1990: 10). Although this can be done more easily through modern anthropological examinations, there are means of questioning cultural understandings of space through archaeological studies. To do so, contextual examinations of artefacts are imperative for understanding how a society understood their architectural and environmental surroundings (Deetz 1977: 25; Kent 1990: 3).

examples demonstrate that even in modern and post-medieval times the bed and sleeping arrangements take on culturally determined forms. One could argue that this does not consider the sleeping arrangements of the ill; however, medieval paintings of hospitals reveal that there was not always a single person in one bed. It has been argued that the scenes of a male and female in the same bed were spouses; however, this argument does not explain paintings with three people placed in the same bed or people of the same sex (Furniss 1970: 3). It is possible, therefore, that Roman soldiers might have had different sleeping arrangements while they were sick or even when healthy in their barracks. The ancient sources do not provide a clear picture of how Roman sleeping arrangements were to be spaced. Recalling the blanket that was ordered for the hospital in Asia Minor, the size is quite large, certainly double, and perhaps it was meant for two people, rather than one. From the Hippocratic writings (Decorum 15)

Conceptions of spatial use have not been considered by Romanists to any great extent, but recently there have been some attempts to take such issues into account (e.g. Allison 1997). If Roman archaeologists had taken greater care to record the context and association of all artefact categories properly it would be easier to make examinations that would enormously benefit our understand of how people organised their space; and this could be reflected in how they cared for their ill, whether it was acceptable to place the sick in the same beds, rooms or buildings as the healthy, or if they should be separated. Bartlett examined the process by which mentally ill patients were taken out of hospitals designated for all types of illness in the 18th and 19th centuries and placed into asylums as a means of segregating them even further from society. If one could use the study of proxemics in Roman medical archaeology attitudes and ideas about certain types of illness or people with illness might become apparent.

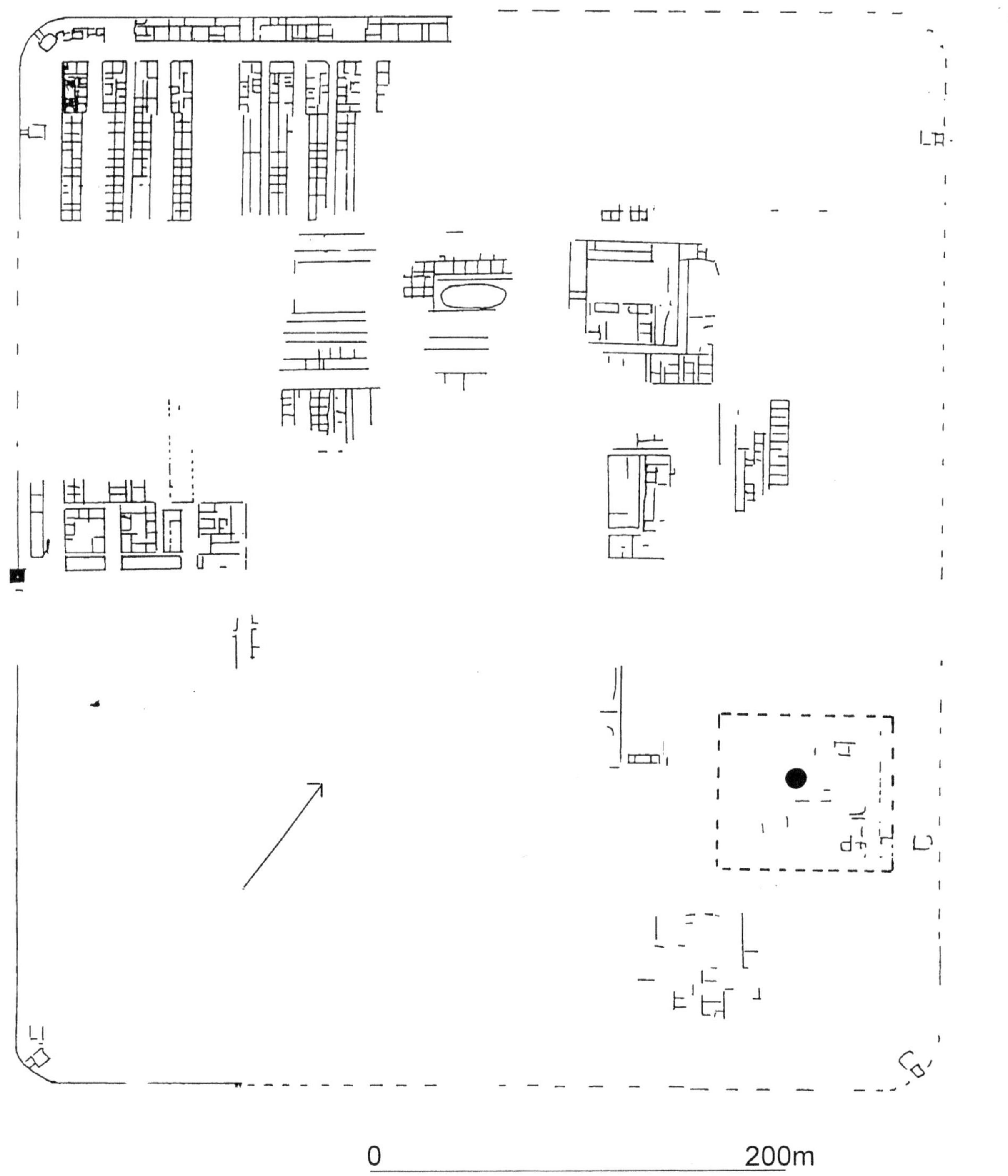

Fig. 61. Plan of Caerleon marking the valetudinarium.
After Johnson 1983: Fig. 197.

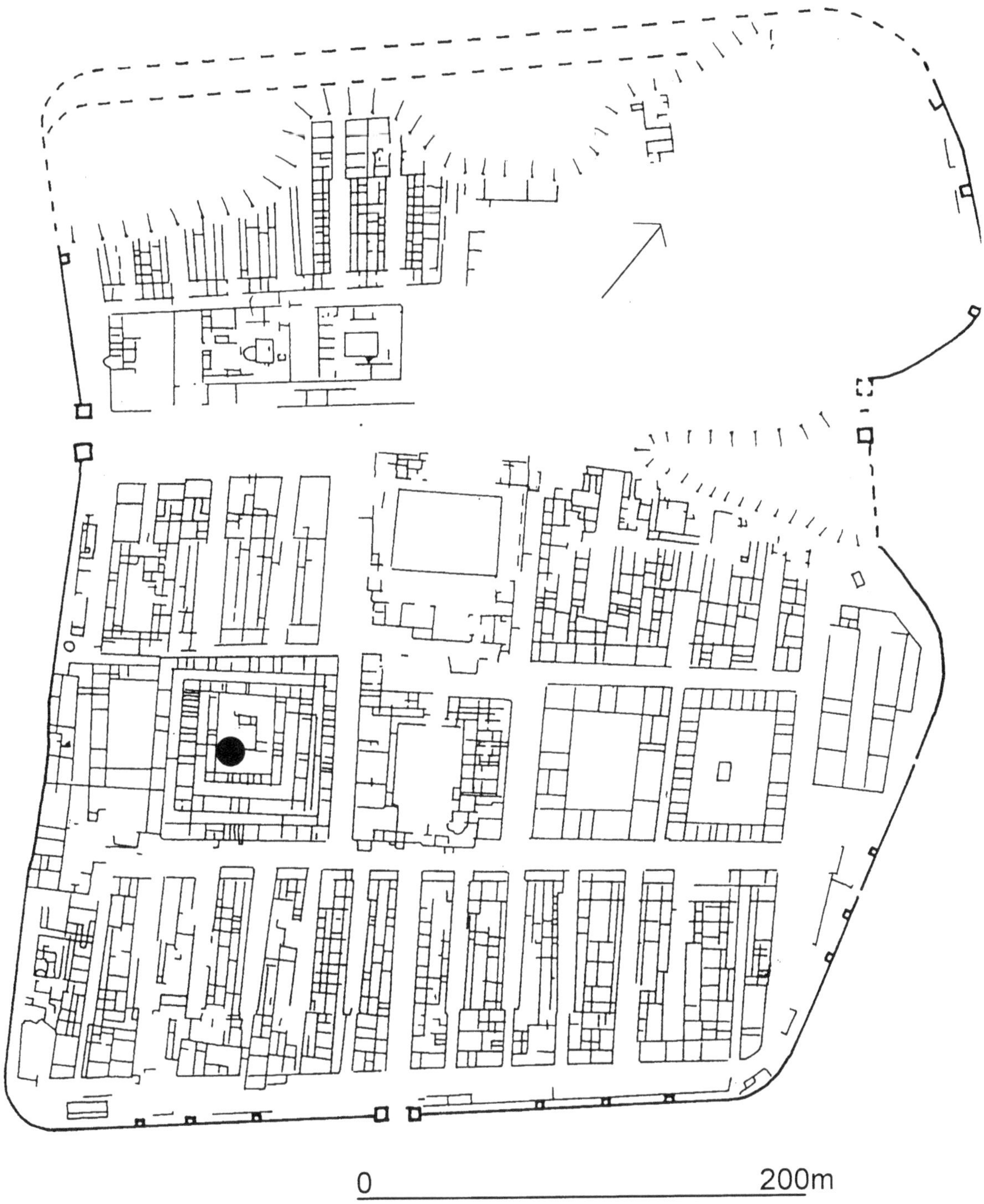

Fig. 62. Plan of Carnuntum marking the valetudinarium. *After Boon 1967.*

There has been one contextual study of the finds from a so-called *valetudinarium*, that at Novae. Although Dyzcek (1995) refers to the building as a *valetudinarium*, if we eliminate the identification of the building and simply look at the arrangement of finds, some interesting patterns begin to appear. Many metal fragments - pieces of armour and a bronze helmet, phalerae, and iron spearhead - along with many fragments of chain were found in the so-called bedrooms of the structure. He also says that in these rooms were also found items possibly related to use in the *valetudinarium*, such as lamps, vessel handles and fibulae (Dyzcek 1995: 200). Yet, it is not explained why these are to be specifically related to *valetudinaria*. Lamps for example were used in most buildings. Being part of normal domestic equipment, fibulae and vessel handles are also found in many areas of fortifications. The small vestibules between the bedrooms had types of tableware and butchered animal bones including a dolphin's rib (Dyzcek 1995: 200-2). Room 48 had a store of broken probes and physicians' caskets (Dyzcek 1995: 202), possibly indicating that health care was offered to the soldiers in this particular room, rather than in the entire building, or it might also indicate storage or deposition. Room 35 was thought to be the room where patients were examined, simply because fragments of two physicians' caskets and a spatula probe were found in the room. The central courtyard of the structure had altars dedicated to Hygia, Aesculapius, Jupiter and Juno, suggesting that there might have been some form of sanctuary in the centre (Dyzcek 1995: 202-3). If one looks at the finds there seem to be specific places where items were kept, or discarded (there is no discussion on whether these finds were from the time of the building's use, abandonment or destruction). Yet, the items tend not to tell us whether the building was a *valetudinarium* because, in addition to the broken instruments, the great variety of other items could relate to a range of functions and other activities, not associated with medicine.

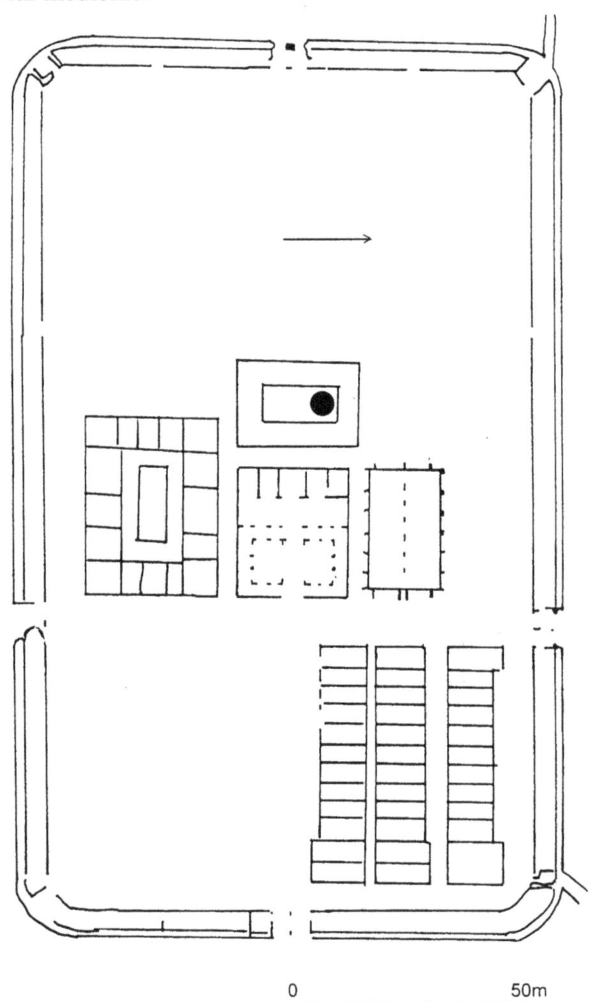

Fig. 63. Plan of Housesteads marking the valetudinarium. *After Johnson 1983: Fig. 190.*

6.6 History of Hospitals

Archaeologists and historians tend to use their present day experiences as a means of explaining how things functioned in the past (e.g. Thomas 1990: 15) – this is a basic form of analogy. As previously mentioned, when looking at the descriptions of Roman hospitals there has been a tendency to describe them as if they were modern hospitals. Koenan made the initial identification of a *valetudinarium* in the early 20th century, at Neuss, and it is quite likely that Koenan's interpretation was heavily influenced by his familiarity with contemporary military and civilian *valetudinaria*. When looking at plans of 19th century German military hospitals we see that they were divided into small wards, and had operating theatres, latrines and baths. Clearly this template has been applied in the identification of Roman military *valetudinaria*, as shown above with the idea that baths, kitchens and latrines should be present, though they do not appear in every structure that has been designated a *valetudinarium*. Behind all of this is the modern expectation that a public building will be definable by its 'institutionalised' architectural form. A tight link is made between form and function. Evans points out in the post-Roman West non-religious institutionalised buildings designed for a specific purpose, as we think of them, tend to be a feature of the 18th century and later (1990: 648). It is clear that there were some buildings in the Roman military that might be classed as institutional, such as the barracks and the headquarters building. However, even these differ from fortification to fortification (Johnson 1983: 105-56). It is possible that the *valetudinarium* was not an institutionalised building in as much as its form was not rigidly perceived. The comparisons shown above indicate that the expectation that all *valetudinaria* were built with the same features is merely an assumption, and the structural evidence shows very little of what is often expected to have been 'typical'.

Since there are many questions raised in this study about the identification of the structure of the Roman *valetudinaria*, and no known contemporary civilian hospital to compare them with, one must look to see if there are any similarities to hospitals of a later date, as seems to be implied with Koenen's identification. The first known hospital outside the Roman world is the Byzantine hospital, or *nosokomeion*. These were not simply places for the sick to receive help, but for the poor to be given food (Miller 1985: 38). From the evidence available thus far, it seems that these hospitals were only found in the East and did not spread to the Latin West (Nutton 1995c: 78). Little information survives about the plan of these structures and whether there were separate military hospitals, as there were in the Roman world.

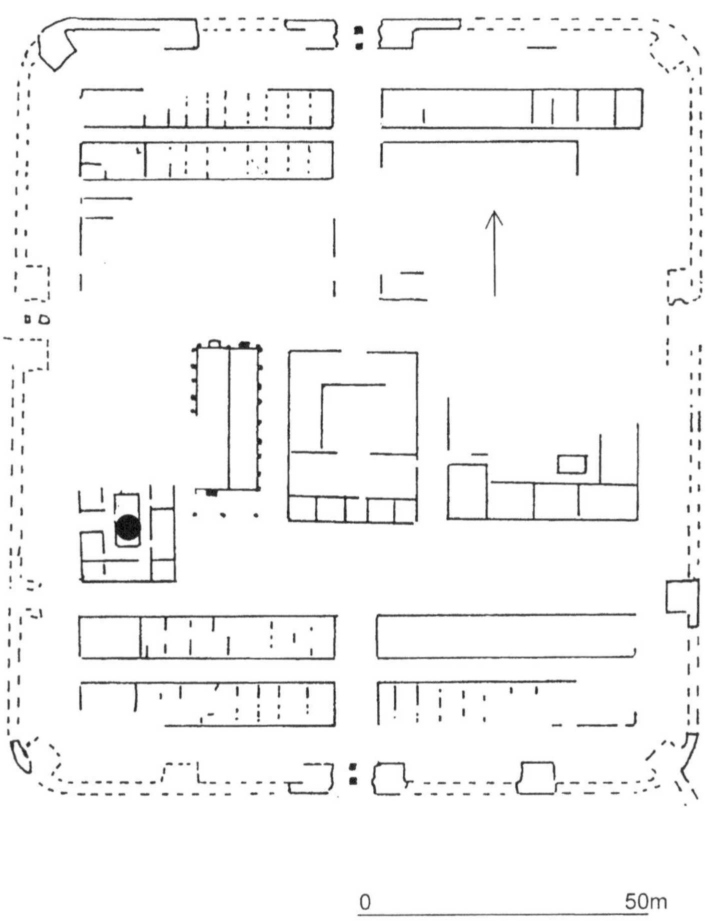

Fig. 64. Plan of Wallsend marking the valetudinarium. *After Johnson 1983: Fig. 201.*

Islamic hospitals were to be constructed in all cities, as the Koran (II, 61) states there is an obligation to aid the poor and help the sick (Houdas 2003: 86). The Islamic hospitals *bímáristán* or *máristán*, Persian meaning place for the sick, also served a number of purposes. Not only were the ill treated in them, but they were places for the poor to receive alms and for scholars to study at because some had libraries built into them (Conrad 1995: 136; Khan 1983: 198-9; Sayili 1980: 112). Soldiers could be treated at these hospitals, but the first military hospital recorded in Islamic medical history was a campaign hospital, not a permanent building. The Selguq kings of Turkey started the mobile hospital units to keep their soldiers in a fit and healthy condition from the 11th to the 13th centuries. The equipment for the hospitals was said to be carried by 200 camels (Elgood 1951: 175; Khan 1983: 200-201). Not all Islamic hospitals were built on the same plan or served the same functions, as they were influenced by more than one type of medicine. Some were constructed as Indian hospitals, which acted as medical dispensaries only, whilst others were influenced by the Greek medical traditions and had the role of places for both medical treatment and scholarship (Sayili 1980: 114-5, 117). Others were large structures with mosques, pharmacies, kitchens, gardens, baths and lecture rooms, as well as having wards for patients (Conrad 1995: 136). They were also constructed in accordance with strict views over the male and female body and separate wards were built for each sex, apparently with separate staff as well (Elgood 1951: 177). Since these hospitals were influenced by a number of medical traditions, there does not seem to have been a direct connection between the expectations of the Roman military *valetudinaria* and those of the Muslims.

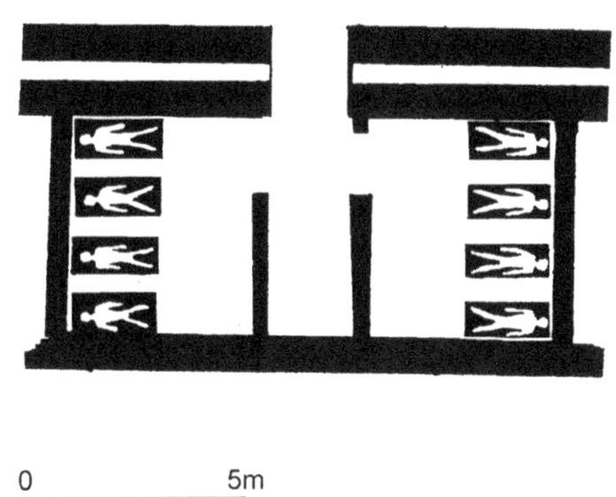

Fig. 65. Plan of conjectured sleeping arrangements in 'hospitals'. After Majno 1975: Fig. 9.39.

If we continue to follow the logic that the Roman *valetudinaria* were expected to have been similar to the 19th - 20th century hospitals, then one would expect the medieval hospital to be based on a similar plan. However, medieval hospitals were designed on an open basilica plan, similar to a church because many were run by the church. Most large medieval buildings follow one of two plans. The first is the church plan or basilica, and the second is the large open hall used in the construction of high status structures: the limited range of both institutionalised and domestic structures can be seen in medieval towns such as Cambridge (RCHME 1959). In medieval basilica hospitals there was usually a chapel or a group of chapels at the end of the nave so patients could witness the daily celebrations. St. Mary's in Newark, Leicestershire, had room for 30 inmates and had room for a single bed each. The beds were supposed to be arranged so that the patients could observe the daily religious services whilst lying in them. There was separate accommodation for hospital staff, usually in an unattached building located off the side of the infirmary. Travellers often lodged with the sick, in the same rooms, and there does not seem to have been a division of genders in all hosptials (Carlin 1989: 28; Furniss 1970: 3; Nutton 1995c: 150-1).

Renaissance Italian hospitals were also based on the basilica plan. In some cases the hospitals were constructed in a cruciform design where everyone could observe the daily religious services taking place in the centre of the building (Henderson 1989: 76). Thus, the medieval hospital, for which there is more evidence than Roman structures, bears little resemblance to that of claimed Roman *valetudinaria*. Perhaps the medieval world rejected the plan of Roman *valetudinaria* if they were aware of it, or perhaps the design does follow the Roman one, and the Roman *valetudinaria* plan has been mis-identified: could large basilica buildings, such as that attached to the bath at Caerleon (Zeinkiewicz 1986) be a contender for a *valetudinarium*? Whatever the case, the comparison of Roman military *valetudinaria* with medieval ones suggests that the model of the Roman *valetudinarium* was probably not carried over into the middle ages.

There are no known particular military hospitals during the medieval period. Furniss observes that soldiers were lucky if they were able to return home and be treated for battle wounds in a public hospital (1970: 2). The Knight's of St. Johns, a military order, set up hospitals but these had grown out of a hospice for the poor in Jerusalem. Traditionally the hospital of St. John's offered many services: alms giving, a place for the lepers to live, maternity care, child care and treatment for soldiers wounded in battle (Luttrell 1994: 64-5). There were no particular architectural structures that defined the building. It could have been a great hall with a chapel, similar to monastic hospitals, or it could have been built in the local architectural tradition of the place where the hospital was being constructed (Luttrell 1994: 75-6).

The idea of a military hospital in the western world does not seem to have come into being until the later middle ages, and the majority of evidence for them only appears in the 18th century. It was mentioned earlier that it is about this time that institutionalised structures begin to become commonplace. One example of this can be found in the development of the Dutch military hospital, which came into being over a long period of time (Langeveld 1989). The Spanish military hospitals, both permanent and field, are known to have come into existence during the reign of Ferdinand of Aragon, in the late 15th century. Being an invading force, the Spanish could not rely on the services of Dutch civilian hospitals for treatment. The army of the Netherlands came into being in the late 16th century during the revolution against Spain, and the soldiers were taken to civilian hospitals for treatment (Langeveld 1989: 90-1). The military hospital system for the Dutch came about because soldiers receiving treatment in civilian hospitals had to pay for their own medical care. By the late 18th century a separate system of medical care with its own buildings was formed (Langeveld 1989: 91-102). The military hospital buildings of the late 19th century in the Netherlands were designed to conform to the Dutch idea of a structure that would promote a cure. The philosophy was 'air - is – life', in other words, the patients were to receive plenty of fresh air. The hospital at Leiden, for example, was constructed around a pavilion. Separate wards were created that could be closed off in case of an outbreak of contagious disease (Langeveld 1989: 122). Both civilian and military German hospitals also follow the same plan and philosophy. The Peter Freidrich Ludwigs Hospital had the necessary components expected by recent scholars in Roman military *valetudinaria*: entrance hall, living rooms for the surgeon, large halls at the entrance with room for about ten beds, toilets, baths and small rooms that could hold six patients (Brat 1966: 8, 22). One wing of the hospital was designated for the military (Brat 1966: 18). The academic hospital in Göttingen had a similar ground plan as well as specific rooms for surgery (Jettner 1966: 144-5).

It cannot be shown that the development of hospitals had a Roman influence (if Koenen and others have described Roman *valetudinaria* properly), but rather what seems clear is that recent northern European military and civilian hospitals have influenced the interpretation of what a Roman hospital should be like. It is more likely that if the Roman *valetudinaria* had been an influence for Byzantine and medieval hospitals then they would not strictly have been used for the treatment of illness and injury, and they would probably have been built on a basilica plan. The main point of discussing hospitals in other historical contexts is to show that they had different forms of structure, function and meanings throughout time, and there is really no reason why Roman *valetudinaria* would have been similar to more modern hospitals as archaeologists have defined them.

6.7 ARTEFACT REMAINS

The final aspect that should be investigated relates to where remains of medical instruments were found in the fortifications, because this might provide a better indication of where the *valetudinaria* were located. The artefacts found in so-called *valetudinaria* will be discussed to see if they can provide any evidence about the intended purpose of the structures. Since many of the fortifications were excavated at the turn of the 20th century the provenance of the instruments was not always recorded with much care (Appendices 4-10). The location of medical instruments in other areas of the fortifications will also be discussed because this might shed some light on where soldiers were receiving treatment.

With the exception of the instruments from Neuss, the contextual evidence for instruments found within fortifications in Germania Inferior has been poorly recorded. The instruments from Neuss (Appendix 6, Table A6.1) are of interest because a number of probes and forceps were found in the so-called *valetudinarium*; four scalpels were also found in the building, although in other rooms. The majority of these came from a single room, room 51, tending to suggest some form of storage rather than a surgical area, especially since they were mainly probes. Nonetheless this structure was not the only building to have yielded instruments. The baths at Neuss had a few instruments as well. The *principia* has seven instruments pointing to the possibility that people were either receiving treatment here, grooming themselves in public, or the instruments might have had another function. Ten instruments were found in the barracks, and it is therefore possible that the fortress doctor could have travelled to the rooms. Eleven instruments were found in other buildings throughout the fortress. Thus the majority of the instruments do not come from the so-called *valetudinarium*, which might indicate that soldiers were able to receive treatment in a variety of places. Of course, the location of the finds need not be a direct reflection of where treatment was taking place – their distribution only reflects a place of loss or final deposition.

In Germania Superior (Appendix 7) the majority of recorded instruments come from auxiliary forts. The fort at Ladenburg has surgical instruments from the bath, located outside of it; however because it is in such close proximity to the fort it was probably used by the soldiers. Evidence from Caerleon suggests that women and children also bathed in military baths (Zienkiewicz 1986: 223), so it is possible that this happened at Ladenburg, implying that the instruments might not have necessarily been used by, or on, the soldiers. The instruments found in the baths included a scalpel, a bone scraper, a serrated spoon or 'wound scoop', an ointment box, a spatula probe and an ointment pallet. Instruments were found in the fort baths at Okarben and Hofheim (Appendix 5, table A5.12 and A5.14). If these finds were a direct reflection of medical activity, it seems that some form of treatment might have been offered in the military baths in Germania Superior. Though some of them could simply have been used for personal hygiene. Nonetheless, hygiene is related to health and the tools demonstrate that people could clean their nails and ears, for example, in the public baths. I mention this because I have attended the Friedricks Bad in Baden Baden, Germany and although following a very similar plan to the Roman baths, I did not see anyone clipping their nails, tweezing their eyebrows or cleaning their ears. The idea was to enjoy the baths for relaxation and therapy for bone and muscle ailments; the idea of cleaning oneself seemed to be a secondary (to me at least) reason for attending them. Having had this experience, my perceptions of Roman bathing would be quite different, as the Romans were preening themselves, when today, public displays of cleaning oneself are often considered vulgar. Any etiquette guide would warn us not to clean our ears, nose or nails in public. So we can see from the instruments that this was probably acceptable behaviour for the Romans.

Perhaps in certain places there was no *valetudinarium,* so the fort doctor was provided with a room or set of rooms to work from wherever there was available space in the fortification. This is not only implied by the instruments found in baths, and the single room of instruments in the *valetudinaria* at Neuss and Novae, but by two instruments found in the west corner tower of the auxiliary fort at Holzhausen (Appendix 5, Table A5.4) and Mainhardt (Appendix 5, Table A5.24). The instruments are probes that could have been used for personal hygiene as well, indicating that soldiers might have been grooming themselves whilst on duty. Alternatively, the location of the instrument in a tower or corner of a structure might suggest an area where trash was discarded, as occurred at Caerleon.

The legionary fortress at Vindonissa (Appendix 5, Table A5.2) has a comparatively high number of instruments that have survived in good condition. Besides the instruments found in the Schutthügel (discussed in Chapter 5), a number of instruments were located in certain structures of the fortification. A large majority of instruments were found in the *principia* and the area of the baths. This might indicate that care was being offered in these buildings, or instruments were being stored or deposited in the structures. The so-called *valetudinarium* had 13 medical tools, but it also had 99 military accoutrements (Unz and Dechler-Erb 1997: 66). Some of the military finds are pieces of scabbards, belt plates, cavalry decorations such as *phalerae*, spear heads, terminals for military aprons and buckles for armour. If one considers these finds, it is not automatically suggested that the building was a *valetudinarium*.

Compared to other provinces, Britain has more instruments with better contextual information. Instruments came from a number of areas throughout the fortress of Caerleon (Appendix 10, Table A10.2). Finds from the amphitheatre illustrate the possibility that the soldiers, or perhaps civilians, had no qualms about cleaning themselves in public, but disposal does not always indicate places of use. The instruments seem to have been clustered in the barracks. The baths have remains a pair of forceps (Appendix 10, Table A10.2, number 5) and milk teeth with indentations that indicate surgical removal (Zienkiewicz 1986: 223). The teeth in the drain provide the strongest indication for surgical treatment in a particular building.

The fortress at Chester (Appendix 10, Table A10.3) has a small number of finds, but they show some clustering as well, especially in the barracks. The amphitheatre, like that at Caerleon, had a pair of forceps. Outside the fortress three ear probes and one set of forceps was found. No *valetudinarium* can be determined on the basis of artefactual finds alone.

At Housesteads no instruments were found in the building claimed to be a *valetudinarium* (Appendix 10, Table A10.9). The few instruments from Birdoswald were mainly found in the area of the granaries (Appendix 10; Table A10.10). One ear probe was discovered in building 197, a granary, whilst the area around building 198, also a granary, contained an ear probe and an ointment pallet. Found on the *via praetoria* was another ear probe, and an ointment pallet was found in the topsoil in section A. There is not enough evidence from either fort to say for certain where the *valetudinarium* might have been located.

Clearly from the evidence of finds, the structures identified as *valetudinaria* do not seem to have been very clean, at least in their final stages of use. It is perhaps more likely that the buildings were used, or also used, for storage or as workshops, which is supported by the evidence supplied by auxiliary structures that the buildings were either *valetudinaria*, *fabrica* or for storage. Thus, the argument that the buildings were meant to have been *valetudinaria* is not strictly supported by the artefactual evidence.

As a final note of caution, although it is important to look at the finds from each structure to attempt to determine its function, it must be remembered that artefacts can be moved from one place to another and are not necessarily found in the locations where they were used or originally deposited (Schiffer 1987). For example certain buildings might have gone out of use, and the objects in them could have been moved to another structure. The obsolete building might then have been used as a place to deposit rubbish brought in from elsewhere. Roman archaeologists sometimes assume that artefacts occur in the same place that they were used, implying they were dropped as 'primary' refuse. Undoubtedly the situation is much more complex (as illustrated in Chapter 5). Thus by looking at the find spots of the instruments it is rather difficult to give a precise idea about where they were intended to be used. The one exception may be with bath buildings where many instruments have been found. The spread of instrument find spots across forts does indicate that the *valetudinaria* cannot be determined from finds alone as the excavator of Neuss and archaeologists who followed have tended to uncritically accept.

6.8 Other Possibilities for *Valetudinaria*

Unfortunately there seems to be little conclusive evidence for specific Roman military buildings serving as *valetudinaria*. The structural evidence appears to fit the early 20th century version of what a *valetudinarium* should be and the artefactual remains are insufficiently recorded to suggest any particular style of building being adopted as a *valetudinarium* throughout the frontiers. On the basis of artefactual material, the barracks and baths seem to have more evidence for medical treatment, and it is only the structures at Neuss, Vindonissa and Novae that have produced remains of surgical tools. There is no reason why the *valetudinarium* had to be based on a strict plan, or that it should conform to what a modern hospital should be. Given that the medieval, Islamic and Byzantine hospitals served a range of other functions, so might Roman *valetudinaria*.

Archaeologists may also have been misled into expecting military *valetudinaria* to comprise separate buildings. There remains a possibility that the *valetudinarium* was one element (perhaps a set of rooms, or a 'doctor's office') within a larger structure or complex. This can be suggested by the fact that the term is mentioned along with the *fabrica* on a Vindolanda tablet discussed above (Bowman and Thomas 1991: 61, 66; Bowman and Thomas 1994: 98). Although the Romans were obviously concerned with personal hygiene, which is evident from the number of public and private baths and chatelaines, they were unaware of the causes of disease through bacteria. Thus they might have placed *valetudinaria* within other buildings if the area appeared clean, but this still does not imply that the area was sterile. The link between *valetudinaria* and *fabrica* implied by the Vindolanda tablet and Hyginus (4), and by the instances of workshop debris and medical instruments occurring in the same structure, suggests another intriguing possibility – that the two were often physically and conceptually linked. Given that often there are embedded links between quite varied and disparate technological practices (e.g. Siller 1999), treatment of the human body, of animals and the repair and manufacture of objects, may have been viewed as closely linked, with all such operations performed in a single area, or even building. The word *valetudinarium* might also be an indication that the *valetudinarium* was physically one part of the workshops, rather than being a separate building itself, as is seen in the terms used for parts of baths such as *frigidarium* and *calidarium*.

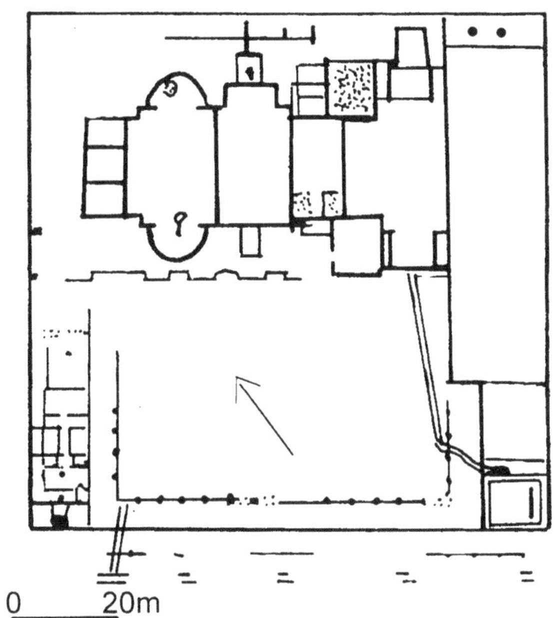

Fig. 66. Plan of the bath at Xanten. After Künzl 1989/90.

Finally there is the possibility that a soldier could choose from a number of places to receive medical treatment within the fortress. It seems that the baths were a likely spot. This is not only supported by evidence of teeth and instruments in military baths, but the civilian bath at Xanten had instruments found in it (Appendix 4, Table A4.9). The area of the bath in which they were found had two rooms adjacent with a small hall dividing them. This arrangement according to Künzl was similar to the wards found in military *valetudinaria* (1986b: 445-6; 1989/90 147), and he believes that this similarity along with the presence of instruments implies that the rooms were used for medical treatment. The two rooms are comparable to those defined as the bedrooms, rather than a place for treatment, but this is based on modern conceptions of the Roman *valetudinarium* (Figs. 66 & 67). Whether the rooms are based on those from the so-called *valetudinaria* is rather difficult to answer because there are many rooms in other buildings that are of similar arrangement to the ones Künzl mentions, but it seems that it might have been a place for a doctor to offer treatment.

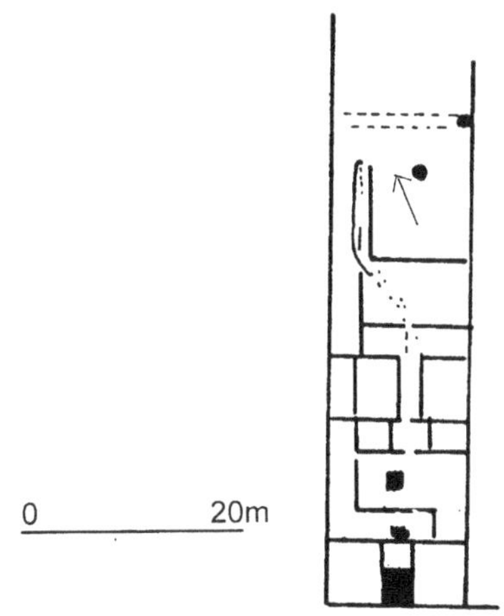

Fig. 67. Close-up of the 'doctor's rooms' in the bath at Xanten. After Künzl 1989/90.

Certain barracks have clusters of instruments, which might be a place where soldiers were treated, or where the doctor resided. So, from the information available in the archaeological record, there seems to be a number of suggestions about where soldiers received treatment, but little can be said about the structures that have been identified as *valetudinaria*. It seems as if there are more questions than answers about their identification.

6.9 Conclusion

It is clear from the evidence presented in this chapter that it is difficult to determine where a *valetudinarium* might have been located in the fortifications, let alone how the structure appeared. It seems the assumptions about their identification have been driven by the anachronistic expectations of how a *valetudinarium* should be arranged, and by the use of archaeological evidence to create a universal explanation for the range of activities and functions contained within them.

It may be, however, that this lack of specifically arranged structures supports part of the argument in chapters 4 and 5 that the organisation of the medical care system in the Roman army was done on a local rather than centralised basis. Even though the structures identified as *valetudinaria* cannot be securely defined as such, the differences within the buildings themselves could be further support for the ideas that there were variations within the army. First of all some fortifications have evidence for the courtyard buildings while others did not. Secondly the structures varied in size and layout. It is likely that most fortifications had some form of health care offered, but in different places depending on the needs of those inhabiting them. Since it is too difficult to define what a *valetudinarium* is, there are problems in determining provincial differences in health care across the frontiers on the basis of the structural evidence alone, even though the information provided by the inscriptions and medical tools tends to support this.

Chapter Seven

Conclusion

7.1. Restating the Questions

The main issue of this examination was to question whether there was a standard system of medical care in the Roman army. This query was raised because it is generally assumed in modern scholarship on Roman military medicine that there was a single system by which all units organised their medical care, rank of doctors and style of treatment. The perception that most aspects of the Roman army were the same throughout the empire has led modern scholars to attempt to deduce the exact specifications of how the medical care system functioned and what the doctors' title indicates about their rank (e.g. Davies 1969; 1970; 1989; Richmond 1952; Wilmanns 1995a & b). Although they are useful studies, and ideas about how the distribution of medical care was offered to the units might have applied to some groups of soldiers, the scholars have not questioned the assumption that medical care was the same throughout the empire. On a broader scale, many arguments in other aspects of Roman military studies are based on little-challenged beliefs formed in the late 19th or early 20th centuries. Although there have been considerable changes in archaeological methods since that time, along with an increasing amount of evidence from excavated material, the interpretation of newly excavated finds often continues to be conducted to fit preconceived ideas, rather than challenge them. The understanding that the Roman army comprised an homogeneous group of soldiers is an idea that is beginning to be challenged in recent scholarship (e.g. Baker 2001; Haynes 1999; James 1999; 2002), and this provides a context for questioning the assumed homogeneity of military medical care.

In order to undertake this study the traditional classical archaeological approach could not be used, because it generally relies on descriptions and typological discussions of material culture, but makes little use of the context and deposition of the material remains as a main source for interpreting the past. Additionally, in studies of classical medicine the archaeological material is frequently tied to the literary sources (Salazar 2000: 230). The narrowness of this approach is obvious because the literature does not tell us everything about past societies, and it seems fair to say that even as a source of material culture literature is open to many conjectures. Furthermore the literature is seen as the only context in which the material culture can be ascribed a meaning; however, if material remains are examined within their own context (their location and associated finds) more can be understood about the functions, meanings and role of objects in social practices. Many parts of the Roman empire do not have much in the way of a literary record, as even extant epigraphic sources only provide us with glimpses into the structures and thoughts of these societies. It is the archaeological material that must primarily be relied upon to gain insights into provincial Roman societies. Since the area of study is essentially proto-historic, broader interpretative methods, used in both post-colonial and prehistoric archaeology, can be used with Roman materials as well, and these methods were used in this study to gain a better understanding of Roman military medicine.

An initial question was raised about the influence of military events and cultural backgrounds of units within the army to see if these aspects might have had an influence on the way the units organised aspects of their official and daily lives. There are some noticeable changes to the frontiers during and after major military events, and it was considered whether these helped influence the way units or the province organised their medical care. It was asked if the auxiliary and legionary units had the same type of medical care made available to them, or if there were differences. There were certainly differences in pay between the units, so there might be evidence for differences in standardisation of organisation. Additionally, asking if there was evidence for civilians being cared for by military doctors raised the question of military and civilian interaction.

Throughout this study the value of incorporating anthropological understandings of medical care was stressed, because the body and its care are culturally defined. The Roman army consisted of multi-cultural units that might not have had the same medical understandings as the Romans from Italy, on whom so many of the assumptions of the army's daily life are based. With very few exceptions, the military and cultural aspects have not been considered in Roman medical archaeology and when they have been it is generally in the context of ideas of 'Romanisation'. It is important to understand that the Roman empire was not culturally homogeneous, but made up of many societies, each with their own beliefs and understandings that had an obvious impact on the way that medical care was provided. The frontier areas in which the Roman army were stationed were complex social systems with many different kinds of interaction taking place, offering opportunities for different medical traditions to mix and develop.

7.2 A Review of the Study

Allason-Jones (1993: 37; repeated in 1999: 144) says in her general discussion on Roman military medical care in the north of Britain that the evidence for health care in the area is very uneven. To balance out the discrepancies she suggests using the finds of instruments to support the paucity of epigraphic and architectural remains, whilst the remaining holes can be filled by comparing the finds from other areas of the empire. This statement shows an expectation that the medical system in one part of the empire must be the same, because certain aspects from one area are expected to compliment another. Yet, with the evidence available the studies made here suggest that there was not a uniform system of medical care in the army. It is possible that there was medical care supplied to all soldiers as suggested, but perhaps one should not expect the same kind of medical treatment to have been offered throughout the frontiers.

Historical processes certainly played their part in shaping the diverse nature of medical provision. For example, evidence for Roman style medical care in Noricum is only present after the Marcommanic wars. Germania Superior has plenty of evidence for medical care, and there were many military conflicts in that area, supporting the possibility that military events might have had an influence on the supply of health care. Yet, there are some complex problems with this. Some provinces with evidence for medical care and warfare only have certain types of fortifications with evidence for treatment. For example, Pannonia Superior only has medical tools and inscriptions from legionary fortifications; with the exception of one tool from an auxiliary fort near the legionary fortress of Vindobona. The province of Pannonia Inferior, although it does have evidence from both auxiliary and its legionary fortification, the finds from auxiliary forts come from ones located close to Aquincum. It seems that these provinces arranged their health care in different manners. Of course military events might not have been the entire reason for health care being offered to soldiers. Germania Inferior has epigraphic evidence for doctors from the 2nd and 3rd centuries, during a time of relative peace, and the same situation applies to Britannia. Therefore, there might be other factors influencing the organisation of health care that are more complicated than simple military events.

Another suggestion that can be made from the evidence available is that individual units chose their own type of medical care rather than the army or provincial administration. This was tested in relation to auxiliary units in order to see if any patterns appeared in the units from specific areas adopting the use of Roman style medical practices. Patterns appeared in the comparisons of both the epigraphic and instrument remains, in that units from Gaul and Spain are associated with the most evidence for the adoption, or perhaps adaptation, of Roman style medical care. Anthropological studies of contact between different groups, undertaken with reference to their medical care, have demonstrated that there are definite reactions by societies when introduced to new medical practices not familiar to their own. In some cases the treatments were rejected outright and in others they were adapted to fit the societies understandings of them. It is highly likely that such processes would have occurred with the units from different cultural groups coming into contact with Roman practices.

Aspects of cultural interaction might also be found in medical evidence relating to women and children. Though not often considered, it is important to explore the possibility that military doctors might have cared for civilians within the area of the fortification, or for the soldiers' wives and children. However, the evidence was fairly slim, as there is only one definite female instrument from Carnuntum and its exact provenance is not known. It is always possible that military doctors could have cared for civilians, which could have allowed for the spread of Roman style medicine in some cases, but there is simply not enough evidence at present to support the argument either way.

It seems more than coincidental, at the moment at least, that certain units were borrowing Roman medical tools and others were not, as well as making inscriptions for doctors. This might suggest that medical care in the Roman army was far more complicated than previously expected.

Very similar patterns began to appear when the range and distribution of medical instruments are examined, in that the provinces with the most evidence of Roman style medical instruments are the ones with the most warfare. As for the comparison of units from the same areas, those using Roman style tools were the same as those erecting inscriptions commemorating Roman style doctors: these are mainly by units from areas in Gaul and Spain. It was in Chapter 5 that the material culture demonstrated that the system of medical care in the military was probably not the same throughout the frontiers, as supported by the epigraphic remains, and that there are complex issues pertaining to various beliefs towards the body and attitudes about medicine which can be deduced through the deposition of instruments. It is clear, from the information at hand, that not all units were using Roman medical tools and this might be evidence for nonconformity on issues relating to the body when the units came into contact with Roman medicine.

One would expect to continue the comparisons of medical care on the frontiers with the buildings identified as *valetudinaria*; however it was necessary to question the correctness of the identity of the structures (Chapter 6). The identification of so-called *valetudinaria* was made at the beginning of the 20th century and has been accepted since that time. However, there is really little evidence to support this. We have little understanding what a *valetudinarium* was, as the Roman *valetudinaria* have traditionally been described as if they were like those in Germany between the 17th and 19th centuries.

For the field of medical history, this study not only has implications for how medical care was organised in the Roman army, but has hopefully contributed to understanding something about the anthropology of the body. Cultural beliefs and feelings about the body can be incorporated into the history of medicine to expand our knowledge of how medicine was practised. Moreover, it has further demonstrated that the notion of 'a Roman army' is becoming more difficult to prove.

APPENDIX ONE PART ONE

A LIST OF FORTIFICATIONS MENTIONED IN THE TEXT

This Appendix (1 part 1) presents basic information about each legionary and auxiliary fortification mentioned in the main text of this examination that has information related to medical care. The dates of occupation, unit types and their names, if known, as well as the Latin names of the fortifications are provided as an easy reference to help the reader in case they should have any basic questions about information not readily available in the text. The fortifications are listed according to their provinces and following the name of each entry is the modern country in which it is located. At the end of each entry is a letter or letters, listed in the abbreviations that represent the type of medical information available from each fortification, such as medical instruments, structural evidence for *valetudinaria* or epigraphic evidence. There is a large number of fortifications not mentioned in this list because no remains of medical instruments were found within them, information about these fortifications can be found in Appendix 1 part 2. More comprehensive descriptions for many of these fortifications mentioned in both parts of Appendix 1 are found in site guides. For German Inferior: Bogaers and Rüger 1974; Germania Superior: von Elbe 1974, Schönberger 1969 and Drack and Fellmann 1988; Raetia: Czysz *et al.* 1995; Noricum: Alföldi 1974 and Genser 1986; Pannonia Superior: Genser 1986 and Mócsy 1974; Pannonia Inferior: Mócsy 1974 and Visy 1988 and for Britannia: Breeze and Dobson 1991.

Abbreviations

V	*Valetudinarium*
M	Medical Implements
I	Inscriptions

Germania Inferior (Figs. 1 & 2)

1. **Valkenburg**. Netherlands. Auxiliary Fort. AD 40 to 260. *Cohors III Galliorum equitata* and *Cohors IIII Thracum equitata* occupied the site at different times (Bogaers and Rüger 1974: 40-3; Bult and Hallewas 1986: 9). **I, M, V**

2. **Alphen aan de Rijn**. *Albaniana*. Netherlands. Auxiliary Fort. AD 50 to the third century. *Cohors III Breucorum* (Bogaers and Rüger 1974: 47). **M**

3. **Bunnik-Vechten**. *Fectio*. Netherlands. Auxiliary Fort. Early 1st century to mid-3rd century. *Cohors II Brittonum milliaria equitata*, *Cohors I Flavia Hispanorum equitata* and *Ala I Thracum* were stationed at the site at different times (Bogaers and Rüger 1974: 63-5). **M**

4. **Kesteren**. *Carvo*. Netherlands. Auxiliary Fort. AD 70 to the 3rd century. Unknown auxiliary troop (Bogaers and Rüger 1974: 70). **M**

5. **Rossum**. *Grinnes*. Netherlands. Auxiliary Fort. 1st century. Unknown troop (Bogaers and Rüger 1974: 74). **M**

6. **Nijmegen**. *Noviomagus*. Netherlands. Legionary Fortress. The Augustan-Tiberian period. to c.175. *Legio X Gemina, Legio VIIII Hispana* and *Legio XXX Ulpia Victrix* (Bogaers and Rüger 1974: 76-9). **M**

7. **Xanten**. *Vetera I and II*. Germany. Legionary Fortress. The reign of Augustus to the 4th century. Vetera I: *Legio XXI Rapax* and *Legio V Alaudae* the former was replaced with *XV Primigenia*. Vetera II was constructed to hold a single legion: *Legio XXII Primigenia pia fidelis*, *Legio VI Victrix* and *Legio XXX Ulpia Victrix* (Horn 1987: 639-44; Lehner 1930: 177, 183; Oelmann 1931: 221; Schultze 1934: 54-63; von Elbe 1974: 65-7). **I, M, V**

8. **Neuss**. *Novaesium*. Germany. Legionary Fortress. Augustus to AD 105. *Legio XX*, *XVI Galica* and *VI Victrix* (Bogaers and Rüger 1974: 139-40; von Elbe 1974: 289-90). **M, V**

9. **Bonn**. *Bonna*. Germany. Legionary Fortress. Augustan period to 3rd century. *Legio I Germanica*, *Legio XXI Rapax* and *Legio I Minerva* (Bogaers and Rüger 1974: 196-8; Horn 1987: 367-73; von Elbe 1974: 72-94). **I, M, V**

Germania Superior (Figs. 1 & 3)

1. **Bingen**. Germany. Auxiliary Fort (?) First half of the 1st century to unknown date. Detachment of *Legio XXII Primigenia* from Mainz (Cuppers and Bernhard 1990: 333; von Elbe 1974: 61-5). **I, M**

2. **Neiderbieber**. Germany. *Numerus* Fort. It was constructed in the 2nd century. It housed a *numerus* unit (Schönberger 1969: fig. 20). **I**

3. **Mainz**. *Mogontiacum*. Germany. Legionary Fortress. 15 BC to the 4th century. The fortress was first constructed to hold two legions. The *Legio Flavian I Adiutrix* and *Legio XIV Gemina* were the first to occupy the site. After the Batavian revolt double legionary fortresses were disbanded and the single legion to occupy the fortress was *the Legio XIV Gemina*, that was replaced by the *Legio XXII Primigenia pia fidelis* which was

stationed at the site from AD 92 to the 4th century (Cuppers and Bernhard 1990: 458-62; Horn 1987: 54; von Elbe 1974: 253-4). **I, M**

4. **Worms**. *Borbetomagus*. Germany. Auxiliary Fort. Augustus' reign to the Flavian period. *Ala I Hispanorum, ala Sebosiana, ala Indiana, ala Agrippiana, cohors Raetorum, cohors I Thracum, cohors VII Breucorum and the cohors Raetorum et Vindelicorum* (Cuppers and Bernhard 1990: 673; Künzl 1982: 78; von Elbe 1974: 464). **M**

5. **Ladenburg**. *Lopodunum*. Germany. Auxiliary Fort. AD 73/4 to Trajan's reign. *Ala I Cannenefatium* (von Elbe 1974: 235-40). **M**

6. **Staden**. Germany. *Numerus* Fort. Unknown unit. **M**

7. **Degenfeld**. Germany. Auxiliary Fort. Unknown Unit. **M**

8. **Windisch**. *Vindonissa*. Switzerland. Legionary Fortress. Tiberian to the 4th century. The units stationed at the site were *Legio XIII Gemina*, *Legio XXI Rapax* and *Legio XI Claudia* (Drack and Fellmann 1988: 540). **I, M, V**

9. **Holzhausen**. Germany. Auxiliary Fort. Late 2nd century to 233. *Cohors II Antoniniana Treverorum* (von Elbe 1974: 154-5). **M**

10. **Zugmantel**. Germany. Auxiliary Fort. AD 90 to 260. *Cohors I Treverorum equitata* (Baatz and Herrmann 1982: 502). **M**

11. **Heftrich**. Germany. Auxiliary Fort. Second century to mid-3rd century. *Numerus Catharensium* (Baatz and Herrmann 1982: 343-5). **M**

12. **Saalburg**. Germany. Auxiliary Fort. It was first constructed during Domitian's reign and it was destroyed by the Alammani in 259/60. Between 125 and 139 the fort was enlarged to occupy the *Cohors II Raetorum civium* (Schönberger 1952: 4; von Elbe 1974: 342-51). **M**

13. **Kapersburg**. Germany. Auxiliary Fort. AD 100 to the mid-3rd century. *Numerus Nidensium* (Beckmann 1975; von Elbe 1974: 164-6). **M**

14. **Obermorlen-Langenhain**. Germany. Auxiliary Fort. The fort was constructed under Trajan and it was occupied until 260. *Cohors I Biturigum Aquitanorum equitata* (Baatz and Herrmann 1982: 456). **M**

15. **Strausbourg**. *Argentorate*. France. Legionary Fortress. **I.**

16. **Oberflorstadt**. Germany. Auxiliary Fort. Trajan to the mid-3rd century. *Cohors XXXII voluntariorum civium Romanorum* (Baatz and Herrmann 1982: 274). **M**

17. **Karben-Okarben**. Germany. Auxiliary Fort. Constructed during the reign of Vespasian and occupied until the 3rd century. *Ala II Flavia Gemina* (Baatz and Herrmann 1982: 367). **M**

18. **Wiesbaden**. *Aquae Mattiacorum*. Germany. Auxiliary Fort. It was built during Gaius' reign and remained in use as a fort to Hadrian's reign. The units that occupied the fort were the *Cohors V Dalmationum*, *Cohors I Pannoniorum*, *Cohors IV Thracurum*, *Cohors III Delmatarum* and the *Cohors II Raetorum* (von Elbe: 1974: 444-55). **M, V**

19. **Hofheim am Taunus**. Germany. Auxiliary Fort. Tiberius' reign until 110. Unknown auxiliary unit (Baatz and Herrmann 1982: 350-1). **M**

20. **Gross-Krotzenburg**. Germany. Auxiliary Fort. It was built by Trajan around 105-110 and it seems to have been occupied until the end of the 2nd or beginning of the 3rd century. *Cohors III Vindelicorum* (Baatz and Herrmann 1982: 325; von Elbe 1974: 139). **I, M**

21. **Stockstadt am Main**. Germany. Auxiliary Fort. It was constructed in AD 90 and remained in use until the mid-3rd century. *Cohors III Aquitanorum equitata civium Romanorum*, *Cohors II Hispania* and the *Cohors I Aquitanorum* occupied the fort at different times (Baatz and Herrmann 1982: 479-81; von Elbe 1974: 374-6). **M**

22. **Obernburg**. *Nemaninga*. Germany. Auxiliary Fort. It was built by Domitian and was abandoned in the mid-3rd century. *Cohors IIII Aquitanorum equitata civium Romanorum* (Baatz and Herrmann 1982: 457; von Elbe 1974: 297-9). **I**

23. **Elzatal-Neckarburken**. Germany. Auxiliary Fort. The fort dates to Trajan's reign to the mid-2nd century. The *numerus* fort was built in AD 100 and was home to the *Brittoni Elantienses*, whilst the cohort fort was built around AD 110 for the *Cohors III Aquitanorum equitata* (Filtzinger *et al.* 1986: 279-82). **M**

24. **Bad-Wimpfen**. Germany. Auxiliary Fort. Built in AD 90 and it was probably abandoned in Pius' reign. *Cohors III Aquitanorum equitata civium Romanorum*, *Cohors II Hispanorum* and the *Cohors I Germanorum* occupied the site at different times (Filtzinger *et al.* 1986: 217-8). **M**

25. **Stuttgart-Bad Cannstatt**. Germany. Auxiliary Fort. It was built during Domitian's reign and was abandoned in the mid-2nd century. *Ala I Scubulorum* (von Elbe 1974: 387). **M**

26. **Köngen**. *Grinario*. Germany. Auxiliary Fort. It was built in Domitian's reign and it was abandoned in the mid-2nd century. Unknown auxiliary unit (von Elbe 1974: 228). **M**

27. **Osterburken**. Germany. Auxiliary Fort. The fort was constructed under Antoninus Pius and was abandoned when the Alammani invaded. *Cohors III Aquitanorum* and a legionary vexillation occupied the site (Filtzinger *et al.* 1986: 470; von Elbe 1974: 307-9). **I**

28. **Öhringen**. Germany. Auxiliary Fort. Two forts were constructed at this site, both during the reign of Antoninus Pius. The western fort was occupied by the *Cohors I Helvetiorum* and two *numeri*. The smaller eastern fort held the *Cohors I Belgarium Septimiana*.

Both were abandoned in c. 259/60 (von Elbe 1974: 305). **M**

29. **Mainhardt**. Germany. Auxiliary Fort. It is constructed in the mid-2nd century as part of the Antonine frontier. It was occupied until the Alammani invasions. *Cohors I Asturum equitata* (Filtzinger *et al.* 1986: 453-7; von Elbe 1974: 251). **M**

30. **Hüfingen**. Germany. Auxiliary Fort. This fort was built during the first years of Vespasian's reign. It was probably abandoned under Domitian's reign. *Cohors I civium Romanorum ingenorum* (Czysz *et al.* 1995: 75). **M**

Raetia (Figs. 1 & 4)

1. **Dambach**. Germany. Auxiliary Fort. The site was first built as a *numerus* fort in the mid-2nd century. Later in the same century it was enlarged and housed the *Cohors II Aquitanorum equitata*. It remained in use until the mid-3rd century (Czysz *et al.* 1995: 432-3). **M**

2. **Gnotzheim**. Germany. Auxiliary Fort. The history of the fort is unclear. It is located on Domitian's line of the Raetian frontier, but it appears to have been rebuilt in stone at the time Antoninus Pius advanced the frontier further north. It was probably occupied until the fall of the Raetian Limes. Two groups are known to have occupied the fort at different times: the *Cohors V Bracaraugustorum* and the *Cohors III Thracum civium Romanorum equitata bis torquata* (Czysz *et al.* 1995: 448-9). **M**

3. **Ellingen**. Germany. Auxiliary Fort. It was probably built during the reign of Trajan and was abandoned in the mid-3rd century. It might have been occupied by a *pedites singulares* (Czysz *et al.* 1995: 436-7). **M**

4. **Weißenburg**. *Bricianis*. Germany. Auxiliary Fort. It was built during the reign of Domitian and remained in use until the mid-3rd century. *Ala I Hispanorum Auriana*. (Czysz *et al.* 1995: 534-5; von Elbe 1974: 442). **M**

5. **Pfünz**. *Vetoniana*. Germany. Auxiliary Fort. It was first constructed under Domitian and it was destroyed during the Marcomannic wars. It was rebuilt and used until the Alamanni invaded in 233. *Cohors I Breucorum civium Romanorum equitata* (Czysz *et al.* 1995: 500-1; von Elbe 1974: 319). **M**

6. **Lonsee-Urspring**. Germany. Auxiliary Fort. The fort is thought to have been constructed under Vespasian's reign. It was probably in use until Antoninus Pius' advance. Unknown auxiliary unit (Filtzinger *et al.* 1986: 430-3). **M**

7. **Heidenheim**. *Aquileia*. Germany. Auxiliary Fort. Built in c. AD 90, the fort was abandoned when the unit moved to Aalen under Antoninus Pius' command. It was occupied by the *Ala II Flavia milliaria* (Filtzinger *et al.* 1986: 321-6; von Elbe 1974: 147). **M**

8. **Munningen**. Germany. Auxiliary Fort. The fort was constructed under Domitian's command, after 110 the fort was changed into a street station. Unknown auxiliary unit (Czysz *et al.* 1995: 484). **M**

9 **Faimingen**. Germany. Auxiliary Fort. The fort was constructed in Antoninus Pius' reign. It remained in use until the mid-3rd century. Unknown auxiliary unit (Czysz *et al.* 1995: 441-4). **M**

10. **Risstissen**. Germany. Auxiliary Fort. The fort was built on the south side of the Danube as part of Claudius' line of forts. It was restored under Vespasian, but was abandoned in c. AD 85 as a result of Domitian's forward advance. Unknown auxiliary unit (von Elbe 1974: 334). **M**

11. **Günzburg**. *Gontia*. Germany. Auxiliary Fort. The foundation date of the fort is uncertain; it may be Claudian or Vespasianic. It was abandoned towards the end of the 1st century. Unknown auxiliary unit (von Elbe 1974: 140). **M**

12. **Oberstimm**. Germany. Auxiliary Fort. The fort was built in the reign of Claudius. It became a policing station in Trajan's reign. Unknown auxiliary unit (Czysz *et al.* 1995: 493-4). **M, V**

13. **Regensburg**. *Castra Regina*. Germany. Legionary fortress. It was first constructed as an auxiliary fort in Vespasian's reign. However, it was rebuilt as a legionary fortress after the Marcomannic wars in 179/80. *Legio III Italica* (von Elbe 1974: 321-2). **I, M**

14. **Straubing**. *Soviodurum*. Germany. Auxiliary Fort. It was built under the reign of Vespasian and was abandoned during the Alamanni invasions. *Cohors II Raetiorum* and *Cohors I Flavia Canathenorum milliaria Sagittariorum* occupied the site at different times (von Elbe 1974: 377). **M**

15. **Künzing**. *Quintana*. Germany. Auxiliary Fort. It was built between AD 90 and 100 and remained in use until the mid-3rd century. It first housed the *Cohors III equitata Thracum civium Romanorum* and then the *Cohors V Bracaraugustanorum* (von Elbe 1974: 233-4). **V**

16. **Wallheim**. Germany. Auxiliary Fort. The fort was constructed during Domitian's reign and was probably occupied until Antoninus Pius moved the frontier past the Neckar. Unknown auxiliary unit (Schönberger 1969: fig. 20). **M**

Noricum (Fig. 5)

1. **Enns-Lorch**. *Lauriacum*. Austria. Legionary Fortress. The fortress was first an auxiliary fort built under the reign of Claudius. It was destroyed under the Marcomannic Wars and was reconstructed as a legionary fortress by the end of Commodus' reign. It was occupied by the *Legio II Italica* (Alföldy 1974: 104, 147, 153, 166, 167, 183; Genser 1986: 128). **I, M, V**

Pannonia Superior (Fig. 6)

1. **Vienna**. *Vindobona*. Austria. Legionary Fortress. The fortress was either built in the late Flavian or early Trajanic period. An inscription was found from the

Legio XIII Gemina from its earliest period. The legion was replaced by the *Legio X Gemina*. (Mócsy 1974: 85, 88, 99, 140; Neumann 1967: 53). **M, V**

2. **Bad Deutsch-Altenburg**. *Carnuntum*. Austria. Legionary Fortress. The fortress was built in the late Augustan or early Tiberian period and remained in use until the late Roman period. It was occupied by the *Legio XX Apollinaris* and was replaced by the *Legio XIII Gemina* during the Dacian Wars. The site had an auxiliary fort located to its west at Petronell, which housed the *Ala I Thracum* (Genser 1986: 685-701; Mócsy 1974: 40). **I, M, V**

3. **Szóny**. *Brigetio*. Hungary. Legionary Fortress. Originally the site was built before the Flavian period. The legionary fortress was built at the turn of the 1st century AD. The final date of occupation is unknown. It was first occupied by the *Legio XXX Ulpia Victrix* and after the Parthian War it was occupied by the *Legio I Adiutrix* (Mócsy 1974: 49, 88, 92, 99, 140, 198, 221). **I, M**

Pannonia Inferior (Fig. 6)

1. **Szentendre**. *Ulcisia Castra*. Hungary. Auxiliary Fort. It was probably built during the Flavian period. It was occupied by a Syrian Cohort in the Severan period (Mócsy 1974: 228). **I**

2. **Budapest**. *Aquincum*. Hungary. Legionary Fortress. There were a number of auxiliary forts built in Budapest before it became a legionary fortress. The first forts date to the reign of Claudius. The location of the Vizivaros fort was discovered at the foot of Buda's Castle Hill and is known from tombstones. The *Ala I Hispanorum* occupied the fort from 50 to 69 and the *Ala I Hispanorum Aurian* occupied the site from 70 to 80. The Emperor Vespasian added a number of new forts along the Danube. Obuda was constructed near the area of the legionary fortress. The *Ala I Tungrorum Frontina* probably constructed Campona located to the south of the city. The first legionary fortress at Aquincum was constructed in 89 for the *Legio II Adiutrix*. It was also occupied by the *Legio XX Gemina* (Korbuly 1934: 5-10; Németh 1994: 140-4; Zsidi 1995: 14-5). **I, M, V**

3. **Dunaújváros**. *Intercisca*. Hungary. Auxiliary Fort. It was built during the reign of Trajan remained in use until the 4th century. It housed the *Ala I Augusta Ituraeorum* and the *Ala I Tungrorum Frontoniana* at different times (Visy 1988: 101-4). **I, M**

Britannia (Figs. 7 & 8)

1. **Caerleon**. *Isca Silurum*. Wales. Legionary Fortress. It was constructed in AD 74/5 during the conquest of South Wales by Julius Frontinus. The fort was occupied into the 4th century. *Legio II Augusta* (Boon and Williams 1967: 1-2; Jarrett 1969: 10, 29, 31). **M, V**

2. **Chester**. *Deva*. England. Legionary Fortress. It was completed in AD 79. The *Legio II Adiutrix* was the first legion to occupy the fortress. They were withdrawn from the province in 86/7 and were replaced with the *Legio XX Valeria Victrix*. The fort remained occupied until the 4th century (Jarrett 1969: 33-42). **I, M, V**

3. **York** *Eboracum*. England. Legionary Fortress. It was constructed under the Flavian reign and remained in use until the 4th century. It was first occupied by the *Legio VIIII Hispana* and was replaced by the *Legio VI Victrix*. **M**

4. **South Shields**. *Arebia*. England. Auxiliary Fort. The fort was an outpost supply fort for Hadrian's Wall and Severus' campaign into Scotland. There may have been a cohors stationed at the fort during the reign of Marcus Aurelius. However, in the 3rd century as a supply fort, the unit stationed at the site was the *Cohors V Gallorum equitata*. In the 4th century a *Numerus barcariorum Tigrisiensium* was stationed at the fort (Breeze and Dobson 1991: 255, 257, 271). **M**

5. **Wallsend**. *Serdunum* or *Segedunum*. England. Auxiliary Fort. It was probably occupied by a *Cohors quingenaria equitata* in Hadrian's reign. During the reign of Marcus Aurelius the fort's garrison was the *Cohors II Nerviorum civium Romanorum*. During the 3rd and 4th centuries the unit was the *Cohors IV Lingonum equitata* (Breeze and Dobson 1991: 54, 142, 243, 271). **M**

6. **Benwell**. *Condecorum*. England. Auxiliary Fort. The fort was probably occupied by an *Ala quingenaria* in Hadrian's reign. Under Marcus Aurelius it was occupied by the *Cohors I Vangionum milliaria equitata*. In the 3rd and 4th centuries it was occupied by the *Ala I Asturum* (Breeze and Dobson 1991: 52, 142, 228, 271). **V**

7. **Halton Chesters**. *Onnum* or *Hunno*. England. Auxiliary Fort. The fort was possibly occupied by a *Cohors quingenaria equitata* under Hadrian's reign. There is no evidence for the unit's name under Marcus Aurelius. In the 3rd and 4th centuries the unit was the *Ala I Pannonionum Sabiniana* (Breeze and Dobson 1991: 142, 271). **M**

8. **Chesters**. *Celunum* or *Cilurnum*. England. Auxiliary Fort. The fort was occupied by the *Ala Augusta ob virtutem appellata* in Hadrian's reign. The *Ala II Asturum* remained stationed at the site from the time of Commodus until the 5th century (Breeze and Dobson 1991: 52, 244, 271). **M**

9. **Housesteads**. *Velurtion* or *Borcovicium*. England. Auxiliary Fort. Under Hadrian's reign the fort was occupied by a *Cohors milliaria peditata*. In the 3rd and 4th centuries the fort was occupied by the *Cohors I Tungrorum milliaria*, *Numerus cuneus Frisiorum* and a *Numerus Hnaudifridi cuneus* (Breeze and Dobson 1991: 271). **I, M, V**

10. **Birdoswald**. *Banna*. England. Auxiliary Fort. In Hadrian's reign the *Cohors I Tungrorum milliaria peditata* occupied the fort. In the 3rd century the *Cohors I Aelia Dacorum milliaria* and the *venatores Banniensis* occupied the fort. *The Cohors I Aelia Dacorum* was the final unit at the site and remained there until the 5th century (Breeze and Dobson 1991: 54, 246, 271). **M**

11. **Bowness-on-Solway**. *Maia* or *Mais*. England. Auxiliary Fort. It probably had a *Cohors milliaria equitata* in Hadrian's reign and in the 3rd century. Its unit names are unknown (Breeze and Dobson 1991: 271). **M**

12. **Corbridge**. *Cambulodunum*. England. Auxiliary Fort. This Stanegate road fort was constructed during Trajan's reign and probably remained occupied until the reign of Marcus Aurelius. The *Cohors I fida Vardullorum equitata milliaria* and the *Ala Petriana* were stationed at the site at different times (Breeze and Dobson 1991: 129-30, 252; Dore 1989: 31). **M**

13. **Chesterholm**. *Vindolanda*. England. Auxiliary Fort. The Stanegate road fort was constructed during the reign of Trajan and remained occupied until the 4th century. The *Cohors II Nerviorum civium Romanorum* and the *Cohors IV Gallorum equitata* occupied the site at different times (Breeze and Dobson 1991: 245, 271). **I**

14. **Carlisle**. England. Auxiliary Fort. This Stanegate road fort was constructed during the reign of Trajan and may have remained in use until the 4th century. The unit names are unknown (Breeze and Dobson 1991: 19, 90). **M**

APPENDIX ONE PART TWO

LIST OF FORTIFICATIONS WITHOUT EVIDENCE FOR MEDICAL CARE

Germania Inferior

1. **Velsen**. *Castellum Flevum* Netherlands. Auxiliary Fort. Unknown Unit. 15 BC-mid-1st century AD (Bogaers and Rüger 1974: 30).

2. **Katwijk-Brittenburg**. *Lugdunum*. Netherlands. Auxiliary Fort. *Cohors I Raetorum civium Romanorum pia fidelis*. First century AD - AD 260 (Bogaers and Rüger 1974: 37-8).

3. **Leiden**. *Matilo* Netherlands. Auxiliary Fort. *Cohors I Lucensium Hispanorum pia fidelis Domitiana, cohors XV voluntariorum civium Romanorum pia fidelis, numerus exploratum Batavorum*. First century AD – 4th century (Bogaers and Rüger 1974: 44).

4. **Alphen aan de Rijn-Zwammerdam**. *Nigrum Pullum*. Netherlands. Auxiliary Fort. Unknown Unit. AD 50 – 4th century (Bogaers and Rüger 1974: 49-52).

5. **Woerden**. *Laurum*. Netherlands. Auxiliary Fort. Unknown Unit. AD 47-3rd century (Bogaers and Rüger 1974: 53).

6. **Vleuten-De Meern**. Netherlands. Auxiliary Fort. *Cohors I classica pia fidelis*. Mid-1st Century AD – mid-3rd century (Bogaers and Rüger 1974: 55).

7. **Utrecht**. *Traiectum*. Netherlands. Auxiliary Fort. *Cohors II Hispanorum peditata pia fidelis*. AD 47 -260 (Bogaers and Rüger 1974: 58).

8. **Wijk bij Duurstede**. *Levefanum*. Netherlands. Auxiliary Fort. *Cohors I Thracum* in the years of 70 to 83. AD 47-270 (Bogaers and Rüger 1974: 67).

9. **Maurik**. *Mannaricium*. Netherlands. Auxiliary Fort. *Cohors II Thracum equitata* from 70 to c. 83, *cohors II Hispanorum equitata* from 70 to c. 83. AD 70 – 260 (Bogaers and Rüger 1974: 68).

10. **Huissen**. Netherlands. Auxiliary Fort. Unknown unit. AD 70 –mid-3rd century (Bogaers and Rüger 1974: 73).

11. **Cuijk**. *Ceuclum*. Netherlands. Auxiliary Fort. Unknown unit. Mid-1st century –c. AD 100 (Bogaers and Rüger 1974: 84).

12. **Herwen en Aerdt-De Bijland**. *Carvium*. Netherlands. Auxiliary Fort. *Cohors II civium Romanorum equitata pia fidelis*. AD 70 –c. 260 (Bogaers and Rüger 1974: 90).

13. **Kleve-Rindern**. *Harentium*. Germany. Auxiliary Fort. Unknown Unit. AD 70 – 3rd century (Bogaers and Rüger 1974: 93; Horn 1987: 458).

14. **Altkalker**. *Burginatium*. Germany. Auxiliary Fort. *Ala Vocontiorum, ala Afrorum*. Flavian – 4th century (von Elbe 1975: 13; Bogaers and Rüger 1974: 101-102; Horn 1987: 452).

15. **Moers-Asberg**. *Asciburgium*. Germany. Auxiliary Fort. *Ala I Tungrorum Frontoniana; ala Moesica felix torquata*. Early 1st century AD – 4th century (Bogaers and Rüger 1974: 128; Horn 1987: 567; von Elbe 1974: 274).

16. **Rheinhausen-Werthhausen**. Germany. Auxiliary Fort. Unknown unit. First Century AD – 2nd century (Bogaers and Rüger 1974: 132).

17. **Neuss-Grimmlinhausen-Reckberg**. Germany. Auxiliary Fort. Unknown unit. First century AD – 2nd century (Bogaers and Rüger 1974: 145).

18. **Dormagen**. *Durnomagus*. Germany. Auxiliary Fort. *Ala Noricum*. Flavian period – 4th century (Bogaers and Rüger 1974: 151; Horn 1987: 397; von Elbe 1974: 111).

19. **Cologne-Bayenthal-Alteburg**. Germany. Naval Fort. *Classis Germanica pia fidelis*. Claudian – 3rd century (Bogaers and Rüger 1974: 166; von Elbe 1974: 184-5).

20. **Wesseling**. Germany. Auxiliary Fort. Unknown unit. First century AD –2nd century (von Elbe 1974)

21. **Remagen**. *Riomagus*. Germany. Auxiliary Fort. *Cohors II Varcianorum equitata civium Romanorum, cohors I Flavia Hispanorum*. Tiberian – 3rd century (Bogaers and Rüger 1974: 208-13; von Elbe 1974: 328-9).

22. **Krefeld-Gellep**. *Gelduba*. Germany. Auxiliary Fort. AD 70 to the late 4th century. *Cohors II Varcianorum equitatae quingenaria* (Bogaers and Rüger 1974: 135-6; Horn 1987: 529-30; von Elbe 1974: 230-2).

23. **Cologne**. *Apud Aram Ubiorum*. Germany. Auxiliary Fort. Augustan period to AD 50. *Legio I Germanica* and *Legio XX Valeria Victrix* (von Elbe 1974: 184).

Germania Superior

1. **Andernach**. *Antunnacum*. Germany. Auxiliary Fort. *Cohors Raetiorum*. Tiberain - Flavian (Cuppers and Bernhard 1990: 304-6; von Elbe 1974: 306).

2. **Koblenz**. Germany. Auxiliary Fort. Unknown unit. Tiberian – Flavian (Cuppers and Bernhard 1990: 418-9; von Elbe 1974: 178-9).

3. **Gross Gerau**. Germany. Auxiliary Fort. Unknown unit. Vespasianic – late 2nd century (Baatz and Herrmann 1982: 322).

4. **Gemersheim**. Germany. Auxiliary Fort. Unknown unit. Early 1st century AD -Flavian (Cuppers and Bernhard 1990: 372-3; von Elbe 1974: 138;).

5. **Rheingoheim**. Germany. Auxiliary Fort. Unknown unit. Claudian - Vepasianic (Cuppers and Bernhard 1990: 455-7).

6. **Heidelberg/Neuenheim**. Germany. Auxiliary Fort. *Cohors XXIIII voluntariorum civium Romanorum, Cohors II Augusta Cyrenaica equitata*. Mid-1st century AD – c. 233 (Filtzinger *et al.* 1986: 316-8; von Elbe 1974: 145).

7. **Speyer**. *Noviomagus*. Germany. Auxiliary Fort. Unknown unit. Late-1st century BC – Flavian (Cuppers and Bernhard 1990: 559-61; von Elbe 1974: 366).

8. **Bendorf**. Germany. Auxiliary Fort. *Cohors I Thracum*. Flavian - ? (Cuppers and Bernhard 1990: 331-2).

9. **Niedernberg**. Germany. Auxiliary Fort. Unknown unit. First century AD - ? (Baatz and Herrmann 1982: 455).

10. **Arzbach**. Germany. Auxiliary Fort. Unknown unit. Early 2nd century AD - ? (Cuppers and Bernhard 1990: 91).

11. **Ems**. Germany. Auxiliary Fort. Unknown unit. Early 2nd century AD - ? (Cuppers and Bernhard 1990: 92).

12. **Hunzel**. Germany. Auxiliary Fort. Unknown unit. Mid-2nd century - ? (Cuppers and Bernhard 1990: 92).

13. **Marienfels**. Germany. Auxiliary Fort. Unknown unit. Mid-2nd century - ? (Cuppers and Bernhard 1990: 92).

14. **Kemel**. Germany. Auxiliary Fort. Unknown units (two forts constructed on the site). Mid-2nd century AD – mid-3rd century (Baatz and Herrmann 1982: 327-73).

15. **Feldberg *(Kleine)***. Germany. *Numerus* fort. *Numerus Alexandriana*. Mid-2nd century AD – mid-3rd century (Baatz 1975; Baatz and Herrmann 1982: 266-9).

16. **Butzbach**. Germany. Auxiliary Fort. *Cohors II Raetiorum Civium Romanorum, Cohors II Augusta Cyrenaica equitata*. Mid-1st century AD – c. 233 (von Elbe 1974: 104).

17. **Arnsburg**. Germany. Auxiliary Fort. *Cohors I Aquitanorum veterana equitatae*. Mid-1st century AD – 3rd century (Baatz and Herrmann 1982: 230).

18. **Hungen-Inheiden**. Germany. Auxiliary Fort. Unknown unit. Trajanic - mid-3rd century (Baatz and Herrmann 1982: 363).

19. **Echzell**. Germany. Auxiliary Fort. *Ala Indiana Gallorum, ala Moesica Felix Torquata, the Ala I Flavia Gemina, Cohors III voluntariorum civium Romanorum*. Mid-1st century AD – mid-3rd century (Baatz and Herrmann 1982: 264).

20. **Bad Nauheim**. Germany. Auxiliary Fort. A garrison of the *Legio XIV Gemina*. AD 83 - ? (von Elbe 1974: 49-50).

21. **Friedburg**. Germany. Auxiliary Fort. *Cohors I Flavia Damascenorum*. Tiberian – mid-3rd century (von Elbe 1974: 133-4).

22. **Altenstadt**. Germany. Auxiliary Fort. Unknown unit. Trajanic – mid-3rd century (Schönberger 1969).

23. **Nidderau-Heldenbergen**. Germany. Auxiliary Fort. Unknown unit. Trajanic – mid-3rd century (Baatz and Herrmann 1982: 450-1).

24. **Marköbel**. Germany. Auxiliary Fort. *Cohors XXX Voluntariorum civium Romanorum*. Trajanic - ? (Baatz and Herrmann 1982: 429-30).

25. **Heidkringen**. Germany. Auxiliary Fort. Unknown unit and date (Baatz and Herrmann 1982: 346).

26. **Frankfurt am Main**. Germany. Auxiliary Fort. Unknown unit. Flavian – late 1st century (von Elbe 1974: 127).

27. **Hannau-Kesselstadt**. Germany. Auxiliary Fort. Unknown unit. Flavian - ? (Baatz and Herrmann 1982: 334-6).

28. **Rückingen**. Germany. Auxiliary Fort. *Cohors III Dalmatorum pia fidelis*. Early-2nd century AD – 3rd century (Baatz and Herrmann 1982: 468; von Elbe 1974: 145).

29. **Hainburg-Hainstadt**. Germany. Auxiliary Fort. Unknown unit. AD 90 – c. 260 (Baatz and Herrmann 1982: 333-4).

30. **Seligenstadt**. Germany. Auxiliary Fort. *Cohors I civium Romanorum Equitata*. Trajanic – 3rd century (Baatz and Herrmann 1982: 477-78).

31. **Niedernberg**. Germany. Auxiliary Fort. Unknown unit and date (Baatz and Herrmann 1982: 455).

32. **Seckmauern**. Germany. Auxiliary Fort. *Cohors I civium Romanorum equitata*. Trajanic – mid- 3rd century (Baatz and Herrmann 1982: 477-8).

33. **Lützelbach**. Germany. Auxiliary Fort. Unknown unit. Mid- 2nd century (Baatz and Herrmann 1982: 424-5).

34. **Michaelstadt-Vielbrunn**. Germany. Auxiliary Fort. Unknown *numerus* unit. c. AD 100 – c. AD 150 (Baatz and Herrmann 1982: 436-37).

35. **Michaelstadt-Eulbach**. Germany. *Numerus* Fort. Unknown *numerus* unit. AD 70 – mid- 2nd century (Baatz and Herrmann 1982: 432).

36. **Würzberg**. Germany. *Numerus* Fort. Unknown *numerus* unit. AD 100 - mid-2nd century (Baatz and Herrmann 1982: 498-500).

37. **Hesseneck-Hesselbach**. Germany. *Numerus* Fort. *Numerus Brittonum*. c.AD 100 – 150 (Baatz and Herrmann 1982: 348-49).

38. **Schlossau**. Germany. Auxiliary Fort. Unknown unit. c.AD 100 – mid-2nd century (Baatz and Herrmann 1982: 410).

39. **Oberscheidental**. Germany. Auxiliary Fort. *Cohors I Sequanorum et Rauracorum equitata*. c.AD 100 – mid-2nd century (Filtzinger *et al.* 1986: 444-6).

40. **Heilbronn-Böckingen**. Germany. Auxiliary Fort. *Cohors V Delmatarum, Cohors I Helvetiorum*. Mid-1st century AD – mid- 2nd century (Filtzinger *et al.* 1986: 332-3).

41. **Walheim**. Germany. Auxiliary Fort. *Cohors I Asturum equitata*. Mid-1st century AD – mid-2nd century (Filtzinger *et al.* 1986: 596-9).

42. **Benningen**. Germany. Auxiliary Fort. Unknown unit. c. AD 85/90 - the reign of Pius. (Filtzinger *et al.* 1986: 239).

43. **Sulz**. Germany. Auxiliary Fort. *Cohors XXIV voluntarium civium Romanorum*. Mid-1st century AD - ? (Filtzinger *et al.* 1986: 597-8).

44. **Rottweil**. Germany. Auxiliary Fort. *Cohors I Biturgium, cohors I Flavia, cohors II Aquitanorum, cohors III Dalmatorum, ala I Flavia Gemina Milliaria*. Vespasianic - Domitianic (Filtzinger *et al.* 1986: 521-3; von Elbe 1974: 336-7).

45. **Alb-Stadt-Lautlingen**. Germany. Auxiliary Fort. Unknown unit. Mid-1st century AD - ? (Filtzinger et. al. 1986: 212-3).

46. **Seckmauern**. Germany. Auxiliary Fort. Unknown unit. Hadrianic – mid-3rd century (Baatz and Herrmann 1982: 476).

47. **Trennfurt**. Germany. Auxiliary Fort. Vexillation of the twenty-second legion from Mainz. Mid-2nd century AD – mid-3rd century (Baatz and Herrmann 1982: 482-3).

48. **Miltenberg-Altstadt**. Germany. Auxiliary Fort. *Cohors I Sequani et Raurici*. Mid-2nd century AD – mid-3rd century (von Elbe 1974: 271-2).

49. **Walldürn**. Germany. Auxiliary Fort. Vexillation of the 22nd legion. Mid-2nd century AD – c. AD 259/60 (Filtzinger *et al.* 1986: 604-6; von Elbe 1974: 439-40).

50. **Jagsthausen**. Germany. Auxiliary Fort. *Cohors I Germanorum civium Romanorum*. Mid-2nd century AD – mid-3rd century (Filtzinger *et al.* 1986: 351-2; von Elbe 1974: 163).

51. **Murrhardt**. Germany. Auxiliary Fort. *Cohors XXI Voluntariorum civium Romanorum*. Mid-2nd century AD – mid-3rd century (Filtzinger *et al.* 1986: 448-51; von Elbe 1974: 280).

52. **Welzheim and Welzheim Ost**. Germany. Auxiliary Fort. *Ala I Scubulorum, numerus Brittonum*. AD 165 – mid-3rd century (Filtzinger *et al.* 1986: 611-7).

53. **Lorch**. Germany. Auxiliary Fort. *Cohors quingenaria equitata*. AD 150 – mid-3rd century (Filtzinger *et al.* 1986: 433-4; von Elbe 1974: 250).

54. **Tuttlingen**. Germany. Auxiliary Fort. Unknown unit. Claudian – Flavian (Czysz *et al.* 1995: 75; Filtzinger *et al.* 1986: 584).

55. **Heddernheim**. Germany. Auxiliary Fort. Late 1st to mid-2nd century occupation. *Ala II Flavia milliaria* (von Elbe 1974: 128).

Raetia

1. **Eislingen**. Germany. Auxiliary Fort. Unknown unit. Flavian (Filtzinger *et al.* 1986: 276-7).

2. **Schwabisch-Gmünd**. Germany. Auxiliary Fort. *Cohors I Raetorum*. Mid-2nd century AD – mid-3rd century (Filtzinger *et al.* 1986: 546-9).

3. **Aalen**. Germany. Auxiliary Fort. The *Ala II Flavia milliaria*. Mid-2nd century AD – 259/60 (Filtzinger *et al.* 1986: 203-8; von Elbe 1974: 5-6).

4. **Buch**. Germany. Auxiliary Fort. Unknown unit. Mid-2nd century AD – 259/60 (Filtzinger *et al.* 1986: 492-5).

5. **Ruffenhofen**. Germany. Auxiliary Fort. *Cohors IX Batavorum equitata milliaria exploratum*. Mid-2nd century AD – mid-3rd century (Czysz *et al.* 1995: 509).

6. **Aufkirchen**. Germany. Auxiliary Fort. Unknown unit. Mid-1st century AD – mid-3rd century (Filtzinger *et al.* 1986: 54, 74).

7. **Unterschwaningen**. Germany. Auxiliary Fort. Unknown unit. Mid-1st century AD – mid-3rd century (Czysz *et al.* 1995: 527).

8. **Gunzenhausen**. Germany. *Numerus* Fort. Unknown *numerus* fort. Mid-2nd century AD – c. AD 243 (Czysz *et al.* 1995: 456).

9. **Theilenhofen**. Germany. Auxiliary Fort. *The Cohors III Bracaraugustanorum equitata* (Czysz *et al.* 1995: 522-23; von Elbe 1974: 388).

10. **Böhming**. Germany. Auxiliary Fort. *Cohors I Breucorum civium Romanorum*. Late-2nd century AD - ? (Czysz *et al.* 1995: 429).

11. **Kösching**. Germany. Auxiliary Fort. *Ala I Flavia Gemelliana*. AD 80 – 259/60 (Czysz *et al.* 1995: 469).

12. **Pförring**. *Celeusum*. Germany. Auxiliary Fort. *Ala I Singularium pia fidelis civium Romanorum*. Trajanic – mid-3rd century (Czysz *et al.* 1995: 499).

13. **Burladingen-Hausen**. Germany. Auxiliary Fort. Unknown unit. AD 80 – early-2nd century (Filtzinger *et al.* 1986: 265-7).

14. **Gomadingen**. Germany. Auxiliary Fort. Unknown unit. c.AD 85/90 – mid-3rd century (Filtzinger *et al.* 1986: 299).

15. **Romerstein-Donstetten**. Germany. Auxiliary Fort. Unknown unit. c.AD 85/90 – mid-2nd century (Filtzinger *et al.* 1986: 508-9).

16. **Bobfingen-Oberdorf**. Germany. Auxiliary Fort. Unknown unit. Late-1st century AD – mid-3rd century (Filtzinger *et al.* 1986: 253-4).

17. **Emerkingen**. Germany. Auxiliary Fort. Unknown unit. Claudian - ? (Filtzinger *et al.* 1986: 285).

18. **Unterkirchberg**. Germany. Auxiliary Fort. Unknown unit. Claudian – Domitianic (Czysz *et al.* 1995: 75, 209).

19. **Aislingen**. Germany. Auxiliary Fort. Unknown unit. Claudian – Domitianic (Czysz *et al.* 1995: 415-6).

20. **Burghöfe**. Germany. Auxiliary Fort. Unknown unit. Claudian – early-2nd century (Czysz *et al.* 1995: 429-30).

21. **Neuburg**. Germany. Auxiliary Fort. Unknown unit. Claudian - Flavian (Czysz *et al.* 1995: 485).

22. **Weltenburg**. Germany. Auxiliary Fort. Unknown unit. Claudian - ? (Czysz *et al.* 1995: 536-7).

23. **Passau**. *Castra Batavia*. Germany. Auxiliary Fort. *Cohors IX Batavorum milliaria equitata*. Second century AD (von Elbe 1974: 311).

24. **Eining**. *Abusina*. Germany. Auxiliary Fort. The fort was constructed c. AD 80 and remained in use for nearly 300 years. *Cohors IIII Gallorum* and *Cohors III Britannorum equitatae* (von Elbe 1974: 114-5).

Noricum

1. **Passau-Innstadt**. *Boiodurum*. Austria. Auxiliary Fort. *Cohors V Breucorum*. Flavian - ? (Alföldy 1974: 58, 104, 147; Genser 1986: 11).

2. **Oberanna**. *Stanacum*? Austria. Auxiliary Fort. Unknown unit and date (Alföldy 1974: 147, 167).

3. **Schlögen**. *Ioviacum?* Austria. Auxiliary Fort. *Cohors V Breucorum*. Hadrianic – early-4th century (Alföldy 1974: 144, 147, 167, 171; Genser 1986: 64).

4. **Eferding**. *Ad Mauros*? Austria. Auxiliary Fort. *Cohors Maurorum*. Hadrianic- ? (Alföldy 1974: 144, 147; Genser 1986: 88).

5. **Linz**. *Lentia*. Austria. Auxiliary Fort. *Ala I Pannoniorum Tampiana*. Claudian - ? (Alföldy: 1974: 75, 104, 144, 146, 167).

6. **Albing**. Austria. Auxiliary Fort. First legionary fortress for the *Legio II Italica*. AD 174 – 177 (Alföldy 1974: 155-6. 165).

7. **Wallsee**. *Adiuvense?* Austria. Auxiliary Fort. Unknown unit. Hadrianic - ? (Alföldy 1974:144, 167, 202).

8. **Mauer ad Url**. *Locus Felicis?* Austria. Auxiliary Fort. *Vexillation of the Legio II Italica*. Hadrianic - ? (Alföldy 1974: 144, 147, 167, 200, 202; Genser 1986: 213).

9. **Ybbs**. Austria. Naval Fort. A detachment for a river fleet. Vespasicanic? – late-2nd century (Alföldy 1974: 144, 148, 167, 202; 203; Genser 1986: 213).

10. **Neumark an der Ybbs**. *Ad Pontum Ises*. Austria. River fleet. Unknown date (Genser 1986: 227).

11. **Pöchlarn**. *Arelape*. Austria. Auxiliary Fort. *Cohors I Flavia Brittonum*. First century AD – 4th century (Alföldy 1974: 148, 150, 167, 202, 259; Genser 1986: 233).

12. **Mautern an der Donau**. *Favianis*. Austria. Auxiliary Fort. *Cohors I Ubiorum, Cohors I Aelia Brittonum milliaria*. First century AD – 4th century (Alföldy 1974: 144, 148, 150, 153, 167, 202, 209, 259; Genser 1986: 271).

13. **Traismauer**. *Augustiana*. Austria. Auxiliary Fort. *Ala I Augusta Thracum*. Claudian – late-Roman period (Alföldy 1974: 104, 145, 148, 150, 153, 167, 202; Genser 1986: 305, 312).

14. **Zwentdorf**. Austria. Auxiliary Fort. *Cohors V Breucorum equitata*. Claudian – 4th century (Alföldy 1974: 104, 148, 149, 153, 168, 200, 259; Genser 1986: 350).

15. **Tulln**. *Commagena*. Austria. Auxiliary Fort. *Ala I Commagenorum, Cohors Flavia Commagenorum*. Flavian – 4th century (Alföldy 1974: 150; Genser 1986: 357).

16. **Zeiselmauer**. *Austuris? Cannabiaca?* Austria. Auxiliary Fort. *Cohors I Asturum*. Late-1st century AD – 5th century (Alföldy 1974: 61, 144, 153, 167, 222, 258).

Pannonia Superior

1. **Klosterneuburg**. *Cannabiaca*? Austria. Auxiliary Fort. Unknown unit. Claudian – mid-3rd century (Mócsy 1974: 88).

2. **Schwechat**. *Ala Nova*. Austria. Auxiliary Fort. Unknown unit and date (Genser 1986: 533).

3. **Fischamend**. *Aequinoctium*. Austria. Auxiliary Fort. Unknown unit and date (Genser 1986: 549).

4. **Rusovce**. *Gerulata*. Hungary. Auxiliary Fort. Unknown unit and date.

5. **Magyaróvár**. *Ad Flexum*. Hungary. Auxiliary Fort. Unknown unit. Flavian – 4th century (Mócsy 1974: 88).

6. **Lébény**. *Quadrata*. Hungary. Auxiliary Fort. Unknown unit. Hadrianic – 4th century (Mócsy 1974: 107).

7. **Gyór**. *Arrabona*. Hungary. Auxiliary Fort. *Ala I Pannoniorum*. Pre-Flavian - ? (Mócsy 1974: 49-50).

Pannonia Inferior

1. **Szazhalombath**. *Matrica*. Hungary. Auxiliary Fort. Unknown unit and date (Mócsy 1974: 106).

2. **Adóny**. *Vetus Salina*. Hungary. Auxiliary Fort. *Cohors I Brittonum milliaria, Cohors I Alpinorum equitata*. Mid-1st century – 4th century (Mócsy 1974: 49, 106; Visy 1988: 97-8).

3. **Baracs**. *Annamatia*. Hungary. Auxiliary Fort. *Cohors I Thracum Germanica*. Second century AD - ? (Visy 1988: 108-9).

4. **Dunakömlod**. *Lussonium*. Hungary. Auxiliary Fort. *Cohors I Alpinorum peditata*. Flavian – 4th century (Visy 1988: 113-4).

5. **Tolna**. *Alta Ripa*. Hungary. Auxiliary Fort. *Ala Siliana Civium Romanorum, ala I Brittonum civium Romanorum*. Early-2nd century AD - ? (Visy 1988: 117).

6. **Ocseny**. *Ad Latus*. Hungary. Auxiliary Fort. *Cohors I Noricum, cohors II milliaria Brittonum*. Unknown dates (Visy 1988: 117).

7. **Vardomb**. *Ad Status*. Hungary. Auxiliary Fort. *Cohors III Lusitanorum, cohors II Asturum et Callaecorum*. Unknown dates (Visy 1988: 120).

8. **Dunaszekcsö**. *Lugio*. Hungary. Auxiliary Fort. *Cohors VII Breucorum*. Second century AD – 3rd century (Visy 1988: 123-4).

9. **Kölked**. *Altinum*. Hungary. Auxiliary Fort. *Cohors I Lusitanorum*. First century AD – 3rd century (Visy 1988: 125-6).

10. **Zmajevac/ Vorosmart**. *Ad Novas*. Serbia. Auxiliary Fort. Unknown unit and date (Visy 1988: 126).

11. **Mursa**. Serbia. Auxiliary Fort. *Ala II Hispanorum, cohors II Alpinorum equitata*. First century AD - ? (Visy 1988: 126).

12. **Dalj**. *Teutoburgium*. Serbia. Auxiliary Fort. *Ala II Hispanorum Arvacorum, ala I civium Romanorum, ala Praetoria civium Romanorum*. First century AD - ? (Visy 1988: 127).

13. **Sotin**. *Cornacum*. Serbia. Auxiliary Fort. *Cohors I Montanorum*. Unknown dates (Visy 1988: 127).

14. **Banostar**. *Bononia*. Serbia. Auxiliary Fort. *Ala I Britannica milliaria civium Romanorum*. Second centuery AD – 3rd century (Visy 1988: 128).

15. **Surduk**. *Rittium*. Serbia. Auxiliary Fort. *Ala I Augusta Ituriaeorum*. Second century AD – 3rd century (Visy 1988: 130).

16. **Novi Banovic**. *Burgenae*. Serbia. Auxiliary Fort. *Cohors I Thracum civium Romanorum equitata*. Second century AD – 3rd century (Visy 1988: 130).

Britannia

1. **Newcastle**. *Pons Aelius*. Auxiliary Fort. *Cohors I Traiana Cugernorum civium Romanorum, cohors prima Cornoviorum*. Second century AD – 4th century (Breeze and Dobson 1991: 59, 142, 243, 271).

2. **Rudchester**. *Vindovala*. Auxiliary Fort. *Cohors prima Frixagorum*. Second century AD – 4th century (Breeze and Dobson 1991: 211, 212, 244, 271).

3. **Carrawburgh**. *Brocolita*. Auxiliary Fort. *Cohors I Batavorum*. Second century AD – 4th century (Breeze and Dobson 1991: 244, 271).

4. **Great Chesters**. *Aesica*. Auxiliary Fort. *Cohors VI Nerviorum, cohors Raetorum, cohors II Asturum*. Second century AD – 4th century (Breeze and Dobson 1991: 54, 245, 271).

5. **Castlesteads**. *Camboglans* (Rudge Cup), *Gabaglanda* (Ravenna Cosmography) and *Amboglanna*. Auxiliary Fort. *Cohors IV Gallorum equitata, cohors II Tungrorum equitata*. Second century AD – 4th century (Breeze and Dobson 1991: 54, 246, 271).

6. **Stanwix**. *Uxelludamo, Petrianis* . Auxiliary Fort. *Ala Petriana; ala Augusta Petriana bis torquata civium Romanorum*. Second century AD – 4th century (Breeze and Dobson 1991: 54, 246, 271).

7. **Burgh-by-Sands**. *Aballaba*. Auxiliary Fort. *Cohors I Nervana Germanorum milliaria equitata, numerus Maurorum Aurelianorum and the cuneus Frisionum Aballavensium*. Second century AD – 4th century (Breeze and Dobson 1991: 54, 241, 246).

8. **Drumburgh**. Auxiliary Fort. Unknown unit. Second century AD –4th century

APPENDIX TWO

THE INSCRIPTIONS

Included within this appendix are the inscriptions mentioning medical personnel found in the area of study. The information is presented according to the province to which it relates. Each entry contains information about the fortification, place of publication, date of the inscription, if known, and the location of the inscription.

Abbreviations

AE *L'Annee Epigraphique*
CIL *Corpus Inscriptorum Latinorum*
ILS *Inscriptiones Latinae Selectae*
PR Provenance

TABLE A2.1: GERMANIA INFERIOR

1. Bonna/Bonn CIL XIII 8011; Wilmanns 1995b: 186, nr. 39 Date second half of the 2nd or first half of the 3rd. PR. Found in the ruins of the Dietkirchen in Bonn. *Herculi/ Victori Cl(audius)/ Edistrus o/ptio valet/udinari(i) et /Aurel(ius) Phil/etus b(ene) f(iciarius) le[g(ati)]/ ex stipibus*	2. Iversheim/ Bonn Kiln Works CIL XIII 7943; Wilmanns 1995b: 185, nr. 38 Date c. AD 145 PR. Kiln works. *Genio/ vexilatio/nis l(egionis) I M(inerviae) p(iae) f(idelis) / M(arcus). Sabinian/ius Quietus miles medicus, /Antonino IIII et Vero / II co(n)s(ulibus)*
3. Valkenburg AE 1975, 634; Wilmanns 1995b: 187, nr. 40 Date Possibly Claudian PR. Unknown *Tul(l)o Loucor(u)m / Albano medico.*	4. Vetera/ Xanten CIL XIII 8606=ILS 4739 Gummerus 95 Date Late Augustan PR. Civil settlement It might not be military, as it was found in close proximity to the fortress. *Alateiviae ex iussu Divos medicus*

TABLE A2.2: GERMANIA SUPERIOR

5. Mogontiacum/ Mainz CIL XIII 6778; Wilmanns 1995b: 255, nr. 95. Date Vespasianic PR. Unknown *Voto su[s]/cepto / L(ucius). Vireius / Dexter se/plesiar(ius) in/ leg(ione) I Ad(iutrice) / v(otum) s(olvit) l(ibens) l(aetus) m(erito).*	6. Mogontiacum/ Mainz CIL XIII 6700; Wilmanns 1995b: 188, nr. 41 Date Between AD 39/43-70/1 PR. It was built into the city wall. *D(is) M(anibus)/ [..].nius Vale(n)s / [me]dicus leg(ionis) IIII / Mac(edonicae)*
7. Niederbieber CIL XIII 11979; ILS 9182; Wilmanns 1995b: 192, nr. 45 Date 3rd Century PR. Unknown *In h(onorum) d(omus) d(ivinae) Genio Capsari/orum n(umeri) Divitiensium/ Gordianorum T(itus) F(lavius) Proces/sus, medicus hordina/rius,sub S(exto) Vibio Vita/le Pr(a)ef(ecto) n(umeri) s(upra) s(cripto) d(e) p(ecunia) s(ua)*	8. Gross-Krotzenburg CIL XIII 7415; Wilmanns 1995b: 196, nr. 47 Date Trajanic PR. Mithraeum *D(eo) Inv(icto)/ L(ucius) Fabi(us)/ Anthi(mus?)/ v(otum) s(olvit) l(aetus) l(ibens) m(erito), / med(icus) [coh(ortis)] IIII (sc. Vindelicorum)*
9. Osterburken CIL XIII 11767; Wilmanns 1995b: 199, nr. 49 Date AD 198 PR. Next to the *Porta Decumana.* *[-]/ [pr]o salu[t]e coh(ortis) III A(quitanorum),/ [Ul]pius Iulianus medicus/ [c]oh(ortis) s(upra) s(cripta), bene merentib[us]/ [d]e suo pos(u)it, Saturn[ino]/ [et] Gal(l)o co(n)s(ulibus) l(ibens) [m(erito)].*	10. Nemaninga/ Obernburg CIL XIII 6621=ILS 2602; Wilmanns 1995b: 197, nr. 48 Date Middle or end of the 2nd century PR. Inside the fort. *I(ovi) O(ptimo) M(aximo),/Apolloni et Aes/culapio, Saluti, / Fortunae, sacr(um)/ pro salute L(ucii) Pe/troni(i) Florenti/ni, praef(ecti) coh(ortis) IIII/ Aq(uitanorum) eq(uitatae) c(ivium) R(omanorum), M(arcus) Ru/brius Zosimus, medicus coh(ortis) s(upra) s(criptae)/ domu Ostia/ v(otum) s(olvit) l(ibens) l(aetus) m(erito)*

11. Vindonissa/ Windisch AE 1953 246b; Wilmanns 1995a: 191, nr. 44 Date 1st century PR. Schutthügel *Prisco medico*	12. Vindonissa/ Windisch CIL XIII (252) 5208; Wilmanns 1995a: 190, nr. 43. Date AD 45/6 PR. Found east of the fortress. *Ti(berio) Claudio Hymno,/medico leg(ionis) XXI,/ Claudiae Quietae (uxori) eius,/ Atticus patronus*
13. Strausburg/ Tilena/Thil Chatel CIL XIII 5623; Wilmanns 1995a: 189, nr. 42 Date 3rd century PR. Unknown. *[In] h(onorem). d(omus) d(ivinae)/ [d]eabus Mair[ab(us)]/[--]ius Regulus m[i]/les legionis VI[II]/ [An]to[n]i[ni]an(a)e A[ug(ustae)]/ [c]absarius ex vo[to]/ pro se et suis/ v(otum) s(olvit) l(ibens) m(erito)*	14. Uncertain CIL XI 3007=ILS 2542; Wilmanns 1995b: 194, nr. 46 Perhaps Upper Germany according to Wilmanns and Africa Date 2nd century? PR. Viterbo, Italy. *D(is) M(anibus)/ M(arco) Ulpio/ [Tele]sporo,/ medico alar(um) / Indianae et tertiae Astorum/ et saliario / civitatis splendidissimae/ Ferentiensium, /Ulpius Protog[e]nes/ lib(ertus) pat(rono) b(ene) m(erenti) f(ecit)*
15. Galen Kühn XIII 604 *ἀγὺμναστος δὲ παντὰπασιν ὢν οὐδὲν ἂν ἐκ τῆς τοιαύτης, εὐπορίας ὠφεληθείης, ὥσπερ οὐδ' οἱ κατὰ τὸν Γερμανικὸν πόλεμον ἰατροὶ ἔχοντες ἐξουσίαν ἀνατομῆς σωμάτων βαρβαρικῶν ἔμαθὸν τι πλέον ὧν οἶ μάγειροι γινώσκουσιν*	16. Bingen Rowland 1977: 175, nr. 407 No Date PR. Unknown. This inscription does not mention a military unit; however, since it was found in the area of Bingen it might be military. *D(is) M(anibus)/ [p]erpetuae secur[ri]/tati Q(uinto) Avitio He[rme] ti medico con[iux]*

TABLE A2.3: RAETIA

17. Uncertain Castra Regina/ Regensburg CIL III 6532; Wilmanns 1995b: 201, nr. 51 Date 178/9 PR. Unknown Wilmanns argues it is a doctor, however there is very little of the inscription surviving to make any specific statements. The underlined portions are all that remain. *[-medico or] dinar(io)/ [leg(ionis) III It]alicae/[-]*	18. Castra Regina/ Regensburg CIL III 5959; Wilmanns 1995b: 200, nr. 50 Date 165/6 PR. Found in the south gate of the city. *Have mihi/ Luciliane!/ Ulp(io) Lucilia/no medico ordinario/ [leg. III Ital./-]*

TABLE A2.4: NORICUM

19. Enns/ Lauriacum CIL V 4367; Wilmanns 1995b: 201, nr. 52 Date 165-191 PR. Brescia, Italy *D(is) M(anibus)/ L(ucii) Caeli(i) Arriani, /medico legionis/ II Italic(ae), qui vix(it) ann(os)/ XXXXVIIII menses VII. /Scribonia Faustina/ co(n)iugi karissimo*

TABLE A2.5: PANNONIA SUPERIOR

20. Carnuntum/ Bad Deutsch-Altenberg ILS 9095; Wilmanns 1995b: 203, nr. 54; Bormann, 1906: 133-6 Date Trajanic? PR. Spolia in wall of the building identified as the *valetudinarium*. *Capsa/riorum /[leg(ionis) X]IIII G(eminae) [-?-]*	21. Carnuntum/ Bad Deutsch-Altenburg AE 1929 (215) No Date PR. The provincial settlement. This might not be a military doctor. *Eucratus Medicus/L Iu[l]i Euthemi/medici Servus An/ XXV H S E/ L. Iulius Euthemis dominus ob/Meritis eius posuit*
22. Adium (West of Brigetio) CIL III 4279; Wilmanns 1995b: 204, nr. 55 Date Late 1st or early 2nd century PR. Gravefield	23. Poetovio CIL III 4061 Gummerus 385 No Date PR. Unknown. Poetovio is not strictly a military site; however this inscription mentions a

D(is) M(anibus)/ Victoriae Verinae, coniugi pientissimae,/ domu Foro Hadrianensi provincia/ Germania Inferiori, vix(it) ann(is) XXX,/ Aemilius Deciminus medicus ordi/ narius leg(ionis) I Adi(utricis) martius bene meritae/ fac(iendum) cur(avit)	military doctor. *Vex(illum) eq(uitum) C/. Rufius C F(ilius) (Tribu) Ouf(entina) med(icus) mile[s]/ leg(ionis) XIII Gem(inae) an(norum)/ XXXVI stip(endierum) XVI /fratre (sic)/ pos(uit) H S E)*

TABLE A2.6: PANNONIA INFERIOR

24. Aquincum/ Budapest AE 1937: 180; Wilmanns 1995b: 207, nr. 57; Kuzsinszky 1934: 7-8, 161 Date-144-147 PR. Central area of the fortress. Wilmanns says it is in the area of the *valetudinarium* based on Kuszinszky (1934); however there is little structural evidence to support the claim. *Aesculapio/ Ti(berius) Martius / Castrensis/ med(icus) leg(ionis) II A(diutricis)/ sub Q(uinto) Fufici/o Cornu/to co(n)s(ule) de(signato)*	25. Aquincum/ Budapest AE 1937: 181; Wilmanns 1995b: 214, nr. 62; Kuzsinszky 1934: 7-8, 161 Date 2nd Century PR. Central area of the fortress. Wilmanns says it is in the area of the *valetudinarium* based on Kuszinszky (1934); however there is little structural evidence to support the claim. *Asculapio et Hygi/ae Aug(ustis) sacrum/ T(itus) Venusius T(iti) f(ilius) Mene(nia tribu) Aper/ [P]raene(ste), opt(io) valetudi(narii), v(otum) s(olvit) l(ibens) l(aetus) m(erito),/[a.d.?] V Kal(endas) Octob(res) posuit.*
26. Aquincum/ Budapest Wilmanns 1995b: 217, nr. 65 Date 2nd or 3rd century PR. Obuda *Telesphoro/ sacrum/ T(itus) Fl(avius) Priscus/ vet(eranus) leg(ionis) IIII Fl(aviae)/ex opt(ione) val(etudinarii)/ d(ono) d(edit).*	27. Aquincum/ Budapest Cod Iustinianus 10, 53 (52); 1; Wilmanns 1995b: 208, nr. 58 Date mid-2nd century PR. Unknown *Imp(erator) Antoninus A(ugustus) Numisio: Cum te medicum legionis Secundae Adiutrix esse dicas,...*
28. Aquincum/ Budapest CIL III 3537; Wilamanns 1995b: 216, nr. 64 Date Mid Second Century PR. Obuda *[- - Cum]/ miae medic[o]/leg(ionis) IIII Fl(avia) m[a]/rito pientis [si]/mo Aur(elia) Ma.[..]/ uxor infe[lic(issima)].*	29. Aquincum/ Budapest CIL III 3413; Wilmanns 1995b: 211, nr. 60 Date mid-2nd century PR. Unknown *Asclepio et/ Hygiae Mar(cius) Marcel/lus med(icus), sub c(ura) a(gens)/ P(ublii) Va[l(erii)] Preasent(is)/ euok(ati), v(otum) s(olvit) l(ibens) m(erito).*
30. Aquincum/ Budapest CIL III 3583; Wilmanns 1995b: 213, nr. 61 Date 2nd or 3rd century PR. Obuda *D(is) M(anibus)/ C(aio) Iul(io) Filetoni{s}, domo/ Africa, medico, qui vi/xit ann(os) XXXV, C(aius) Iul(ius) Filet/us et Iul(ia) Euthenia, parentes,/ filo karrisimo f(aciendum) c(uraverunt)/ et Iul(io) Athenodoro fratri eius,/ qui vixit ann(os) XXXV Euthe/nia. Is ad quem sepultura(m)/ coll(egium) cent(onariorum) (denarios) CCC contulit*	31. Aquincum/ Budapest AE 1986; Wilmanns 1995b: 215, nr. 63 Date Hadrianic PR. South of the legionary fortress in the *vicus*. *I(ovi) O(ptimo) M(aximo) D(olicheno)/ Ulpi[us Flo]/ren[t]in/us, mi(les) ca/ps(arius) leg(ionis) II/ Ad(iutricis) v(otum) s(olvit) l(ibens) m(erito).*
32. Aquincum/ Budapest CIL III 14347, 5; Wilmanns 1995b: 217, nr. 66 Date 3rd century PR. Obuda *D(is) M(anibus)/ T(ito) Aur(elio)/ Numeri(o)/ militi/medico/ leg(ionis) XXII/ Pr(imigeniae) p(iae) f(idelis),/ et G(aio) Iul(io)/Me<r>catori,/ militi leg(ionis)/eiiu[sdem-].*	33. Aquincum/ Budapest AE 1923, 14; Wilmanns 1995b: 209, nr. 59 Date 146-150 PR. Carthage *D(is) M(anibus)/ Marcius Calli/nicus pat(er). medi[c(us)]/ leg(ionis) II Adi(utricis), et Tette/dia Hygia mater fili(o)/ b(ene) m(erenti) peregr(e) posue(runt), /qui vix(it) ann(um) (unum) mene(es) V*
34. Ulcisia Castra/ Szent-Endre CIL III 13386; Wilmanns 1995b: 219, nr. 67 Date Severan? PR. Unknown *[I(ovi)] O(ptimo) M(aximo)/ dis deab/usque Sep(timius)/ Bauleus eq(ues)/ caps(arius) v(otum) s(olvit) l(ibens) m(erito).*	35. Interciscia/ Dunaújváros ILS 9169; Wilmanns 1995b: 220, nr. 68 Date 3rd century PR. Unknown *D(is) M(anibus)/Ael(io) Munatio/ caps(ario) coh(ortis) (milliariae) Hem[e]s(enorum)/ stup(endiorum) XXVIII, dom(o)/ Sam(osata) Aur(elia) Cansa/una con Ant(onio)/*

	Basso vex(illario), sec(undo) her(ede),/ sanctiss(imo) coniug[i]/ con se natib(us)q(ue) suis /fecit m(onumentum) m(emoriae)

TABLE A2.7: BRITANNIA

36. Deva/ Chester CIL VII p. 48; RIB 461; IG XIV; Wilmanns 1995b: 175 nr. 30 No Date PR. Found in possible area of the *principia*; however Wilmanns argues that it is the *valetudinarium*, but one has not been identified with any certainty (Mason 2000: 410). *[Θεοῖς/ σωτ] ῆρσιν / ὑπερμενέσιν/Ερμογένης/ ἰατρὸς βωμὸν/ τόνδ' ἀνέθηκα*	37. Deva/ Chester AE 1969/70: 291; ; Nutton 1972: 7-13; Wilmanns 1995b: 176, nr. 31; Wright: 1969: 235, Nr. 3. No Date PR. Found in possible area of the *principia*; however Wilmanns argues that it is the *valetudinarium*, but one has not been identified with any certainty (Mason 2000: 410). *Πανυπειρόχα/σ 'Ανθρώπων /σωτῆρας ἐν ἀθα/ νατοῖσιν / 'Ασκληπιὸν ἠ/πιοχεῖρα 'Υγεί/ην Πανάκει/ αν ειἠτρος/ [Α]ντί [ο]χος/*
38. Binchester RIB 1028; Wilmanns 1995b: 178, nr. 33 Date 2nd or 3rd AD PR. Unknown. *[Aesc]ulapio / [et?] Saluti,/ [pro salu]te alae Vet/[tonum] c(ivium) R(omanorum) M(arcus) Aure/[lius- - -] ocomas me/[dicus v(otum) s(oluti)] l[ibens m(erito).*	39. Housesteads CIL VII 690=RIB 1618; Wilmanns 1995b: 178, nr. 32; Glison 1978: 162-5. 3rd Century PR. Unknown. *D(is) M(anibus)/ Anicio/ Ingenuo,/ medico ord(inario) coh(ortis) / I Tungr(orum), /vix(it) an(nos) XXV*
40. Britain Galen (K) XII 786 12; Wilmanns 1995b: 181, nr. 35 No Date Before or during Galen's lifetime. Late 1st or early 2nd century AD. PR. Unknown, Wilmanns suggests Gallia Belgica, but this is uncertain. *Κινναβάριον ἀξίου ὀφθαλμικοι Στόλου Βρεττανιοῦ, ...*	

TABLE A2.8: DACIA

41. Drobetae CIL III 14216, 9=ILS 7150a; Wilmanns 1995b: 222, nr.70. No Date PR. Unknown *D(is) M(anibus)/ M(arcus) Val(erius) M(arci) F(filus) /Longinu[s]/ med(icus) leg(ionis)/ VII Cl(audiae), / ornat(us) orna/ment(is) decu[r(io-nalibus)] / a splendid(issimo)/ordin(e) m(unicipii) H(adriani) D(robetae), /vix(it) an(nos) XXIII, M(arcus) Victorius/ [L]anio et Victoria/ [Ge]mina fil(io) pien[t(issimo)]/ p(osuerunt).*

TABLE A2.9: MOESIA SUPERIOR

42. Mantissa Addendorum/ Stojnik CIL III 14537=ILS 9147 Date AD 179 PR. Unknown *Valetu/dinarium/ Coh(ortis) II Aur(aliana)/Nov Equit(ata)/ CRT Bebeni/us Iustus praef(ectus)/Imp(erato). Co[mmodo]*

Appendix Three

Modern descriptions of medical tools

The following descriptions of medical implements are arranged in alphabetical order. They are based on those provided by a number of scholars who have written on the functions of medical tools (e.g. Bliquez 1981b; 1988; Braadbaart 1994b; Jackson 1990; 1994b; 2002; Künzl 1983; 1996; Milne 1907). It must be remembered that these tools might have had other purposes not related to medicine. Nonetheless, the descriptions provided are specifically related to the medical uses of the tools, and not even all of those are mentioned because most of the tools could be used in many surgical and pharmaceutical procedures. This is not the complete list of instrument types, as other instruments are known of in the archaeological and literary record, but they are rare and have not been found in the areas in question and are, therefore, not described in the text. Illustrations are given of the basic instrument type. All instruments are slightly different from one another, either through size, decoration, material and/or design and the catalogue of instruments examined (Appendices 4-10) has descriptions of the more unusual ones. Overall, however, the instruments discussed in the main text conform to the types described below.

Cauteries (*ferrum cadens, καυτήριον, καυτήρ*). Very few cauteries are known in the archaeological record because, according to Jackson, few probably would have been purpose made since they were simply a vehicle for transferring heat (1994b: 177-8). Most were probably made of iron as their Latin name suggests, many would have corroded, explaining the small numbers in the archaeological record. A special implement was developed for cauterisation of areas that were difficult to reach. A tube was placed over the hot cautery so that the skin of a non-infected area would remain unharmed:

> "*Apud quosdam tamen positum est vel fictilem fistulam vel enodem scriptorium calamum in narem esse coiciendum, donec susum ad os perveniat*" (Cels. 7. 11).

There are a few general reasons for the use of a cautery. It was used for haemostasis, or the stoppage of bleeding, and to remove unhealthy tissue or bone. The cauterisation of unhealthy tissue was done to allow for the healthy tissue to remain undamaged whilst the unhealthy area was being treated (Jackson 1994b: 178). Finally it could be used on boils and gangrene (Albucasis 1. 51-52). Since there were many shapes and sizes referred to in the written sources it is likely that doctors could have used a variety of instruments, such as double ended probes, and double simple probes as well as the spatula from a spatula probe to fit the size and shape of the area in need of treatment (Braadbaart 1994b: 54; Künzl 1983: 25-6; Milne 1907: 116-20).

Cupping Vessels (*cucurbitula, σικύα, κύαθος*). (Fig. 68) Celsus says that there is scarcely any malady in which blood may not be let,

> "*Sanguinem incisa vena mitti novum non est: sed nullem paene esse morbum, in quo non mittatur, novum est*" (2. 10. 1).

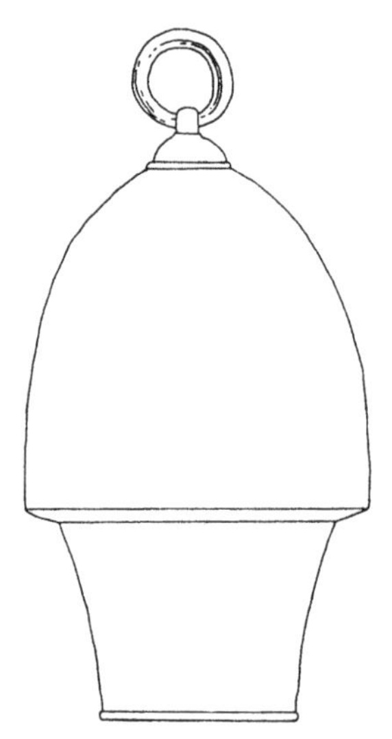

Fig. 68. Cupping Vessel (height 144mm). After Jackson 1994b: Fig. 3:12.

According to Albucasis the vessels came in different sizes: large, medium and small depending on the specific areas of the body that might have required different shapes and sizes (Spink and Lewis 1973: 46). They were also made of various materials. The cupping vessels made of horn had a hole on the top that was used for creating a vacuum effect. Those manufactured in copper alloy were solid and a piece of burning lint was placed inside them to create a vacuum. Milne quotes Oribasius, who says that they could also be made of glass to measure the amount of blood that was removed from the body (1907: 102-3). Oribasius said that sometimes the lips of the vessel were flat, "*ἐπίπεδα τὰ χείλεα*" and other times concave, "*σεσιμωμένα τὰ χείλεα*" (*Med. Coll.* 7. 16; Milne 1907: 102). These instruments were used for both wet and dry cupping. For wet cupping a knife was used to make a small incision and then the vessel was placed over it, drawing out the tainted blood or infected matter. Dry cupping was used in the release of bad humours and was suggested for headache and painful joints (Jackson 1994b: 182-4).

Forceps (*vulsella, τριχολαβίς*) This instrument has many functions and basically acts as an extension of the fingers. It could have been used for personal hygiene and depilation. A variety of forceps have been found in the archaeological record and are mentioned in the literature. Most of the simple tweezers were made of a single strip of metal bent in the middle with straight edges (Fig. 69) or slightly turned-in edges, come of them are cast with finial decorations (Figs. 70, 71, 72). Those with smooth jaws were recommended for epilation in granular conjunctivitis (Paul Aeg. 6. 13; Milne 1907: 91). They could also be used in the removal of bone splinters (Jackson 1994b: 174). They could also be used in the seizure of an ulcerated foreskin,

> "*Quae si cutem occupavit, protinus specillum subiciendum, eaque incidenda est; deinde orae vulsella prendendae*" (Cels. 6. 18. 3).

Fig. 69. Forceps made of one strip of metal with toothed edges (length 107mm). After Jackson 1990: Fig. 3:9.

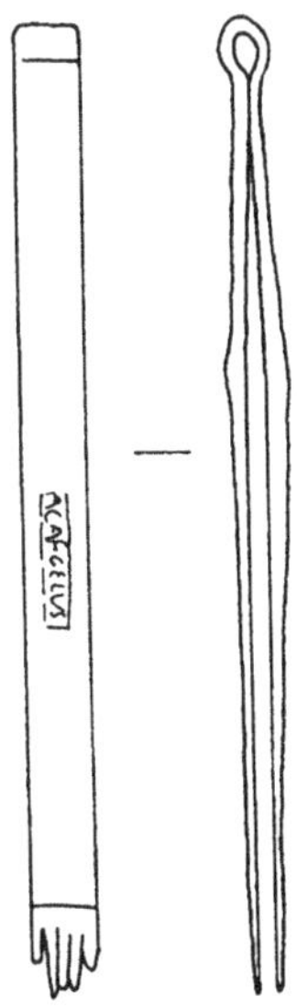

With the exception of size, they are similar to many that have been found on chatelaines. Bliquez (1988: 50-1) believes that the size of the instrument is the key to its function whether it is surgical or toilet. In general anything under 6 centimetres was personal and anything over was surgical; however, this is a modern interpretation, and one really cannot say, unless the tool was obviously part of a chatelaine. The instrument might also have served other purposes.

Toothed edges with fixation clamps are found on some types of forceps (myzon, vulsella, *μύδιον, σαρκολαβίς*). The teeth were designed to make traction on an object. They were applied to the removal of warts and partial excision of the uvula, or on tumours found on other areas of the body, "*tum vulsella tuberculum adprehensum iuxta radices praeciditur*" (Celsus *de med* 7. 30. 2; Künzl 1983: 18-19).

Some forceps have jaws that come out at an angle, rather than being placed straight on the end of the forcep handles (Fig. 73).

These usually have concave jaws on the interior of the instrument and convex jaws on the exterior. Sometimes there are fine teeth at the end of the jaws. Although Paul of Aegina does not provide a separate name for these forceps, it is suggested by Milne that these were the type used when Paul of Aegina was discussing the plastic operation for an eyelid with trichiasis.

> "*βλεφαροκατόχῳ μυδίῳ. τοῦτ' ἔστι πρὸς τὴν περιφέρειαν τοῦ βλεφάρου ἐσχατισμένῳ ἀνατείναντες τὸ περιττὸν δέρμα σμιλίῳ ἀποκόπτουσι*" (Paul Aeg. 6. 8).

Fig. 70. Two forceps with straight edges (lengths 177 and 143mm). After Jackson 1990: Fig. 2:2.

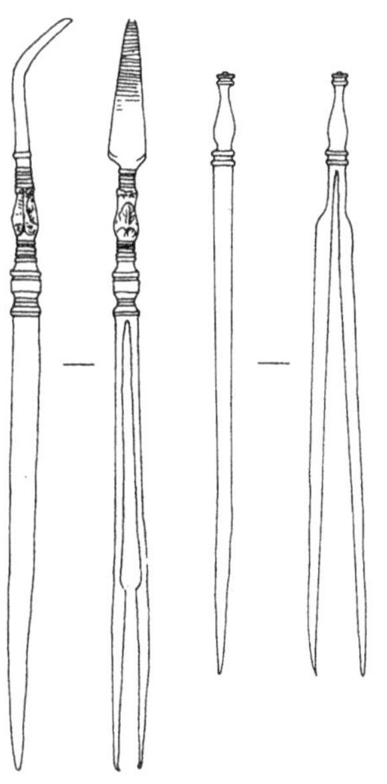

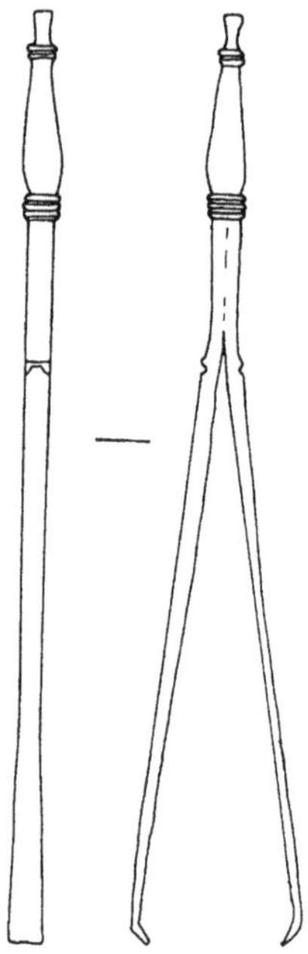

Fig. 71. Forceps with edges turned inwards (length 134mm). After Jackson 1990: Fig. 2:3.

Dental forceps (*forfex, ὀδοντάγρα, ῥιζάγρα*) are designed more specifically for the task of tooth removal. They have powerful jaws sometimes with an indentation for the tooth, so the tooth would not be crushed during removal, which would have caused greater problems (Fig. 74). To create a stronger hold on the tooth the arms of the dental forceps were crossed in the centre and attached with a bolt (Jackson 1994b: 175-6).

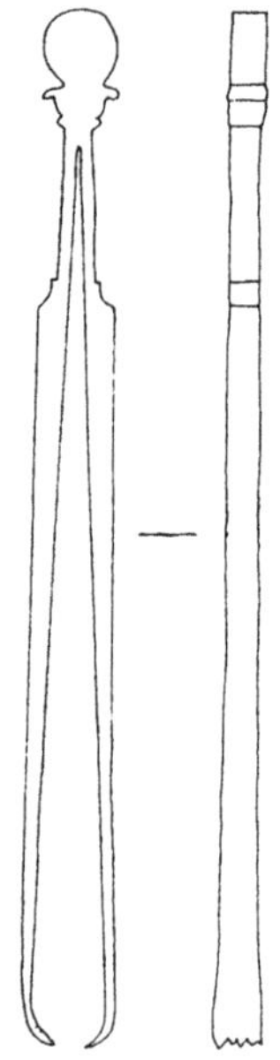

Fig. 72. Forceps with toothed edges turned inwards (length 153mm). After Jackson 1990: Fig. 3:5.

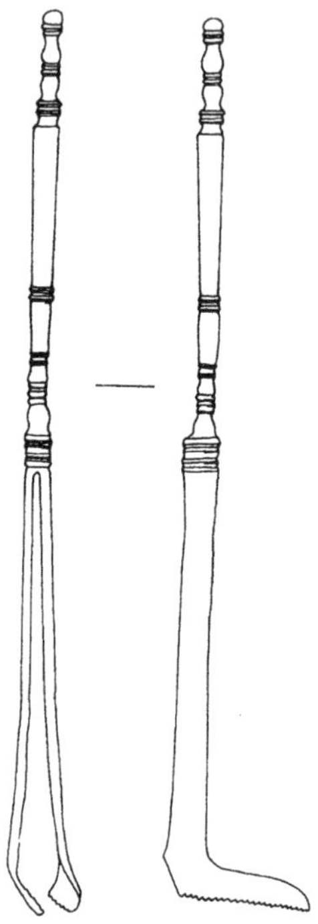

Fig. 73. Angle-edged toothed forceps (length 167mm). After Jackson 1990: Fig. 3:6.

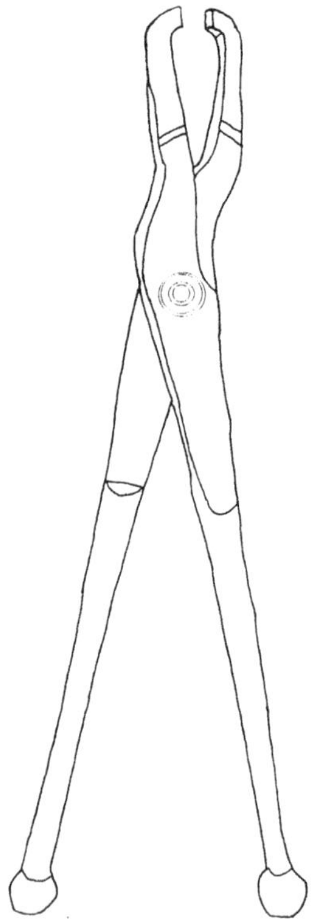

Fig. 74. Dental forceps (length 180mm). After Matthäus 1989: Fig. 13.

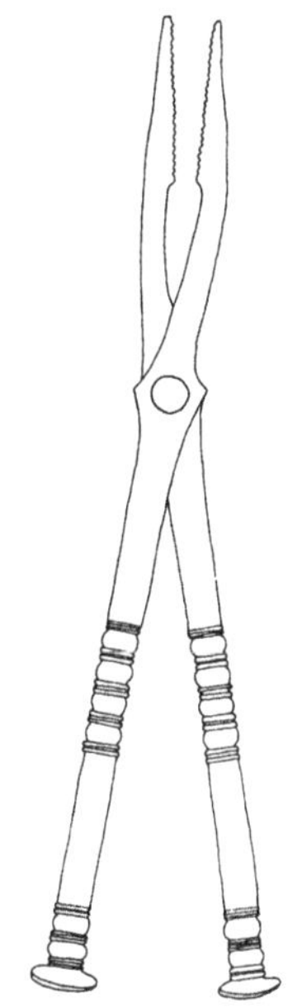

Fig. 75. Straight-edged bone forceps (length 222mm). After Jackson 1990: Fig. 5:4.

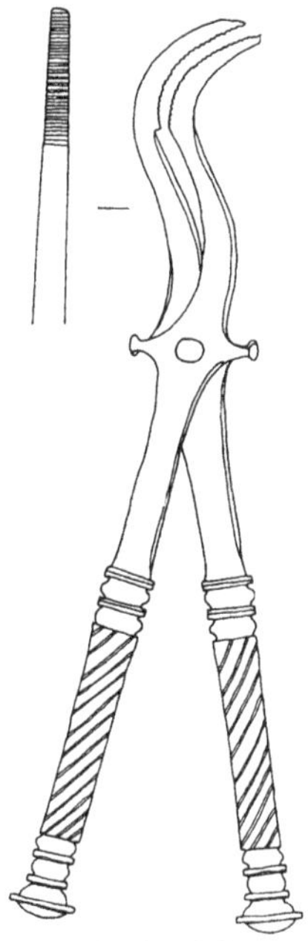

Fig. 76. Curved-edged bone forceps (length 212mm). After Jackson 1990: Fig. 5:3.

For the removal of bone and missiles, such as arrow and spearheads, forceps were made with strong arms crossed in the centre and for an even greater grip the head of the forceps had serrated teeth (Fig. 75). In some cases the utility end of the tool was curved (Fig. 76).

The removal of the uvula was a common operation in the Roman period, so a specific type of forceps was designed to aid in its removal, called the *staphylagra*. These could also be used in a haemorrhoidectomy (Jackson 1994a: 168). The *staphylagra* (Fig. 77) were made of two arms joined in the centre and the jaws of the instrument were toothed in order to crush the uvula and clamp it down while another set of forceps was employed to twist the uvula off the soft pallet of the throat. If

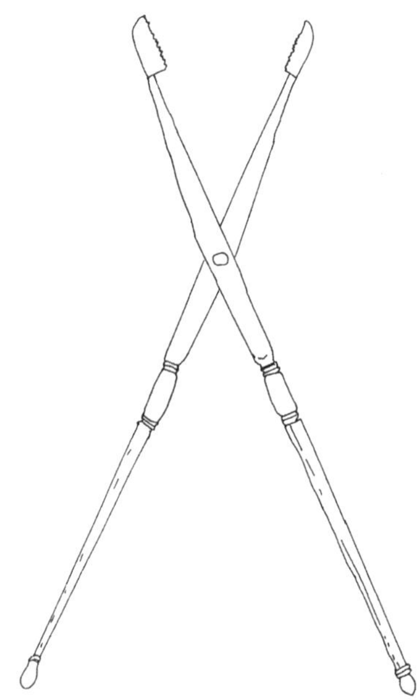

Fig. 77. Staphylagra (length 192mm). After Jackson 1990: Fig. 3:7.

a patient was unable to handle the pain of the forceps, staphylocaustes (Fig. 78) were suggested for both the removal of the uvula (Paul Aeg. 6. 31) and for haemorrhoids, (Paul Aeg. 6. 79). These forceps were similar in design to the staphylagra, but rather than having toothed forceps they had ends with hollowed out centres in which to place a caustic medicament, used to burn the uvula or haemorrhoid. The uvula would die and eventually come off the back of the throat (Jackson 1994a: 169-70). The extant varieties of these have both straight and bowed arms; the straight arms are suggested for the throat and the bowed for external haemorrhoids (Jackson 1994b: 172).

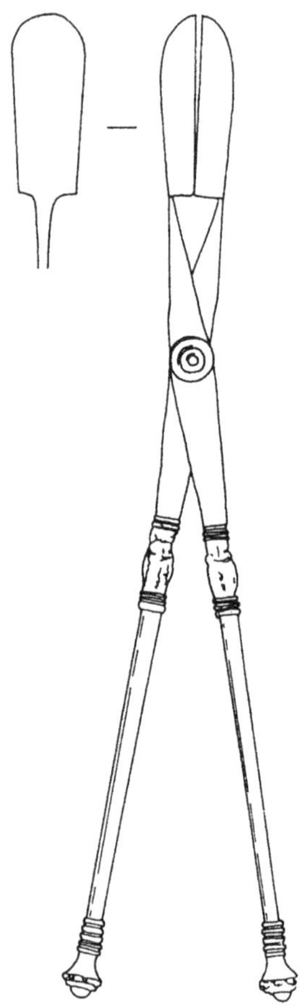

Fig. 78. Staphylochaustes (length 210mm). After Jackson 1990: Fig. 3:8.

Gynaecological and Gender-specific instruments. Some instruments were specifically designed for the male and female bodies. The catheter, discussed under syringes and tubes, was designed specifically for each sex. Soranus mentioned a number of implements developed specifically for gynaecological treatments and childbirth: the vaginal speculum (Fig. 79), uterine dilator, decapitating knife and a foetal hook (Fig. 80) to name a few. These instruments, however, could be used to treat both the male and female bodies, as seen with the rectal spculum (*ἑδροδιασταλεύς, μικρὸν*) (Braadbaart 1994a: 164; 1994b: 52). The design of the instrument had a handle and two prongs that would separate when the handle was squeezed (Fig. 81). This tool could have been used for the removal of weapons, to treat problems in the rectum, and it was also recommended for small women and girls as a vaginal speculum.

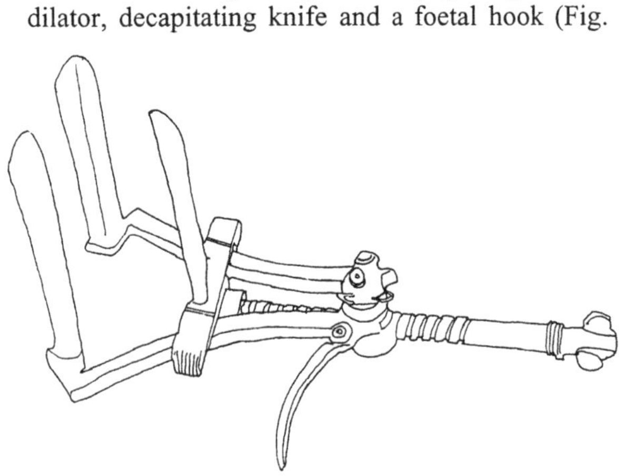

Fig. 79. Vaginal speculum. After Matthäus 1989: Fig. 27.

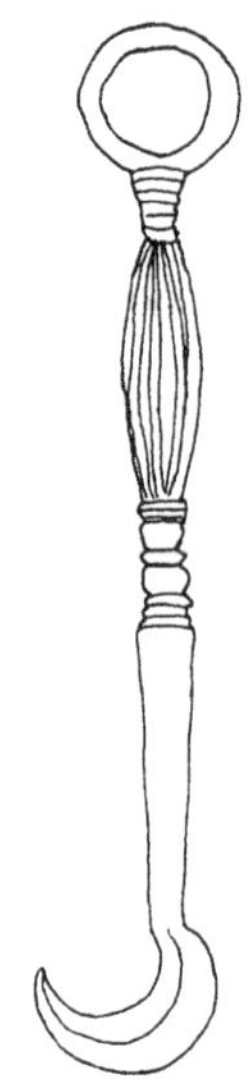

Fig. 80. Foetal hook (length 150mm). After Milne 1907: Pl. 5.

Fig. 81. Rectal speculum. After Matthäus 1989: Fig. 27.

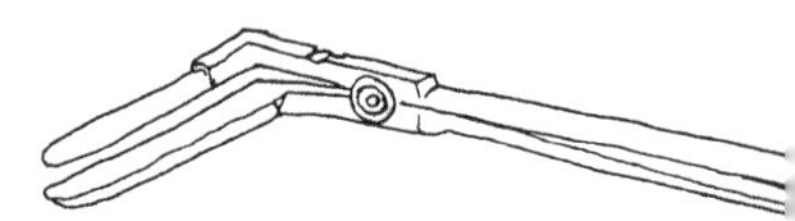

Hooks. These were used for seizing and holding tissue, boils and tonsils (Milne 1907: 85-7). The two most common hooks were sharp and blunt forms. The sharp hooks (Fig. 82) (*hamulus acutus, uncus, ἄγκιστρον*) were made of a copper-alloy and used to hold open the margins of a wound, giving the surgeon room to operate (Jackson 1994b: 172; Milne 1907: 87). Blunt hooks (*hamus retusus, τυφλάγκιστρον*) were used in more delicate operations such as raising veins (Figs 83-84). In some instances the instrument has been found to have hooks on both ends (Fig. 85). The lithotomy hook (*uncus)* was a blunt hooked spoon or scoop roughened on one side and designed for removing stones from the bladder or urethra. The hook (Fig. 86) was rough on one side so that it could grab the calculus and a smooth side that would not harm the body. Some handles had slotted sockets for a knife that could be used for the first incision (Jackson 1994b: 173). Forked, or bifurcated, hooks (Fig. 87) were also used for this purpose because they have blunt ends, rather than sharp ones.

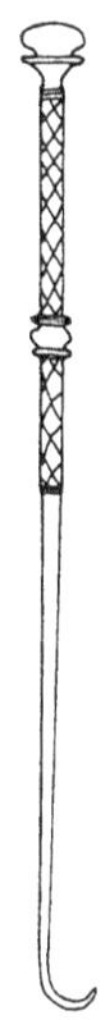

Fig. 82. Sharp hook (length 14 2mm). After Jackson 1990: Fig. 2:2.

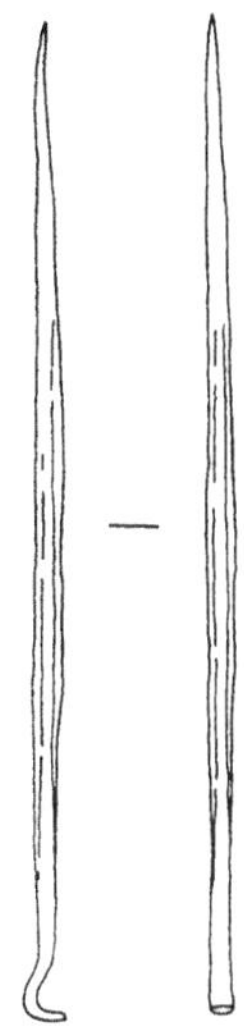

Fig. 83. Blunt hook (length 133mm). After Jackson 1990: Fig. 2:8.

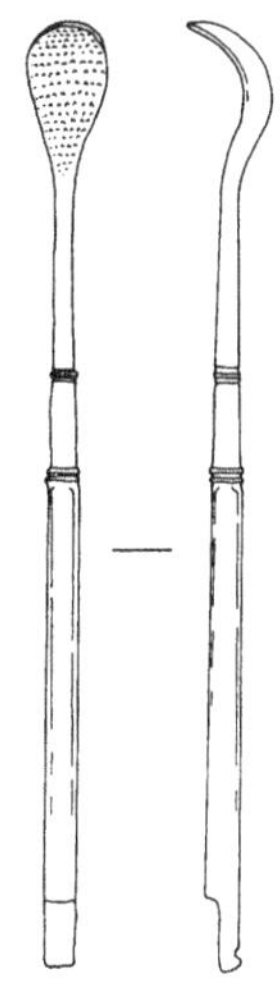

Fig. 86. Double-ended lithotomy scoop with a slot for a blade (length 175mm). After Jackson 1990: Fig. 6:7.

For stone extraction Oribasius mentions two hooks: the λίθουλκος (45.6.2 and 6 in Bliquez 1984: 120) was used like a miniature crow-bar, and the Κιρσουλκός (45.18.5 in Bliquez 1984: 121) was shaped like the Greek letter gamma. There is a variety of shapes, but generally one must question whether all of these more specialised instruments were necessary for the doctor's kit, or if they could have functioned adequately with a sharp and blunt hook.

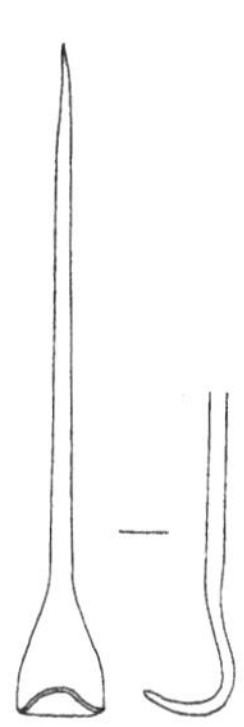

Fig. 84. Wide blunt hook (length 122mm). After Jackson 1990: Fig. 2:9.

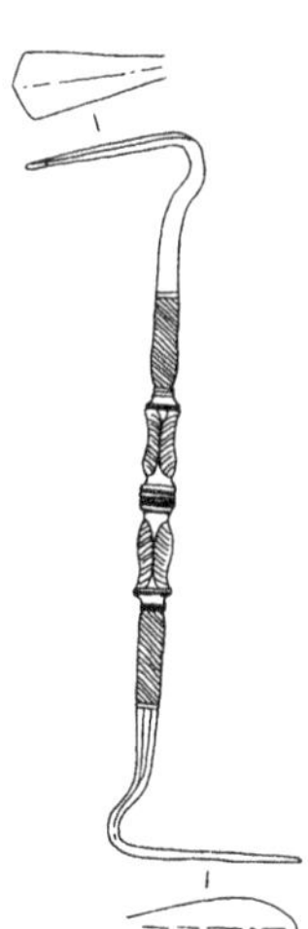

Fig. 85. Double-ended blunt hook (length 159mm). After Jackson 1990: Fig. 2:7.

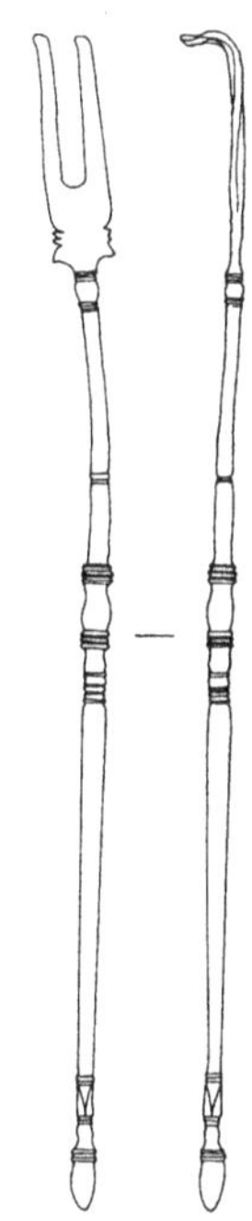

Fig. 87. Birfurcated hook (length 226mm). After Jackson 1990: Fig. 2,5

Medical Boxes (Fig. 88). The boxes used by doctors to carry medicaments are sometimes found in fortifications. It is difficult to say whether these were all meant for a doctor's use, as they could also have been used as paint cases, or for cosmetics and jewellery, for example. They were made out of a number of materials such as copper-alloy, ivory and wood. The wood ones were probably the least expensive to make, but also quite perishable, so very few remain. They were rectangular in shape ranging from seven to eight centimetres in length and about five centimetres wide and two centimetres deep. They had separate compartments covered with individual tops (Milne 1907: 170; Sobel 1991: 121-2). Another doctor's case was the cylindrical instrument case, about 20 centimetres long and one to two centimetres wide. These could only contain small number of instruments (Milne 1907: 168-9). There are representations of folding boxes used for containing surgical knives and scalpels. One example is on an inscription from the temple of Aesculapius from the Acropolis in Athens. The relief has an open box with scalpels and bone lifters carved on it (Milne 1907: 170).

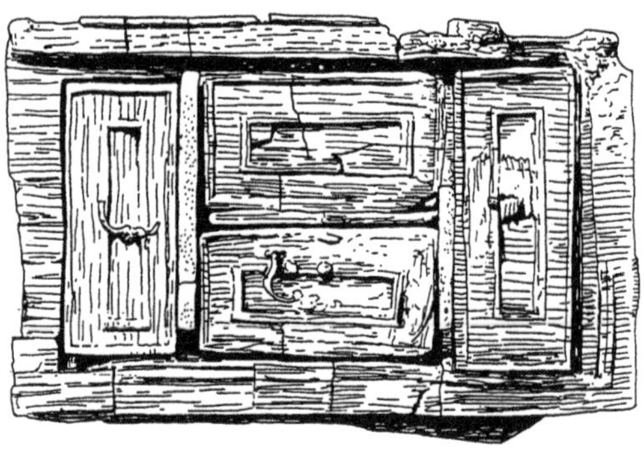

Fig. 88. Medical box. After Künzl 1983: Fig. 76.

Needles. Needles are important in a number of surgical procedures. There are two types known of through literature, those with eyes used for suturing wounds and lacerations and for sewing bandages and those with cylindrical handles that are made of copper-alloy with a hole in one end for a steel needle. Only the latter was examined in the study because it would be too difficult to make an identification between the surgical eyed-needles and those used for domestic purposes. Suturing needles would need a cutting edge so they would

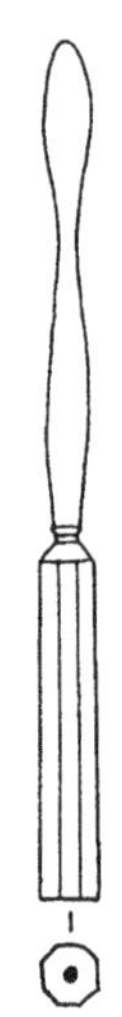

Fig. 89. Needle handle (length 92mm). After Jackson 1990: Fig. 4:5.

have been made of steel. Many would have corroded, making it even more difficult to determine what they looked like (Braadbaart 1994b: 54; Jackson 1994b: 177). The handled needle (Fig. 89) was examined in this study because it is more substantial in design and easier to identify, and it was used for more varied procedures than suturing. There were a number of proposed uses for the handled needle: puncturing skin, perforating pustules and raising the skin off the eyeball (Cels. 5. 28. 19C; 5. 28. 4D; 6. 18. 9C).

The cataract needle (*acus*) (Fig. 90), was said to be pointed sufficiently to penetrate the eye, but not so narrow as to be unable to break up the cataract: "*Tum acus admovenda est, sic acuta, ut foret, non nimium tenuis*" (Cels. 7. 7. 14D; Jackson 1994b: 177; Künzl: 1983: 26-7; Milne 1907: 74-5). The operation seems to have been common, or at least known about, as Martial accuses one doctor of

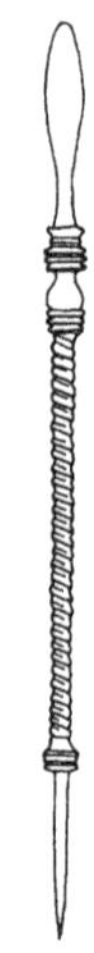

Fig. 90. Cataract needle (length 144mm). After Jackson 1990: Fig. 4:1.

being very careless by stating that a gladiator had formally been an eye doctor, but technically he was still performing the same job, "*Oplomachus nunc es, fueras opthalmicus ante. Fecisti medicus quod facis oplomachus*" (8. 74).

Oculist Stamps (Fig. 91). These stamps are found in a number of sites throughout the empire, though

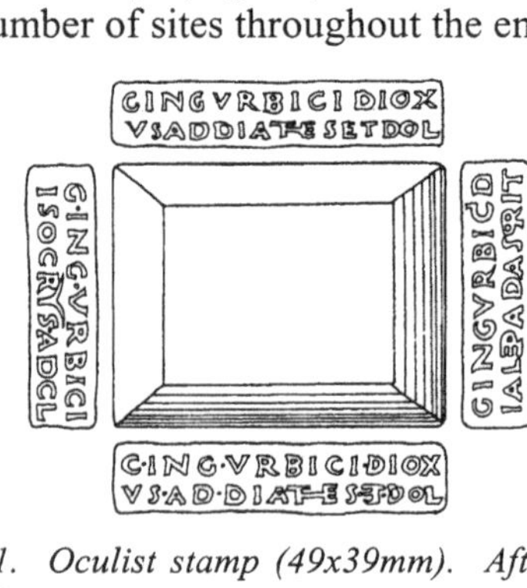

Fig. 91. Oculist stamp (49x39mm). After Künzl 1983: Fig. 48.

the majority come from the north-western provinces. They are made of stone and have the name of the doctor, illness and the ointment inscribed on the sides. As for their size and shape, the oculist stamps are generally square and about one or two centimetres wide and a few millimetres in depth. They were used more for pharmaceutical procedures, as a stamp to mark medicines for eye diseases (Jackson 1996: 2,240-3).

Ointment Pallet. (Fig. 92) Although this is not a surgical instrument, it does have associations with pharmaceutical procedures and is found frequently in the archaeological record. The pallets are made of stone and often found worn down on one side, due to the grinding it was used for (Milne 1907: 171). It is also possible that they were used for make-up and paints.

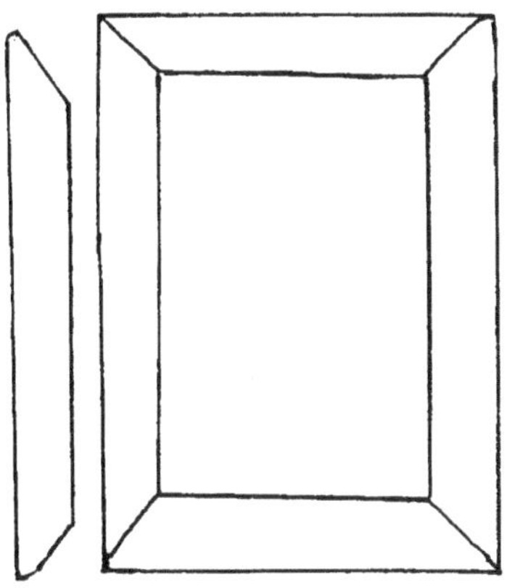

Fig. 92. Ointment pallet (150x120mm). After Matthäus 1989: Fig. 7:100.

Probes. These instruments, also referred to as sounds, are the most common type of instruments overall. The probes were fabricated as a multi-purpose instrument that could be utilised in a number of surgical procedures, minor operations, pharmaceutical preparations, personal hygiene as well as non-medical procedures such as mixing paints.

Double Olivary End Probe (*διπύρηνος μήλη, ἀμφίσμιλος*). This was also a simple instrument that had an olivary end placed on both terminations of its thin handle (Fig. 93). The olivary ends could be used in pharmaceutical procedures to mix ointments. It was also possible to use it to create a drip effect much like a modern eye-dropper by placing a piece of cloth soaked in a liquid medicament above the olivary end, and squeezing the cloth so that the ointment would slide down over the termination and drip onto the area in need of the medicine. As a surgical implement the olivary end could be used to explore fistula, "*Ante omnia autem demitti specillum in fistulam convenit*" (Cels. 5. 28. 12 C), and for examining carious bone,

> "*..in carie quidem expedita cognito est. Specillum tenue in foramina demittitur, quod magis minusve intrando vel in summo cariem esse vel altius descendisse testatur*" (Cels. 8. 2. 3).

Many (Fig. 93) have been found with a hole drilled through one of the olivary probes (in some cases both). The probe was used in the removal of anal fistula whereby an incision was made beneath the fistula. The probe with a drilled hole was used for holding string, much like the eye of a sewing needle. This probe was drawn up to its end in the incision, and the string was drawn through the incision when the probe was being removed (Jackson 1994b: 180; Künzl 1983: 27-8; Milne 1907: 55).

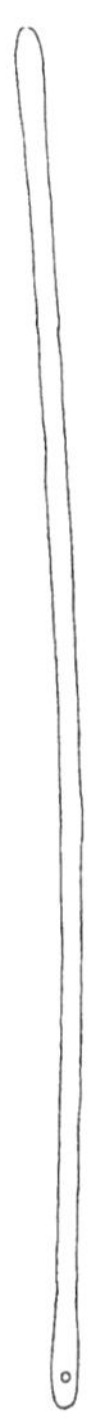

Fig. 93. Double-ended olivary probe with eye (length 280mm). After Jackson 1990: Fig. 4:7.

> "*Propriam etiamnum animadversionem desiderant eae, quae in ano sunt. In has demisso specillo ad ultimum eius caput incidi cutis debet, dein novo foramine specillum educi lino sequente, quod in aliam eius partem ob id ipsum perforatam coniectum sit*" (Cels. 7. 4. 4A).

Few of these were found in the examination, but a number of probes have been found broken where only the olivary end survives; perhaps some of these were actually part of double olivary probes rather than spatula or spoon probes. The probe could also serve the same function as the single olivary end of the other probes.

Double Simple Probe (*specillum, ἀπυρηνομήλη*). This instrument is not recognised often in the archaeological record possibly because its simple design, consisting of a thin rod with two blunt ends (Fig. 94), can have easily been transfigured or mistaken for another object. They were used in delicate probing and may even have served as a tiny cautery. Paul of Aegina suggests using the olivary end of a probe to cauterise eyelashes in the treatment of trichiasis or granular conjunctivitis, where the eyelid turns in upon itself and the lashes then scratch the eyeball (6. 14). It is possible that an olivary end to a probe might have been too large in certain instances for probing, so perhaps the double simple probe was employed. Furthermore, the pointed end of an ear probe could probably serve the same function, perhaps being another reason these are not found often in the archaeological record. Similar to this is the dipyrene, which looks like a double-ended olivary probe, but without the eye for thread (Fig. 95). It too was multi-functional acting as an ointment drip, cautery and even probe.

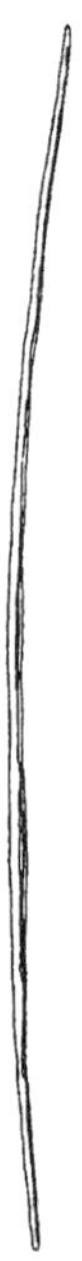

Fig. 94. Double simple probe (length 131mm). After Gilson 1981: Fig. 4.

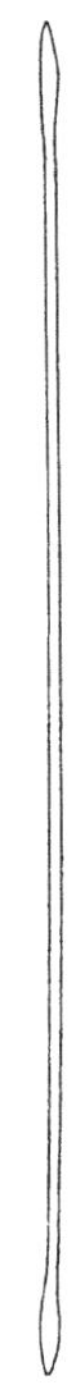

Fig. 95. Dipryene (length 165mm). After Jackson 1990: Fig. 4:8.

Ear Probe (*oricularium speculum, μηλωτίς*). These instruments are generally called ligulae; however, many museums also label spoon probes as ligulae, so to be more specific they shall be referred to as ear probes in this study. There are two types those with flat ends (Fig. 96) and those with small round spoon-scoped ends (Fig. 97) (Braadbaart 1994b: 54; Jackson 1994b: 181; Künzl 1983: 27-8; Milne 1907: 63). They have thin handles that terminate in blunt points on one end, whilst the utility end has a small, flat slanted circular head which is generally quite small, but does sometimes measure to five or six millimetres in width, but can still fit into the ear. For medical purposes they were dipped in resin and could have been used to remove foreign bodies from the ear such as maggots, "*Ubi vero vermes orti sunt, si iuxta sunt, protrahendi oriculario specillo sunt*" (Cels. 6. 7. 5). They were suggested to aid in the removal of linen placed in the incision of a haemorrhoid removal operation, "*Interpositis quinque aut sex diebus oriculario specillo linamenta educenda*" (Cels. 7. 30. 3D).

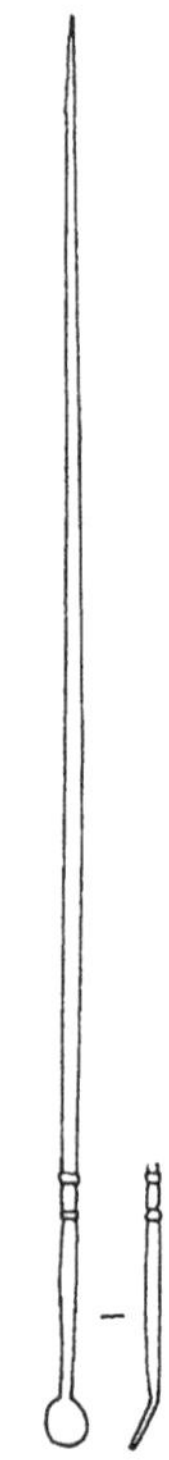

Fig. 96. Flat-headed ear probe (length 161mm). After Jackson 1990: Fig. 4:9.

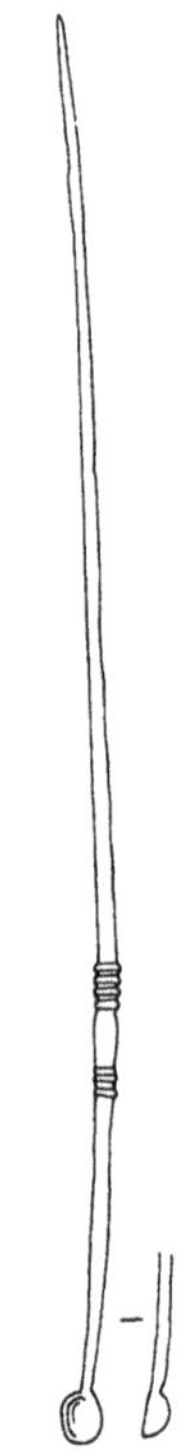

Fig. 97. Spoon-headed ear probe (length 178mm). After Jackson 1990: Fig. 4:10.

Spatula probe (*spathomele, σπαθομήλη*). The instrument consists of a long thin handle and tends to range in size from roughly 6 to 15 centimetres with a spatula on one end of its handle and an olivary probe on its other end, indicating its multi-functionality. The spatula is usually leaf-shaped and tends to be flat on one side and slightly rounded on the other (Fig. 98). Some spatula ends are quite thin, perhaps five or six millimetres in width, whilst others are short and blunt. Some have more of a rectangular shape to them (Fig. 99) and others have a spatula blade on both ends (Fig. 100). It could be used for spreading medicaments on infected areas of the body as well as mixing medicines on an ointment pallet. Sometimes the spatula could be used as a cautery, as Soranus mentions using it on the umbilical cord "*τοῦ πλάτεος τῆς μήλης*" (*Gyn* 3. 27; Milne 1907: 60). It could also be used as a tongue depressor (Milne 1907: 59) and as a blunt dissector (Milne 1907: 60). The olivary end could be used in the same way as many already suggested for the double-ended olivary probe. These are only some of the medical uses for the tool, and they are also known to have been found with painting and writing materials.

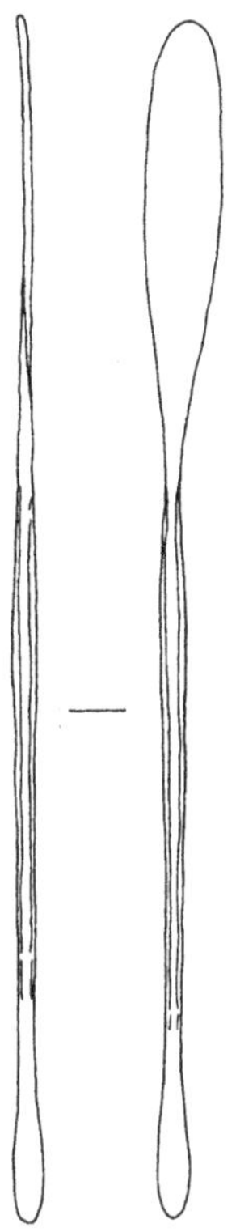

Fig. 98. Leaf-shaped spatula probe (length 190mm). After Jackson 1990: Fig. 4:15.

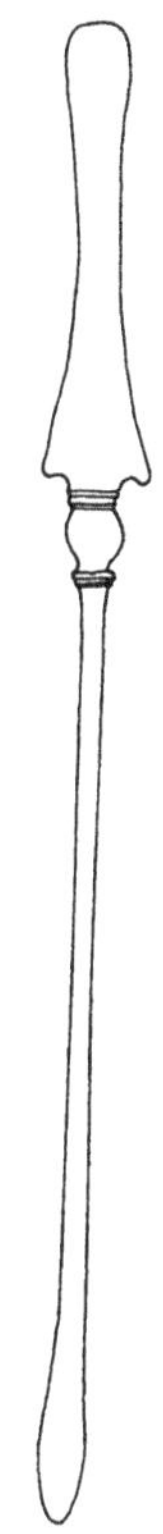

Fig. 99. Rectangular spatula probe (length 184mm). After Jackson 1990: Fig. 4:14.

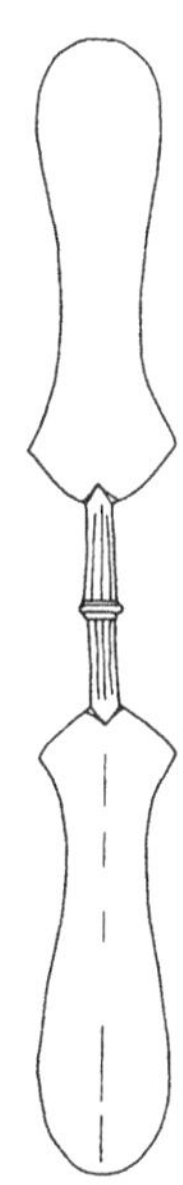

Fig. 100. Double-ended spatula probe (length 175mm). After Jackson 1990: Fig. 4:16.

Spoon Probe (*cyathiscomele*). This is similar to the spatula probe, but has a narrow leaf shaped spoon in place of the spatula (Fig. 101). They also have the same olivary end as spatula probes. For pharmaceutical purposes the spoon was used to remove medicines from their flasks, explaining the many different sizes of the spoon and handle. It might have been used to mix ointments as well. For surgery Milne suggests it might have been used as a curette (1907: 62). There is also the possibility that it was applied in lithotomy operations to help remove stones from the urethra; although there were special spoons made for this procedure which did not have an olivary end and had a deeper more rounded and sharper spoon already discussed (Jackson 1994b: 181; Milne 1907: 62).

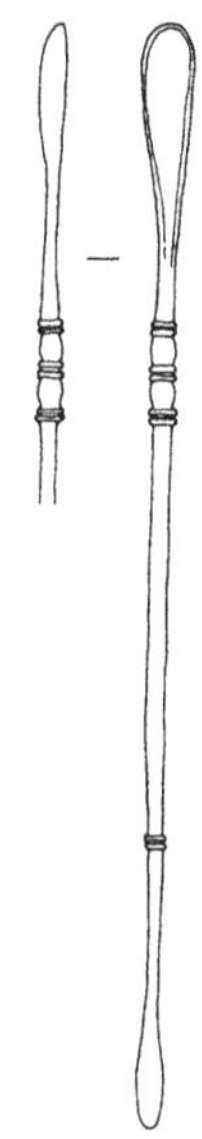

Fig. 101. Spoon probe (length 168mm). After Jackson 1990: Fig. 4:11.

Scalpel (*scalpelus, σμίλη*). This is one of the tools recommended most often in Roman surgical procedures (Braadbaart 1994b: 52; Jackson 1994b: 169-71; Künzl 1983: 15-16; Milne 1907: 27). The remains of the instrument, usually just the handle, are found throughout the empire (Figs. 102-104). The handles are usually rectangular, with a blunt leaf shaped blade on one end that was recommended in operations requiring blunt dissections. The opposite end had a slot for a steel blade, or perhaps iron. The steel from Noricum was said to be of the highest quality for blades (Galen 2. 682 K). There were a number of different shapes to the blade but the most common seems to have been the bellied or convex form (Jackson 1994b: 170). Amongst numerous applications, it could be used to incise skin that had become badly infected:

> "*Luxata igitur, in quacumque parte corporis sunt, quam primum sic curari debent, ut, qua dolor est, ea scalpello cutis crebro incidatur*" (Cels. 7. 1. 1).

With anything that needed a sharp incision the scalpel was recommended. The instrument could also have other non-medical purposes, such as the possibility of leather working.

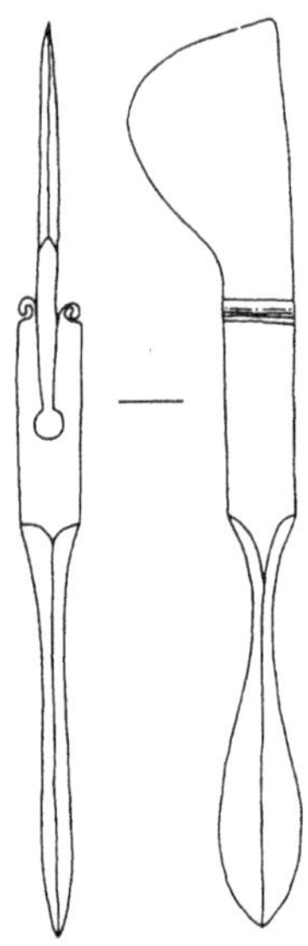

Fig. 102. Scalpel (length 153mm). After Jackson 1990: Fig. 1:6.

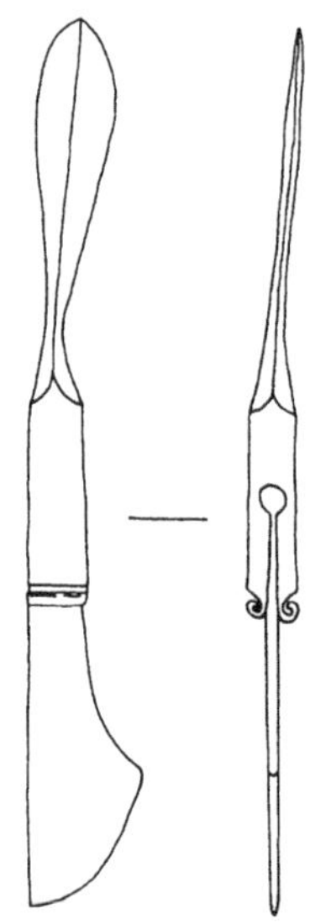

Fig. 103. Scalpel (length 131mm). After Jackson 1990: Fig. 1:7.

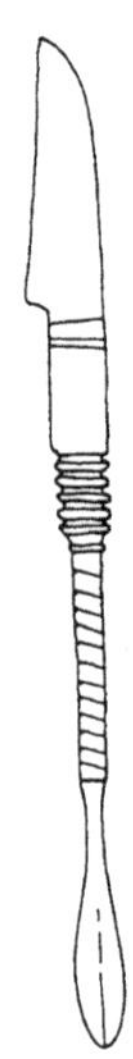

Fig. 104. Scalpel (length 124mm). After Jackson 1990: Fig. 1:8.

Shears (*forfex, ψάλις*) (Braadbaart 1994b: 55). Overall these were not dealt with in this study because they could also have served a non-surgical function, even when they are found in relation to doctor's kits, as doctors would have needed them for cutting bandages and hair (Fig. 105). Celsus informs us that they could be used in a surgical manner for cutting mortified omentum in an abdominal wound:

> "*His conditis, omentum quoque considerandum est, ex quo, si quid iam nigri [emortui] est, forfice excidi debet* (7. 16. 3); *Fuerunt etiam qui omentum forfice praeciderent*" (Cels. 7. 21. 1C; Jackson 1994b: 171).

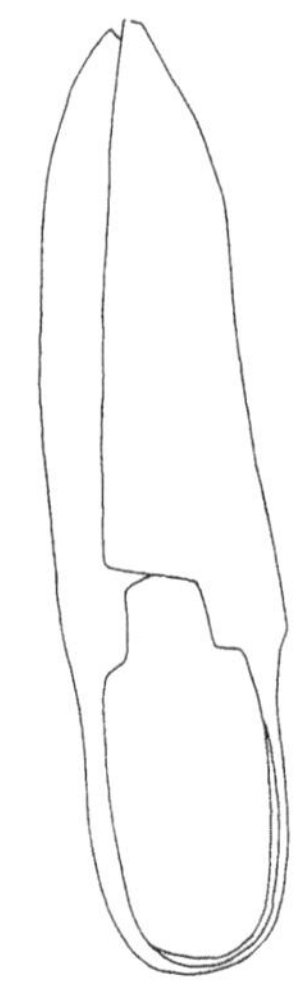

Fig. 105. Shears (length 202mm). After Jackson 1990: Fig. 1:5.

Surgical Knives (Fig. 106). Along with scalpels these are mentioned frequently through the medical literature, but very few survive in the archaeological record. One knife that has been identified is the lithotomy knife, a form with a

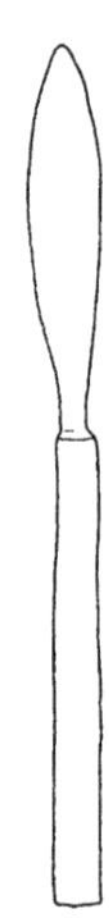

Fig. 106. Surgical knife. After Deringer 1954: Fig. 81: 2.

hook on one end and a sharp knife on the other (Jackson 1994b: 170-1). Nonetheless, Celsus states that a scalpel could also be used for removing a stone (Cels. 7, 26, 2 N-O). Overall, however, there is a smaller number of surgical knives in the archaeological record and this might be because the scalpel had a number of blades and could have been used in the same capacity as the knife. Another knife that had a distinct function was the lancet (*phlebatom*) that was used in scarification during wet cupping (Fig. 107).

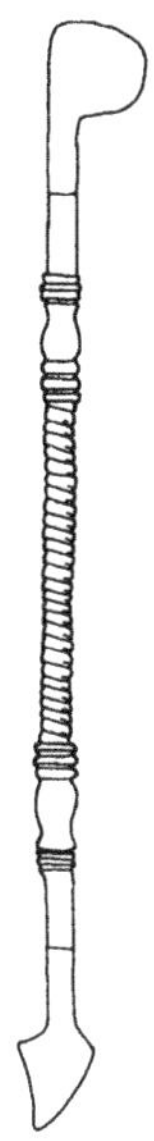

Fig. 107. Lancet (length 128mm). After Jackson 1990: Fig. 1:4.

Syringes and Tubes. These are not commonly found because they are hollow and could quite easily have been misshapen, making them difficult to identify in the archaeological record. Celsus says that the tube either had upturned lips on one end or a collar around the middle so that the instrument would not become lost within the body:

> "*vel recurvatis in exteriorem partem labris,*
> *vel in media circumsurgente quandam mora*
> *ne tota intus delabi possit*" (7. 15. 2).

This might have been a problem with a dropsical patient who had tubes placed in his abdomen for draining water. Catheters are also found within the confines of military sites; these are important for helping aid urination when the bladder was blocked by a calculus. The catheters were designed for both the male and the female body, thereby making them gender specific instruments. The males' were more "S" shaped and long (Fig. 108), whilst the females' (Fig. 109) were shorter and straighter (Jackson 1994b: 185). Three sizes were recommended for men and two for women. For men they were 15, 12 and 9 fingerbreadths, while women were 9 and 6 fingerbreadths in length. The differences in the male and female body designated the need for a gender specific design for the catheters. The instruments are basically hollow tubes with one end open like a straw and the other, which is to be inserted in the urinary tract, had a small hole on the side of the tube, rather than on the top, because this would allow for the top to have been rounded and inserted with more care.

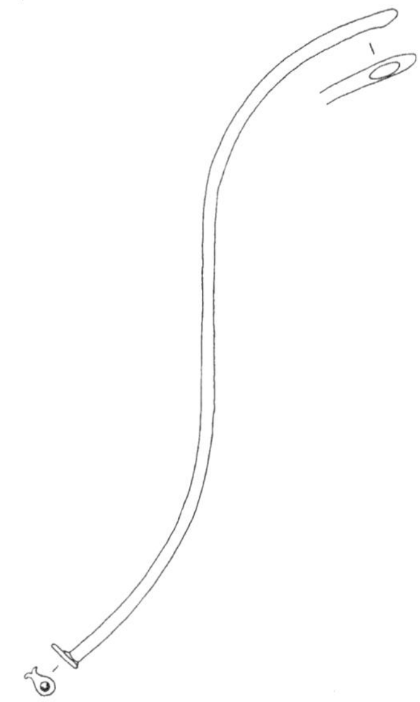

Fig. 108. Male catheter (length 285mm). After Jackson 1990: Fig. 6:2.

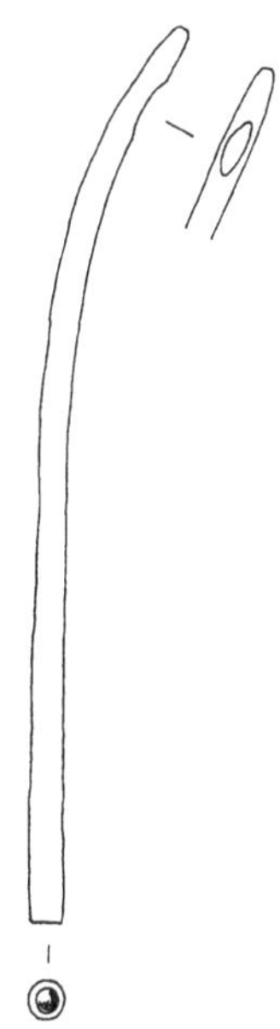

Fig. 109. Female catheter (length 143mm). After Jackson 1990: Fig. 6:3.

The tube could also have been used as a clyster or syringe by attaching a bag or pouch to one end and squeezing it to introduce medicines into the body (Figs. 110-111). Sometimes an ear syringe is mentioned or *clyster oricularis*. It seems that this may have been worked by a plunger rather than a bladder. The medicament would have been placed in the tube in this instance and then a solid plunger would push the medicament through a small hole at the opposite end (Jackson 1994b: 187; Milne 1907: 105). There was a *pyoilkos* mentioned by Heron in his *Pneumatica* (2. 18). It was a hollow injection pipe that was attached to a reservoir tube equipped with a close fitting plunger, itself a plugged tube. It was recommended for inserting liquids into an orifice of the body and also for drawing out infectious liquids from the body. It seems, however, that the *cannula* (hollow tube) with a stopper was more commonly used (Bliquez and Oleson 1994: 83-103).

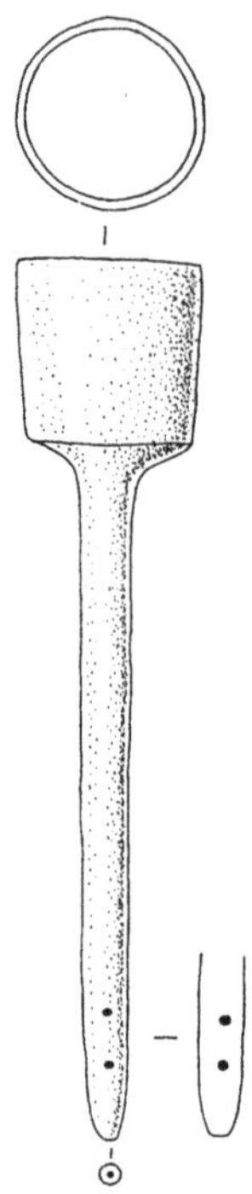

Fig. 110. Clyster (length 157mm). After Jackson 1990: Fig. 6:5.

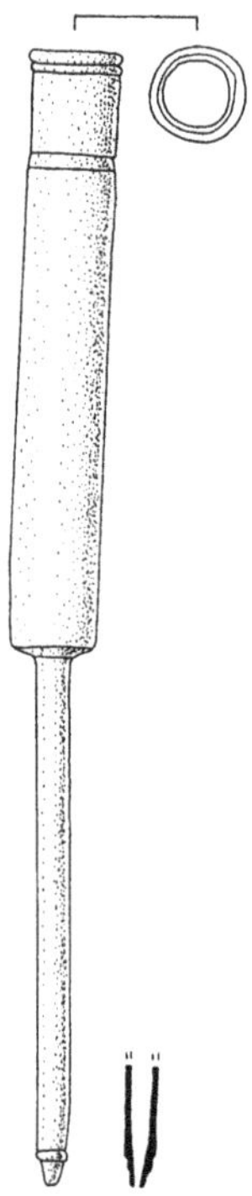

Fig. 111. Clyster or syringe (length 203 mm). After Jackson 1990: Fig. 6:6.

Tools for battle wounds. There were special instruments designed for the removal of missiles and arrowheads, but these too are not very common because other instruments, knives, probes and forceps, are also recommended for battle wound operations. The trepan with straps was developed for trepanation (Fig. 112); however, the instruments could also be used for the removal of missiles from the bone. If the weapon had become lodged in a bone, the bone was drilled around the outer edges of the missile to make a larger area around the weapon, which could be removed without damaging or splintering the bone, something that posed a threat if the weapon was pulled directly out of the bone. Furthermore, a bone cut with smooth edges would heal more easily. Another suggestion for avoiding further tissue damage was to place reeds around the barbed edges of the missile head, thereby protecting the tissue from being damaged even further when the missile was removed.

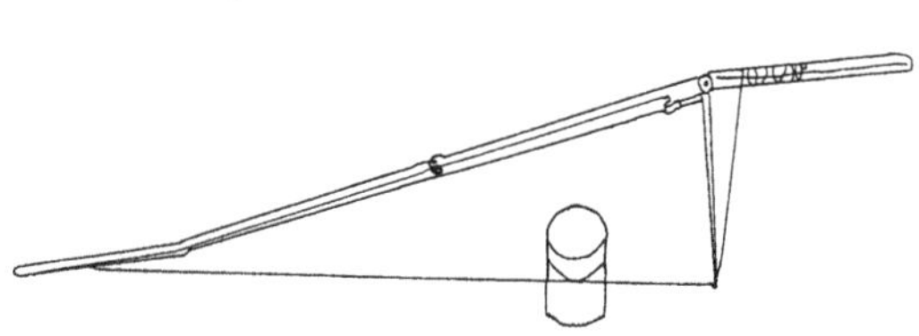

Fig. 112. Trepanning blade with bow (length 340mm). After Jackson 1990: Fig. 5:8.

Two other instruments developed for the removal of implements were mentioned by Celsus. The spoon of Diocles is a much discussed instrument but no positively identifiable example is extant. No examples exist in the archaeological record. Celsus says this instrument was developed to remove wide barbed missiles. According to Celsus the tool was constructed in two parts; one side had a long narrow scoop with a hole in the bottom to catch the pointed end of the missile and the sides of the instrument were turned inwards to keep the barbed ends of the arrow or spear from damaging the flesh upon removal of the weapon. The second part was a smooth blade basically placed behind the unprotected side of the spoon:

> "*Evellendum est ergo genere quodam ferramenti, quod Diocleum cyathiscum Graeci vocant, quonicam auctorem Dioclen habet*" (Cels. 7. 5. 3 A-B).

The second instrument mentioned by Celsus is said to have been shaped like a Greek letter; however there is a lacuna in the text that states which Greek letter it is. It is possible that the letter Celsus was describing was an upsilon (Y) because the description of how the instrument functioned sounds as if it might have been a speculum. The tool was supposed to spread the skin so the doctor could extract the weapon with greater ease:

> "*Sed inde aperta via, caro diduci debet ferramento ad similitudinem facto Graecae litterae ... deinde*" (Cels. 7. 5. 2 B; Jackson 1994b: 189-90).

He also suggests pushing missiles through the rest of their course or through a counter-opening, rather than pulling the missile out through the place where it entered the body:

> "*Saepius itaque ab altera parte, quam ex qua venit, recipienda et praecipue quia fere spiculis cingitur, quae magis laniant, si retrorsus quam si contra eximatur*" (Cels. 7. 5. 2 A-B).

This, he felt, might cause less damage, but how often this procedure was practised cannot be said (Jackson 1994b: 189). It may be expected that these more intricate tools would be found on military sites; however, with the exception of a rectal specula from Vechten, no other has been found, implying that surgeons could probably rely on their standard kit for more procedures.

Tools for bone operations. Operations in relation to broken bones were treated like a craft such as carpentry. Celsus described in book eight of his *de Medicina* the tools used for bone surgery. The tools recommended are often like carpentry tools and Jackson says that there may have been tools for bone surgery made to order, carpentry tools acquired by medical personnel, or carpentry tools used by doctors to make splints (Jackson 1994b: 190-5; Milne 1907: 121-36). The only tool that was found in a military context was the crown trephine, already mentioned for missile removal, from Bingen (Como 1925), and some tools to lift bones (Fig. 113). The crown trephine was used to saw out small discs of carious bone. There were also a few others from the tomb at Bingen four bone levers and an elevator rasp.

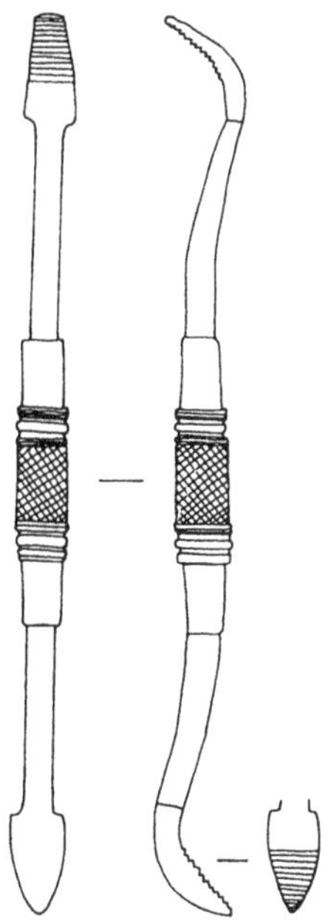

Fig. 113. Bone lever (length 160mm). After Jackson 1990:Fig. 5:6.

The saw was a necessary tool used in amputations, but this practice was only recommended as the final choice in medical emergencies. Overall the tools for bone work are hard to identify because they were more likely to have been made of iron and mistaken for carpentry tools.

APPENDICES FOUR-TEN

TABLES OF MEDICAL INSTRUMENTS FROM EACH OF THE RELEVANT PROVINCES

The following six appendices are lists of medical tools discussed in the main text that were gathered through field-work and publications. The appendices are divided by province. Each is sub-divided further into tables according to fortification, and each instrument has its own entry. The instrument entry provides information about its inventory number, followed by an abbreviation for the museum in which it is located. This is followed by its size and material. Certain fortifications in the main text have a distribution map showing the location of the instrument finds: of Chester, Caerleon, Neuss, Oberstimm, Birdoswald, Housesteads and Vindonissa, The number for these is listed after the provenance. Additional publication information and descriptions are provided when necessary.

Abbreviations for Appendices Four-Ten

CA Copper Alloy
Inv. No. Museum Inventory Number
L Length of the Instrument
Il. Illustration number
PR. Provenance
NA Not Available
E Espérandieu, *Signacula medicorum oculariorum. Corpus Inscriptionum Latinarum* vol. 13, pars 3, fasc 2.
V Voinot, J. 1984. *Inventaire des cachets d'oculistes gallo-romains.*

APPENDIX FOUR

MEDICAL INSTRUMENTS FROM GERMANIA INFERIOR

Abbreviations for Museums

GI 1 Clemens-Sels Museum, Neuss, Germany
GI 2 Rijks Museum van Oudheden, Leiden, The Netherlands
GI 3 Rijks Museum van Oudheden, Nijmegen, The Netherlands
GI 4 Rheinisches Landesmuseum, Bonn, Germany
GI 5 Rheinisches Landesmuseum, Trier, Germany

TABLE A4.1: NEUSS, NOVAESIUM, LEGIONARY FORTRESS (FIG. 22)

1. Scalpel Inv. No. 6024, GI 1, L. NA, CA PR. South Section of the camp Lehner 1904: 401, Nr. 11-Tab. 25 Fig. 31	2. Scalpel Inv. No. 10952, GI 1 L. NA, CA PR *Valetudinarium* Lehner 1904: 401, Nr. 11-Tab 25 Fig. 32	3. Scalpel Inv. No. 11846, GI 1 L. NA, CA PR. NA Lehner 1904: 401, Nr. 11-Tab. 25 Fig. 33
4. Scalpel Inv. No 12660, GI 1 L. NA, CA PR. *Valetudinarium,* Fig. 22, Nr. 1 Lehner 1904: 401	5. Scalpel Inv. No 1365, GI 1 L. 8.5, CA PR. *Valetudinarium,* Fig. 22, Nr. 1 Watermann 1978: Nr. 1 -Tab. 3 Nr. 33	6. Scalpel Inv. No. 1366, GI 1 L. 7.5, CA PR. *Valetudinarium,* Fig. 22, Nr. 1 Watermann 1978: Nr. 2-Tab. 3 Nr. 31
7. Surgical Knife Inv. No. NA, GI 1 L. 12.5, CA PR. NA Watermann 1978: Nr. 20	8. Pterygotom Inv. No. 1383. GI 1 L. NA, CA PR. NA Watermann 1978: Nr. 18-Fig. 7	9. Spatula Probe Inv. No. 8037, GI 1 L. 7.7, CA PR. Barrack 30, Fig. 22, Nr. 7 Lehner 1904: 400, Nr. 1-Tab. 25 Fig. 1
10. Spatula Probe Inv. No. 12607, GI 1 L. NA, CA PR. Building 125, Fig. 22, Nr. 8 Lehner 1904: 400, Nr. 2-Tab. 25 Fig. 2	11. Spatula Probe Inv. No. 12608, GI 1 L. NA, CA PR. Building 125, Fig. 22, Nr. 8 Lehner 1904: 400, Nr. 2-Tab. 25 Fig. 2	12 Spatula Probe Inv. No. 12497, GI 1 L. NA, CA PR. *Valetudinarium,* Fig. 22, Nr. 1 Lehner 1904: 400, Nr. 2-Tab. 25 Fig. 3
13 Spatula Probe Inv. No. 12498, GI 1 L. NA, CA PR. *Valetudinarium,* Fig. 22, Nr. 1 Lehner 1904: 400, Nr. 2-Tab. 25 Fig. 4	14 Spatula Probe Inv. No. 12500, GI 1 L. NA, CA PR. *Valetudinarium,* Fig. 22, Nr. 1 Lehner 1904: 400, Nr. 2 –Tab. 25 Fig.	15 Spatula Probe Inv. No. 12502, GI. 1 L. NA, CA PR. *Valetudinarium,* Fig. 22, Nr. 1 Lehner 1904: 400, Nr. 2-Tab. 25 Fig. 6

Lehner 1904: 400, Nr. 2-Tab. 25 Fig. 4	Lehner 1904: 400, Nr. 2 –Tab. 25 Fig. 5	Lehner 1904: 400, Nr. 2-Tab. 25 Fig. 6
16. Spatula Probe Inv. No. 12503, GI 1 L. NA, CA PR. *Valetudinarium,* Fig. 22, Nr. 1 Lehner 1904: 400, Nr. 2 –Tab. 25 Fig. 7	17. Spatula Probe Inv. No. 10992, GI 1 L. 33.5, CA PR. *Valetudinarium,* Fig. 22, Nr. 1 Lehner 1904: 400, Nr. 5-Tab. 25 Fig. 11	18 Spatula Probe Inv. No. 13272, GI 1 L. NA, CA PR. Hackenberg, outside the fortress Lehner 1904: 400
19. Spatula Probe Inv. No. 6020, GI 1 L. NA, CA PR. NA Lehner 1904: 400	20 Spatula Probe Inv. No. 6610, GI 1 L. NA, CA PR. NA Lehner 1904: 400	21 Spatula Probe Inv. No 9969, GI 1 L. NA, CA PR. NA Lehner 1904: 400
22. Spatula Probe Inv. No 1368, GI 1 L. 14.1, CA PR. NA Watermann 1978: Nr. 13	23. Spatula Probe Inv. No. 1367, GI 1 L. 15.4, CA PR. NA Watermann 1978: Nr. 14	24 Spatula Probe Inv. No. 1364, GI 1 L. 14.3, CA PR. NA Watermann 1978: Nr. 15
25 Spoon Scoop Inv. No. 13749, GI 1 L. 18.3, CA PR. Tribune's House, Fig. 22, Nr. 9 Lehner 1904: 400, Nr. 4-Tab. 25 Fig. 10	26. Spoon Probe Inv. No. 5308, GI 1 L. NA, CA PR. NA Lehner 1904: 400, Nr. 5-Tab. 25	27. Spoon Probe Inv. No. 5405, GI 1 L. NA, CA PR. NA Lehner 1904: 400, Nr. 5
28. Spoon Probe Inv. No. 6021, GI 1 L. NA, CA PR. NA Lehner 1904: 400, Nr. 5	29. Spoon Probe Inv. No. 6022, GI 1 L. NA, CA PR. NA Lehner 1904: 400, Nr. 5	30 Spoon Probe Inv. No 6934, GI 1 L. NA, CA PR. Building 41?, Fig. 22, Nr. 5? Lehner 1904: 400, Nr. 5
31 Spoon Probe Inv. No. 6936, GI 1 L. NA, CA PR. Building 41?, Fig. 22, Nr. 5? Lehner 1904: 400, Nr. 5	32 Spoon Probe Inv. No. 7837, GI I L. NA, CA PR. Barracks 46-52, Fig. 22, Nr. 2 Lehner 1904: 400, Nr. 5	33. Spoon Probe Inv. No. 9670, GI 1 L. NA, CA PR. Provincial Settlement Lehner 1904: 400, Nr. 5
34 Spoon Probe Inv. No. 9671, GI 1 L. NA, CA PR. Provincial Settlement Lehner 1904: 400, Nr. 5	35. Spoon Probe Inv. No. 9968, GI 1 L. NA, CA PR. NA Lehner 1904: 400, Nr. 5	36 Spoon Probe Inv. No. 10627, GI 1 L. NA, CA PR. *Valetudinarium,* Fig. 22, Nr. 1 Lehner 1904: 400, Nr. 5
37 Spoon Probe Inv. No. 12499, GI 1 L. NA, CA PR. *Valetudinarium,* Fig. 22, Nr. 1 Lehner 1904: 400, Nr. 5	38. Spoon Probe Inv. No. 12274, GI 1 L. NA, CA PR. Building 90 *Principia,* Fig. 22, Nr. 3 Lehner 1904: 400, Nr. 5	39 Spoon Probe Inv. No. 13813, GI 1 L. NA, CA PR. N-W Barracks, Fig. 22, Nr.10 Lehner 1904: 400, Nr. 5
40. Spoon Probe Inv. No. 1412, GI I L. 7.0, CA PR. NA Watermann 1978: Nr. 16	41. Spoon Probe Inv. No. NA, GI 1 L. 6.8, CA PR. NA Watermann 1978: Nr. 17	42 Forceps Inv. No. 7929, GI 1 L. 6.4, CA PR. Building 46-52, Fig. 22, Nr. 2 Lehner 1904: 400, Nr. 8-Tab. 25 Fig. 18
43 Forceps Inv. No. 6919, GI 1 L. NA, CA PR. NA Lehner 1904: 400	44. Forceps Inv. No. 10611. GI 1 L. 12.0, CA PR. Building 44, Fig. 22, Nr. 11 Lehner 1904: 400, Nr. 8-Tab. 25 Fig. 19	45. Forceps Inv. No. 1999, GI 1 L. 8.6, CA PR. NA Watermann 1978: Nr. 3
46. Forceps Inv. No. NA, GI 1 L. 8.0, CA PR. NA Watermann 1978: Nr. 4	47. Forceps Inv. No. 1397, GI 1 L. 12 CA PR. NA Watermann 1978: Nr. 5	48. Forceps Inv. No. NA, GI I L. 10.0, CA PR. NA Watermann 1978: Nr. 6
49. Ear Probe Inv. No. 5379, GI 1 L. NA, CA PR. South Section, 1888	50. Ear Probe Inv. No. 5403, GI 1 L. NA, CA PR. South Section, 1888	51 Ear Probe Inv. No. 5404, GI 1 L. NA, CA PR. South Section, 1888

Lehner 1904: 400, Nr. 9	Lehner 1904: 400, Nr. 9	Lehner 1904: 400, Nr. 9
52 Ear Probe Inv. No. 6023, GI 1 L. NA, CA PR. *Principia*, Fig. 22, Nr.3 Lehner 1904: 400, Nr. 9	53. Ear Probe Inv. No. 6226, GI 1 L. NA, CA PR. *Principia*, Fig. 22, Nr. 3 Lehner 1904: 400, Nr. 9	54 Ear Probe Inv. No. 6229, GI 1 L. NA, CA PR. *Principia*, Fig. 22, Nr. 3 Lehner 1904: 400, Nr. 9
55. Ear Probe Inv. No. 6612, GI 1 L. NA, CA PR. *Principia*, Fig. 22, Nr. 3 Lehner 1904: 400, Nr. 9	56 Ear Probe Inv. No. 6613, GI 1 L. NA, CA PR. *Principia*, Fig. 22, Nr. 3 Lehner 1904: 400, Nr. 9	57 Ear Probe Inv. No. 6935, GI 1 L. NA, CA PR. *Principia*, Fig. 22, Nr. 3 Lehner 1904: 400, Nr. 9
58 Ear Probe Inv. No. 7836, GI 1 L. NA, CA PR. Building 46-52, Fig. 22, Nr. 2 Lehner 1904: 400, Nr. 9	59. Ear Probe Inv. No. 7837, GI 1 L. NA, CA PR. Building 46-52, Fig. 22, Nr. 2 Lehner 1904: 400, Nr. 9	60. Ear Probe Inv. No. 8172, GI 1 L. NA, CA PR. Building 46-52, Fig. 22, Nr. 2 Lehner 1904: 400, Nr. 9
61 Ear Probe Inv. No. 8298, GI 1 L. NA, CA PR. NA Lehner 1904: 400, Nr. 9	62. Ear Probe Inv. No. 9275, GI 1 L. NA, CA PR. Building 55, Fig. 22, Nr. 12 Lehner 1904: 400, Nr. 9	63. Ear Probe Inv. No. 9903, GI 1 L. NA, CA PR. Building 88, Fig. 22, Nr. 6 Lehner 1904: 400, Nr. 9
64. Ear Probe Inv. No. 9907, GI 1 L. NA, CA PR. Building 88, Fig. 22, Nr. 6 Lehner 1904: 400, Nr. 9	65 Ear Probe Inv. No. 10622, GI 1 L. NA, CA PR. *Valetudinarium,* Fig. 22, Nr. 1 Lehner 1904: 400, Nr. 9	66. Ear Probe Inv. No. 10623, GI 1 L. NA, CA PR. *Valetudinarium,* Fig. 22, Nr. 1 Lehner 1904: 400, Nr. 9
67 Ear Probe Inv. No. 11778, GI 1 L. NA, CA PR. NA Lehner 1904: 400, Nr. 9	68. Ear Probe Inv. No. 11845, GI 1 L. NA, CA PR. NA Lehner 1904: 400, Nr. 9	69. Ear Probe Inv. No. 12275, GI 1 L. NA, CA PR. Building 60, Fig. 22, Nr. 13 Lehner 1904: 400, Nr. 9
70. 'Scratcher' Inv. No. 1402, GI 1 L. 32.0, CA PR. NA Watermann 1978: Nr. 19	71. Olivary End Probe Inv. No. 1396, GI 1 L. 9.0, CA PR. NA Watermann 1978: Nr. 7	72. Olivary End Probe Inv. No. 1370, GI 1 L. 12.2, CA PR. NA Watermann 1978: Nr. 8
73. Olivary End Probe Inv. No. 1369, GI 1 L. 13.4, CA PR. NA Watermann 1978: Nr. 9	74. Olivary End Probe Inv. No. 1371, GI 1 L. 12.4, CA PR. NA Watermann 1978: Nr. 10	75 Olivary End Probe Inv. No. 1361, GI 1 L. 10.4, CA PR. NA Watermann 1978: Nr. 11
76. Olivary End Probe Inv. No. 1363, GI 1 L. 14.2, CA PR. NA Watermann 1978: Nr. 12	77. Olivary End Probe Inv. No. 7838, GI 1 L. 11.1, CA PR. Building 46-52, Fig. 22, Nr. 2 Lehner 1904: 400, Nr. 7-Tab. 25 Fig. 17	78 Olivary End Probe Inv. No. 6524, GI 1 L. NA, CA PR. NA Lehner 1904: 400, Nr. 3-Tab. 25 Fig. 8
79 Olivary End Probe Inv. No. 11335, GI 1 L. NA, CA PR. NA Lehner 1904: 400, Nr. 3-Tab. 25 Fig. 9	80. Ointment Pallet Inv. No. 5344, GI 1 7.0 x 6.0, Stone PR. NA Lehner 1904: 402, Nr. 13-Tab. 25 Fig. 35 and Watermann 1978: Nr. 21-Fig. 3 Nr. 36	81. Ointment Pallet Inv. No. 6237, GI 1 8.0x5.5, Stone PR. Building 143, Fig. 22, Nr. 14 Lehner 1904: 402, Nr. 13-Tab. 25 Fig. 35 and Watermann 1978: Nr. 22-Fig. 3 Nr. 37
82 Ointment Pallet Inv. No. 6705, GI 1 L. NA, Stone PR. NA Lehner 1904: 402, Nr. 13	83 Ointment Pallet Inv. No. 7736, GI 1 L. NA, Stone PR. Buildings 46-52, Fig. 22, Nr. 2 Lehner 1904: 402, Nr. 13	84 Ointment Pallet Inv. No. 11857, GI 1 8.0 x 6.0 Stone PR. Buildings 18-20, Fig. 22, Nr. 15 Lehner 1904: 402, Nr. 13 and Watermann 1978: Nr. 23-Fig. 3 Fig. 3 Nr. 38

TABLE A4.2: NIJMEGEN, NOVIOMAGUS, LEGIONARY FORTRESS

1. Scalpel	2. Scalpel	3. Scalpel

Inv. No. Nr 2452, NA L. 25.0, CA PR. Hunnerberg Grave 4 Vermeulen 1932: 134-144	Inv. No. Nha 14a, GI 2 L. 10.7, CA PR. Hunnerberg Sarcophagus 1 Künzl 1983: 93, Fig. 74-75	Inv. No. NHa 14b, GI 2 L. NA, CA PR. Hunnerberg Sarcophagus 1 Künzl 1983: 93, Fig. 74-75
4. Scalpel with Iron Blade Inv. No. Nr 16, GI 2 L. NA, CA PR. Nijmegen Sarcophagus Grave 1 Künzl 1983: 93, Fig. 74-75	5. Scalpel with Iron Blade Inv. No. Nr. 17, GI 2 L. NA, CA PR. Nijmegen Sarcophagus Grave 1 Künzl 1983: 93, Fig, 74-75	6. Sharp Hook Inv. No. Nr 11, GI 2 L. NA, CA PR. Nijmegen Sarcophagus Grave 1 Künzl 1983: 93, Fig. 74-75
7. Bifurcated Hook Inv. No. Nr 12, GI 2 L. NA, CA PR. Nijmegen Sarcophagus Grave 1 Künzl 1983: 93, Fig. 74-75	8. Handle for a Double Needle Inv. No. Nr 13, GI 2 L. NA, CA PR. Nijmegen Sarcophagus Grave 1 Künzl 1983: 93, Fig. 74-75	9. Oculist Stamp Inv. No. ID 3, GI 2 3.7 x 3.4, Slate PR. Environs of Nijmegen Braadbaart 1994a: 165, Nr, 1-Pl. 3; Feugère et al 1985: 479, Nr. 9
10. Oculist Stamp Inv. No. NA L. NA PR. NA Feugère, *et al.* 1986: 479, Nr. 10	11. Forceps Inv. No. Nha 10, GI 2 L. NA, CA PR. Hunnerberg 1840, Sarcophagus 1 Künzl 1983: 93, Fig. 74-75	12. Spoon Probe Inv. No. Nr. 367, GI 2 L. NA, CA PR. Hunnerberg, Grave 60 Vermeulen 1932: 134
13. Spoon Probe Inv. No. 235, GI 3 L. NA, CA PR. Nijmegen Sarcophagus Grave 1 Künzl 1983: 97	14. Spoon Probe Broken Inv. No. Nr 14, GI 2 L. 10.7, CA PR. Nijmegen Sarcophagus Künzl 1983: 93, Fig. 74-75	15 Spatula Probe Inv. No. NA, NA L. 11.1, CA PR. Hunnerberg, Grave 8 Vermeulen 1932: 146
16. Spatula Probe Inv. No. NS 273, GI 3 L. 15.8, CA PR. River Waal Braadbaart 1994a: 165. Nr.1-Pl. 4	17. Spatula Probe Inv. No. NAVVY 6, GI 2 L. 15.5, CA PR. Environs of Nijmegen Braadbaart 1994a: 165	18. Medical Box Inv. No. Nr 21, GI 2 L. NA, wood PR. Nijmegen Sarcophagus Grave 1 Künzl 1983: 93, Fig, 74-75
19. Ointment Pallet Inv. No. 235, GI 3 L. NA, Stone PR. Nijmegen Sarcophagus Künzl 1983: 97		

TABLE A4.3: BONN, BONNA, LEGIONARY FORTRESS

1. Scalpel Inv. No. 20840, GI 4 L. 9.5, CA PR. Fabrica Bonner Berg outside fortress van Driel-Murray and Gechter 1984: 62, Nr. 69, Tab. 17	2. Oculist Stamp Inv. No. 2345 a-c, GI 4 3.5x 2.9 Stone PR. Grave on the Heerstrassel Künzl 1983: 86, Pl. 61-62	3. Uvula Forceps Inv. No. NA, GI 4 L. 18.6, CA PR. NA Lindenschmit 1889: Tab. 22 Nr. 7
4. Forceps Inv. No. 22039, GI 4 L. 10.0, CA PR. Stiftplatz Künzl 1986b: 507, C 10	5. Spatula Probe Inv. No. 7291, GI 4 L. 17.75, CA PR. Bonn Künzl 1986b: 507, C 9	6. Spoon Probe Inv. No. 20837, GI 4 L. 16.0, CA PR. Fabrica Bonner Berg outside fortress van Driel-Murray and Gechter 1984: 62, Nr. 70, Tab. 17
7. Ear Probe Inv. Nr. 20841, GI. 4 L. 11.8, CA PR. Fabrica Bonner Berg outside fortress van Driel-Murray and Gechter 1984: 62, Nr. 71, Tab. 18	8. Ear Probe Inv. No. 20842, GI 4 L. 15.7, CA PR. Fabrica Bonner Berg outside fortress van Driel-Murray and Gechter 1984: 62, Nr. 72, Tab. 18	9. Medical box Inv. No. 4786, GI 4 13.9x 7.8x 2.2 PR. Bonn Künzl 1986b: 506, C5

TABLE A4.4: VECHTEN, AUXILIARY FORT

1. Rectal Speculum Inv. No. VF 735, GI 2	2. Scalpel Inv. No. f 1940/5, 11, GI 2	3. Shears Inv. No. VF 687, GI 2

15.5 x 8.2, CA PR. Vechten 1870 Braadbaart 1994a: 164, Nr. 1-Pl. 1	L. 8.8, CA PR. NA Braadbaart 1994a: 164	L. 7.2, CA PR. NA Braadbaart 1994a: 165
4. Spatula Probe Inv. No. VF 674, GI 2 L. 12.4, CA PR. NA Braadbaart 1994a: 165	5. Spatula Probe Inv. No. VF 722, GI 2 L. 17.0, CA PR. NA Braadbaart 1994a: 165	6. Spatula Probe Inv. No. VF 725, GI 2 L. 16.8, CA PR. NA Braadbaart 1994a: 165
7. Spoon Probe Inv. No. VF 679, GI 2 L 16.1, CA PR. Vechten, 1869 Braadbaart 1994a: 166	8. Spoon Probe Inv. No. VF 730, GI 2 L. 13.5, CA PR. Vechten 1870 Braadbaart 1994a: 166	9. Spoon Probe Inv. No. VF 731, GI 2 L. 12.3, CA PR. Vechten 1870 Braadbaart 1994a: 166
10 Spoon Probe Inv. No. VF 732, GI 2 L. 13.4, CA PR. Vechten 1870 Braadbaart 1994a: 166	11 Spoon Probe Inv. No. VF 738, GI 2 L. 16.7, CA PR. Vechten 1871 Braadbaart 1994a: 166	12 Ear Probe Inv. No. VF 677, GI 2 L. 12.0, CA PR. Vechten 1869 Braadbaart 1994a: 167
13. Ear Probe Inv. No. VF 678, GI 2 L. 7.4, CA PR. Vechten 1869 Braadbaart 1994a: 167	14. Ear Probe Inv. No. VF 737, GI 2 L. 7.2, CA PR. Vechten 1870 Braadbaart 1994a: 167	15. Ear Probe Inv. No. f 1940/5 134, GI 2 L. 13.9, CA PR. Vechten 1937 Braadbaart 1994a: 167
13. Ear Probe Inv. No. VF 678, GI 2 L. 7.4, CA PR. Vechten 1869 Braadbaart 1994a: 167	14. Ear Probe Inv. No. VF 737, GI 2 L. 7.2, CA PR. Vechten 1870 Braadbaart 1994a: 167	15. Ear Probe Inv. No. f 1940/5 134, GI 2 L. 13.9, CA PR. Vechten 1937 Braadbaart 1994a: 167
16. Ear Probe Inv. No. f 1940/5. 142, GI 2 L. 14.3, CA PR. Vechten 1937 Braadbaart 1994a: 167. There is a small perpendicular hook on the opposite end of the probe rather than the typical straight blunt point.	17 Olivary End Probe Inv. No. VF 670, GI 2 L. 15.9. CA PR. Vechten 1869 Braadbaart 1994a: 166	

TABLE A4.5: VALKENBURG, AUXILIARY FORT

1. Spatula Probe Inv. No. h 1991/9. 6086, GI 2 L. 22.0, CA PR. NA Braadbaart 1994a: 166	2. Spoon Probe Inv. No. h1991/9.4888, GI 2 L. 18.5, CA PR. NA Braadbaart 1994a: 166
3. Olivary End Probe Inv. No. h 1991/9.5217, GI 2 L. 16.0, CA PR. NA Braadbaart 1994a: 166	4. Ointment Pallet Inv. No. h 1991/9.3686, GI 2 8.9 x 5.7, Lydite PR. NA Braadbaart 1994a: 165

TABLE A4.6: ROSSUM, GRINNES, AUXILIARY FORT

1. Spoon Probe Inv. No. RM 252, GI 2 L. 17.4, CA PR. Rossum 1881 Braadbaart 1994a: 165	2. Ear Probe Inv. No. RM 253, GI 2 L. 11.0, CA PR. NA Braadbaart 1994a: 166

TABLE A4.7: ALPHEN AAN DE RIJN, ALBANIANA, AUXILIARY FORT

1. Spatula Probe Inv. No. h 1991/ 5.808, GI 2 L. 17.0, CA PR. NA

Braadbaart 1994a: 165

TABLE A4.8: KESTEREN, CARVO, AUXILIARY FORT

1. Double Simple Probe Inv. No. e 1892/5.8, GI 2 L. 7.7, CA PR. NA Braadbaart 1994a: 166

TABLE A4.9: XANTEN, CIVILIAN SETTLEMENT

1. Bone Knife Inv. No. NA, GI 5 L. 13.4, Iron and CA PR. Room in the bath Künzl 1986b: 494, 4; Künzl 1989/90: 147	2. Bone Knife Inv. No. NA, GI 5 L. 13.4, Iron and CA PR. Room in the bath Künzl 1986b: 494, 5; Künzl 1989/90 147	3. Scalpel Handle Inv. No. NA, GI 5 L. 9.9 PR. Room in the Bath Künzl 1986b: 493, 1; Künzl 1989/90: 147. The instrument has silver inlay
4. Scalpel Handle Inv. No. NA, GI 5 L. 9.2 PR. Room in the Bath Künzl 1986b: 493, 2; Künzl 1989/90: 147	5. Scalpel Handle Inv. No. NA, GI 5 L. 9.8 PR. Room in the Bath Künzl 1986b: 493, 3; Künzl 1989/90: 147. The instrument has silver inlay	6. Spoon Probe Inv. No. 8561, GI 4 L. 17.5, CA PR. Room in the Civilian Bath Kunzl 1986b: 507, C8. The spoon has Corpirtus fec(it) inscribed on it.

APPENDIX FIVE

MEDICAL INSTRUMENTS FROM GERMANIA SUPERIOR

ABBREVIATIONS FOR MUSEUMS

GS 1 Archäologische Sammlungen im Reiß-Museum der Stadt Mannheim, Germany
GS 2 Römisch-Germanisches Zentralmuseum, Mainz, Germany
GS 3 Vindonissa Museum, Brugg, Switzerland
GS 4 Lobdengau-Museum, Ladenburg, Germany
GS 5 Kurpfälzisches Museum, Heildelberg, Germany
GS 6 Limeskastell und Museum, Saalburg, Germany
GS 7 Städtisches Museum, Wiesbaden, Germany
GS 8 Hessisches Landesmuseum, Darmstadt, Germany
GS 9 Heimatmuseum der Stadt, Bingen, Germany
GS 10 Museum der Stadt, Worms, Germany

TABLE A5.1: MAINZ, MOGONTIACUM, LEGIONARY FORTRESS

1. Scalpel Inv. No. NA, GS 1 L. 11.7, CA PR. NA	2. Scalpel Inv. No. 1, GS 1 L. 9.0, CA PR. NA	3. Surgical Knife Inv. No. NA, GS 2 L. 8.2, CA PR. NA Lindenschmitt 1889: Nr. 12-Tab. 22
4. Bifurcated Hook Inv. No. NA, GS 1 L. 19.8, CA PR. NA	5. Foetal Hook Inv. No. NA, GS 2 L. 7.8, CA PR. NA Lindenschmitt 1889: Nr. 13-Tab. 22	6. Forceps Inv. No. NA, GS 2 L. 12.8, CA PR. NA Lindenschmitt 1889: Nr. 16-Tab. 22
7. Spoon Probe Inv. No. D-339-AV-SLG, GS 1 L. NA, CA PR. NA	8. Spoon Probe Inv. No. NA, GS 1 L. 11.6, Bone PR. NA	9. Spoon Probe Inv. No. D-337-AV-SLG, GS 1 L. NA, CA PR. NA
10. Spoon Probe Inv. No. N 298 D 333, GS 1 L. 15.0, CA PR. NA	11. Spoon Probe Inv. No. NA, GS 2 L. 16.0, CA PR. NA Lindenschmitt 1889 Nr. 10-Tab. 22	12. Spatula Probe Inv. No. D-334-AV-SLG, GS 1 L. 7.61, CA PR. NA
13. Spatula Probe Inv. No. 11530 (27), GS 1 L. 16.5, CA PR. NA	14. Spatula Probe Inv. No. 50, D-338, GS 1 L. 17.8, CA PR. NA	15. Spatula Probe Inv. No. NA, GS 1 L. 14.9, CA PR. NA
16. Spatula Probe Inv. No. NA, GS 2 L. 18.6, CA PR. NA Lindenschmitt 1889: Nr. 15-Tab. 22	17. Needle Inv. No. DI 159, GS 1 L. 17.2, CA PR. NA	18. Needle Inv. No. D 385-AV-SLG, GS 1 L. 15.9, CA PR. NA
19. Needle Inv. No. D 384-AV-SLG, GS 1 L. 14.2, CA PR. NA	20. Needle Inv. No. D 386-AV-SLG, GS 1 L. 8.9, CA PR. NA	21. Needle Inv. No. D-381, GS 2 L. 11.0, CA PR. NA
22. Ear Probe Inv. No. NA, GS 2 L. 8.7, CA PR. NA Lindenschmitt 1889: Nr. 8-Tab. 22	23. Oculist Stamp Inv. No. NA L. NA PR. NA Feugère *et al.* 1985: 479, Nr. 18; E. 163; V. 8	24. Oculist Stamp Inv. No. NA L. NA PR. NA Feugère *et al* 1985: 479, Nr. 19; E. 32; V. 72
25. Oculist Stamp Inv. No. NA L. NA PR. NA Feugère *et al* 1985: 479, Nr. 20; E. 150; V. 164	26. Oculist Stamp Inv. No. NA L. NA PR. NA Feugère *et al* 1985: 479, Nr. 21; V. 226	27. Oculist Stamp Inv. No. NA L. NA Il. 32 PR. NA Feugère *et al* 1985: 479, Nr. 22; V. 278
28. Oculist Stamp Inv. No. NA	29. Oculist Stamp Inv. No. NA	30. Broken Olivary End Probe Inv. No. NA

L. NA PR. NA Feugère *et al* 1985: 479, Nr. 23; V. 279	L. NA PR. NA Feugère *et al* 1985: 481, Nr. 264	L. 11.0, CA PR. NA Behrens and Brenner 1911: 110 Nr. 119
31. Broken Olivary End Probe Inv. No. NA L. 8.2, CA PR. NA Behrens and Brenner 1911: 110 Nr. 123	32. Handle of a Probe Inv. No. NA L. 5.5, CA PR. NA Behrens and Brenner 1911: 110 Nr. 124	33. Broken Spoon Probe Inv. No. NA L. 9.4, CA PR. NA Behrens and Brenner 1911: 110 Nr. 125
34. Broken Forceps Inv. No. NA L. 8.0, CA PR. NA Behrens and Brenner 1911: 110 Nr. 129		

TABLE A5.2: WINDISCH, VINDONISSA, LEGIONARY FORTRESS (FIG. 26)

1. Forceps Inv. No. 3853, GS 3 L. 15.5, Iron PR. Schutthügel, Fig. 26, Nr. 1 Forceps joined together with one screw placed below the forceps' jaws. Döderlein 1973: 410, Pl. 4	2. Forceps Inv. No. 4196, GS 3 L. 17.0, Iron PR. Schutthügel, Fig 26, Nr. 1 Forceps joined together with one screw placed below the forceps' jaws. Frolich 1910: 127, Fig. 17	3. Surgical Knife Inv. No. 31:1341, GS 3 L. 5.0, CA PR. Dätweiler, Fig 26, Nr. 13
4. Scalpel Inv. No. 36:493, GS 3 L. 10.4, CA PR. Breite Fig 26, Nr. 5 The scalpel has a spoon on its handle, rather than a blunt dissector.	5. Scalpel Inv. No. 35:1121, GS 3 L. 10.0, CA PR. Breite, Fig 26, Nr. 8	6. Scalpel Inv. No. 35:1313, GS 3 L. 7.5, CA PR. Breite, Fig 26, Nr. 8
7. Scalpel Inv. No. 18:08, GS 3 L. 9.4, CA PR. Meier Excavation, NA	8. Scalpel Inv. No. 32:2738, GS 3 L. 7.8, CA PR. Breite, Fig 26, Nr. 6	9. Scalpel Inv. No. 33:801, GS 3 L. 7.11, CA PR. NA
10. Scalpel Inv. No. 1938:64, GS 3 L. 7.0, CA PR. Breite, Fig 26, Nr. 4	11. Forceps Inv. No. 28:1882, GS 3 L. 9.6, CA PR. Breite, Spillmann, Fig 26, Nr. 16 There are jagged teeth on the forceps.	12. Forceps Inv. No, 22:08, GS 3 L. 11.7, CA PR. Schutthügel, Fig 26, Nr. 1
13. Forceps Inv. No. 36:433, GS 3 L. 14.6, CA PR. Breite, Fig 26, Nr. 5	14. Forceps Inv. No. 2190 g, GS 3 L. NA, CA PR. Schutthügel, Fig 26, Nr. 1	15. Forceps Inv. No. 13:810, GS 3 L. 13.0, CA PR. Schutthügel, Fig 26, Nr. 1 There is an ear probe attached to the top of the forceps
16. Forceps Inv. No. 3369, GS 3 L. 12.5, CA PR. Schutthügel, Fig 26, Nr. 1 There is an ear probe attached to the top of the forceps	17. Forceps Inv. No. KAA 369.1, GS 3 L. NA, CA PR. NA	18. Forceps Inv. No. KAA 369.4, GS 3 L. NA, CA PR. NA
19. Forceps Inv. No. 23:365, GS 3 L. 12.6, CA PR. Schutthügel (west), Fig 26, Nr. 1 There is a clamp to hold the ends together; it has jagged teeth that are turned inwards.	20. Spoon Probe Inv. No. 2183, GS 3 L. 18.2, CA PR. Schutthügel, Fig 26, Nr. 1	21. Spoon Probe Inv. No. 1937:3087, GS 3 L. 14.6, CA PR. Breite, Fig 26, Nr. 3
22. Spoon Probe Inv. No. 34:1910, GS 3 L. 17.4, CA	23. Spoon Probe Inv. No. 35:600, GS 3 L. 17.8, CA	24. Spoon Probe Inv. No. 33:5945, GS 3 L. 14.2, CA

PR. Breite, Fig 26, Nr. 10	PR. Breite, Fig 26, Nr. 10	PR. Breite, Fig 26, Nr. 9
25. Spoon Probe Inv. No. NA, GS 3 L. 18.4, CA PR. NA	26. Spoon Probe Inv. No. NA, GS 3 L. 17.0, CA PR. NA	27. Spoon Probe Broken Inv. No. 23:529, GS 3 L. NA, CA PR. Schutthügel, Fig 26, Nr. 1
28. Spoon Probe Broken Inv. No. 2183, GS 3 L. NA, CA PR. Schutthügel, Fig 26, Nr. 1	29. Spoon Probe Broken Inv. No. 2183.41, GS 3 L. NA, CA PR. Schutthügel, Fig 26, Nr. 1	30. Spoon Probe Broken Inv. No. 2183.39, GS 3 L. NA, CA PR. Schutthügel, Fig 26, Nr. 1
31. Spoon Probe Broken Inv. No. 23:1145, GS 3 L. NA, CA PR. Schutthügel, Fig 26, Nr. 1	32. Spoon Probe Broken Inv. No. 23:361, GS 3 L. NA, CA PR. NA	33. Spoon Probe Broken Inv. No. 23:433, GS 3 L. 17.2, CA PR. Schutthügel (west), Fig 26, Nr. 1
34. Spoon Probe Broken Inv. No. 23:407, GS 3 L. 14.3, CA PR. Schutthügel (east), Fig 26, Nr. 1	35. Spoon Probe Broken Inv. No. 23:399, GS 3 L. 15.9, CA PR. Schutthügel (west), Fig 26, Nr. 1	36. Spoon Probe Broken Inv. No. 23.395, GS 3 L. 15.3, CA PR. Schutthügel (east), Fig 26, Nr. 1
37. Spoon Probe Broken Inv. No. 23.395, GS 3 L. NA, CA PR. Schutthügel (east), Fig 26, Nr. 1	38. Spoon Probe Broken Inv. No. 23.5, GS 3 L. 12.9, CA PR. Schutthügel, Fig 26, Nr. 1	39. Spoon Probe Broken Inv. No. 36.479, GS 3 L. NA, CA PR. Breite, Fig 26, Nr. 5
40. Spoon Probe Broken Inv. No. 38.459, GS 3 L. NA, CA PR. NA	41. Spoon Probe Broken Inv. No. 35.511, GS 3 L. NA, CA PR. NA	42. Spoon Probe Broken Inv. No. 17.553, GS 3 L. NA, CA PR. NA
43. Spoon Probe Broken Inv. No. 21.78, GS 3 L. NA, CA PR. Schutthügel, Fig 26, Nr. 1	44. Spoon Probe Broken Inv. No. 19670, GS 3 L. NA, CA PR. Schutthügel, Fig 26, Nr. 1	45. Spoon Probe Broken Inv. No. 21:79, GS 3 L. NA, CA PR. Schutthügel, Fig 26, Nr. 1
46. Spoon Probe Broken Inv. No. 13.831, GS 3 L. NA, CA PR. Schutthügel, Fig 26, Nr. 1	47. Spoon Probe Broken Inv. No. 14.81, GS 3 L. NA, CA PR. NA	48. Spoon Probe Broken Inv. No. 16.361, GS 3 L. NA, CA PR. Schutthügel, Fig 26, Nr. 1
49. Spoon Probe Broken Inv. No. 2193b, GS 3 L. 15.9, CA PR. NA	50. Spoon Probe Broken Inv. No. 2193c, GS 3 L. 14.1, CA PR. NA	51. Spoon Probe Broken Inv. No. 2193I, GS 3 L. NA, CA PR. Schutthügel, Fig 26, Nr. 1
52. Spoon Probe Broken Inv. No. 2193d, GS 3 L. 13.8, CA PR. Schutthügel, Fig 26, Nr. 1	53. Spoon Probe Broken Inv. No. 2193f, GS 3 L. NA, CA PR. Schutthügel, Fig 26, Nr. 1	54. Spoon Probe Broken Inv. No. 2193h, GS 3 L. NA, CA PR. NA
55. Spoon Probe Broken Inv. No. KAA 370.7, GS 3 L. NA, CA PR. NA	56. Spoon Probe Broken Inv. No. KAA 370.11, GS 3 L. NA, CA PR. NA	57. Spoon Probe Broken Inv. No. 2193g, GS 3 L. NA, CA PR. NA
58. Spoon Probe Broken Inv. No. 2193e, GS 3 L. NA, CA PR. Schutthügel, Fig 26, Nr. 1	59. Spoon Probe Broken Inv. No. 575, GS 3 L. NA, CA PR. NA	60. Spoon Probe Broken Inv. No. 61.1733, GS 3 L. NA, CA PR. Königsfelden, Fig 26, Nr. 19
61. Spoon Probe Broken Inv. No. 61.2087, GS 3 L. NA, CA PR. Königsfelden, Fig 26, Nr. 19	62. Spoon Probe Broken Inv. No. 63.1622, GS 3 L. NA, CA PR. Königsfelden, Fig 26, Nr. 20	63. Spoon Probe Broken Inv. No. 66.522, GS 3 L. NA, CA PR. Breite, Fig 26, Nr. 21
64. Spoon Probe Broken Inv. No. 67.5104, GS 3 L. NA, CA PR. NA	65. Spoon Probe Broken Inv. No. 27.25, GS 3 L. NA, CA PR. NA	66. Spoon Probe Broken Inv. No. 28:2302, GS 3 L. NA, CA PR. Schutthügel, Fig 26, Nr. 1
67. Spoon Probe Broken Inv. No. 29:979, GS 3 L. NA, CA PR. Breite, Spillmann, Fig 26, Nr. 18	68. Spoon Probe Broken Inv. No. 25:240, GS 3 L. NA, CA PR. Breite, Spillmann, Fig 26, Nr. 15	69. Spoon Probe Broken Inv. No. 31:1587, GS 3 L. NA, CA PR. Dätweiler, Fig 26, Nr. 13

70. Spoon Probe Broken Inv. No. 52.63, GS 3 L. NA, CA PR. Schutthügel, Fig 26, Nr. 1	71. Spoon Probe Broken Inv. No. 52.78, GS 3 L. NA, CA PR. Schutthügel, Fig 26, Nr. 1	72. Spoon Probe Broken Inv. No. 52.92, GS 3 L. NA, CA PR. Schutthügel, Fig 26, Nr. 1
73. Spoon Probe Broken Inv. No. 52.99, GS 3 L. NA, CA PR. Schutthügel, Fig 26, Nr. 1	74. Spoon Probe Broken Inv. No. 55.9, GS 3 L. NA, CA PR. Schutthügel, Fig 26, Nr. 1	75. Spoon Probe Broken Inv. No. 55.105, GS 3 L. NA, CA PR. Schutthügel, Fig 26, Nr. 1
76. Spoon Probe Broken Inv. No. 59.8, GS 3 L. NA, CA PR. NA	77. Spoon Probe Broken Inv. No. 59.1867, GS 3 L. NA, CA PR. NA	78. Spoon Probe Bent Inv. No. 1879, GS 3 L. NA, CA PR. Portier Haus I, NA
79. Spoon Probe Bent Inv. No. 995, GS 3 L. NA, CA PR. NA	80. Spoon Probe Bent Inv. No. 507, GS 3 L. 13.1, CA PR. NA	81. Spoon Probe Bent Inv. No. 13.809, GS 3 L. NA, CA PR. NA
82. Spatula Probe Inv. No. 23:307, GS 3 L. 19.5, CA PR. Schutthügel (east), Fig 26, Nr. 1	83. Spatula Probe Inv. No. 36:1038, GS 3 L. 18.2, CA PR. Breite, Fig 26, Nr. 5	84. Spatula Probe Inv. No. 2345, GS 3 L. 18.5, CA PR. Schutthügel, Fig 26, Nr. 1
85. Spatula Probe Inv. No. 52.102, GS 3 L. 17.9, CA PR. Schutthügel, Fig 26, Nr. 1	86. Spatula Probe Inv. No. 4176, GS 3 L. 14.4, CA PR. Schutthügel, Fig 26, Nr. 1	87. Spatula Probe Inv. No. 1940.4, GS 3 L. 16.9, CA PR. NA
88. Spatula Probe Inv. No. 36.49.4, GS 3 L. 18.7, CA PR. Breite, Fig 26, Nr. 5	89. Spatula Probe Inv. No. 2945, GS 3 L. 18.5, CA PR. NA	90. Spatula Probe Inv. No. 260E, GS 3 L. 13.9, CA PR. Wernly-Acker Windisch, NA
91. Spatula Probe Inv. No. 23:324, GS 3 L. 19.9, CA PR. Schutthügel (west), Fig 26, Nr. 1	92. Spatula Probe Inv. No. 56:204, GS 3 L. 19.8, CA PR. Breite, Fig 26, Nr. 12 The handle is hollow and has a circular opening (4 mm wide) instead of an olivary probe.	93. Spatula Probe Inv. No. 23:427, GS 3 L. 14.6, CA PR. Schutthügel (west), Fig 26, Nr. 1
94. Spatula Probe Inv. No. 35:1063, GS 3 L. 11.0, CA PR. Breite, Fig 26, Nr. 8	95. Spatula Probe Inv. No. 996, GS 3 L. 12.3, CA PR. NA	96. Spatula Probe Inv. No. 23:2894, GS 3 L. 16.4, CA PR. NA
97. Spatula Probe Broken Inv. No. 36:530, GS 3 L. 10.9, CA PR. Breite, Fig 26, Nr. 5	98. Spatula Probe Broken Inv. No. 55.83, GS 3 L. NA, CA PR. Schutthügel, Fig 26, Nr. 1	99. Spatula Probe Broken Inv. No. 55.85, GS 3 L. NA, CA PR. Schutthügel, Fig 26, Nr. 1
100. Spatula Probe Broken Inv. No. 52:297, GS 3 L. 3.0, CA PR. Schutthügel, Fig 26, Nr. 1	101. Spatula Probe Broken Inv. No. 1376, GS 3 L. 5.0, CA PR. NA	102. Spatula Probe Broken Inv. No. 1373, GS 3 L. 6.0, CA PR. NA
103. Spatula Probe Broken Inv. No. 1370, GS 3 L. 4.9, CA PR. NA	104. Spatula Probe Broken Inv. No. 1377, GS 3 L. NA, CA PR. NA	105. Spatula Probe Broken Inv. No. 1374, GS 3 L. 4.5, CA PR. NA
106. Spatula Probe Broken Inv. No. 1375, GS 3 L. NA, CA PR. NA	107. Spatula Probe Broken Inv. No. 263 g, GS 3 L. 5.9, CA PR. NA	108. Spatula Probe Broken Inv. No. 262 g, GS 3 L. 5.0, CA PR. NA
109. Spatula Probe Broken Inv. No. NA, GS 3 L. 13.5, CA PR. NA	110. Spatula Probe Broken Inv. No. 55.51, GS 3 L. 23.2, CA PR. Schutthügel, Fig 26, Nr. 1	111. Spatula Probe Broken Inv. No. 69.221, GS 3 L. 13.9, CA PR. Windisch, Friedhof, Fig 26, Nr. 22 It has AeICO FECIT inscribed on it.
112. Spatula Probe Broken Inv. No. 62.1006, GS 3	113. Spatula Probe Broken Inv. No. 31:1687, GS 3	114. Spatula Probe Broken Inv. No. 61.2737, GS 3

L. NA, CA PR. NA	L. 14.4, CA PR. Dätweiler, Fig 26, Nr. 12	L. NA, CA PR. Königsfelden, Fig 26, Nr. 19
115. Spatula Probe Broken Inv. No. 35:1101, GS 3 L. 5.0, CA PR. Breite, Fig 26, Nr. 8	116. Spatula Probe Broken Inv. No. 35:669, GS 3 L. 6.0, CA PR. Breite, Fig 26, Nr. 8	117. Spatula Probe Broken Inv. No. 35:819, GS 3 L. 7.6, CA PR. Breite, Fig 26, Nr. 8
118. Spatula Probe Broken Inv. No. KAA 370.9, GS 3 L. NA, CA PR. NA	119. Spatula Probe Broken Inv. No. 27:209, GS 3 L. NA, CA PR. Breite, Spillmann, Fig 26, Nr. 19	120. Spatula Probe Broken Inv. No. 23.361, GS 3 L. NA, CA PR. Schutthügel, Fig 26, Nr. 1
121. Spatula Probe Broken Inv. No. 28:3646, GS 3 L. NA, CA PR. Breite, Spillmann, Fig 26, Nr. 16	122. Spatula Probe Broken Inv. No. 5455, GS 3 L. NA, CA PR. Schutthügel, Fig 26, Nr. 1	123. Spatula Probe Broken Inv. No. 6846, GS 3 L. NA, CA PR. Schutthügel, Fig 26, Nr. 1
124. Spatula Probe Bent Inv. No. 35:765, GS 3 L. 16.5, CA PR. Breite, Fig 26, Nr. 8	125. Spatula Probe Bent Inv. No. 52.563, GS 3 L. 16.8, CA PR. Schutthügel, Fig 26, Nr. 1	126. Ear Probe Inv. No. KAA 365.5, GS 3 L. 15.9, CA PR. NA
127. Ear Probe Inv. No. KAA 365.7, GS 3 L. 15.5, CA PR. NA	128. Ear Probe Inv. No. KAA 365.6, GS 3 L. 15.6, CA PR. NA	129. Ear Probe Inv. No. KAA 367.1, GS 3 L. NA, CA PR. NA
130. Ear Probe Inv. No. KAA 367.2, GS 3 L. NA, CA PR. NA	131. Ear Probe Inv. No. KAA 367.8, GS 3 L. NA, CA PR, NA	132. Ear Probe Inv. No. KAA 367.4, GS 3 L. NA, CA PR. NA
133. Ear Probe Inv. No. KAA 367.5, GS 3 L. NA, CA PR. NA	134. Ear Probe Inv. No. KAA 367.9, GS 3 L. NA, CA PR. NA	135. Ear Probe Inv. No. KAA 367.10, GS 3 L. NA, CA PR. NA
136. Ear Probe Inv. No. KAA 367.11, GS 3 L. NA, CA PR. NA	137. Ear Probe Inv. No. KAA 367.7, GS 3 L. NA, CA PR. NA	138. Ear Probe Inv. No. 55:100, GS 3 L. NA, CA PR. NA
139. Ear Probe Inv. No. NA, GS 3 L. NA, CA PR. NA	140. Ear Probe Inv. No. NA, GS 3 L. NA, CA PR. NA	141. Ear Probe Inv. No. NA, GS 3 L. NA, CA PR. NA
142. Ear Probe Inv. No. NA, GS 3 L. NA, CA PR. NA	143. Ear Probe Inv. No. NA, GS 3 L. NA, CA PR. NA	144. Ear Probe Inv. No. NA, GS 3 L. NA, CA PR. NA
145. Ear Probe Inv. No. NA, GS 3 L. NA, CA PR. NA	146. Ear Probe Inv. No. NA, GS 3 L. NA, CA PR. NA	147. Ear Probe Inv. No. NA, GS 3 L. NA, CA PR. NA
148. Ear Probe Inv. No. NA, GS 3 L. NA, CA PR. NA	149. Ear Probe Inv. No. 34:2844, GS 3 L. NA, CA PR. Breite, Fig 26, Nr. 10	150. Ear Probe Inv. No. 33:1667, GS 3 L. NA, CA PR. Breite, Fig 26, Nr. 7
151. Ear Probe Inv. No. 35:1333, GS 3 L. NA, CA PR. Breite, Fig 26, Nr. 8	152. Ear Probe Inv. No. 35:672, GS 3 L. NA, CA PR. Breite, Fig 26, Nr. 8	153. Ear Probe Inv. No. 35:327, GS 3 L. NA, CA PR. Breite, Fig 26, Nr. 8
154. Ear Probe Inv. No. 35:1129, GS 3 L. NA, CA PR. Breite, Fig 26, Nr. 8 It has a hook on its end rather than a point.	155. Ear Probe Inv. No. 52:562, GS 3 L. NA, CA PR. NA	156. Ear Probe Inv. No. 38:44, GS 3 L. NA, CA PR. Breite, Fig 26, Nr. 2
157. Ear Probe Inv. No. 40.12, GS 3 L. NA, CA	158. Ear Probe Inv. No. 42.193, GS 3 L. NA, CA	159. Ear Probe Inv. No. 42.195, GS 3 L. NA, CA

PR. NA	PR. NA	PR. NA
160. Ear Probe Inv. No. 42.196, GS 3 L. NA, CA PR. NA	161. Ear Probe Inv. No. 52.96, GS 3 L. NA, CA PR. NA	162. Ear Probe Inv. No. 52.87, GS 3 L. NA, CA PR. NA
163. Ear Probe Inv. No. NA, GS 3 L. NA, CA PR. NA	164. Ear Probe Inv. No. NA, GS 3 L. NA, CA PR. NA	165. Ear Probe Inv. No. NA, GS 3 L. NA, CA PR. NA
166. Ear Probe Inv. No. NA, GS 3 L. NA, CA PR. NA	167. Ear Probe Inv. No. NA, GS 3 L. NA, CA PR. NA	168. Ear Probe Inv. No. NA, GS 3 L. NA, CA PR. NA
169. Ear Probe Inv. No. NA, GS 3 L. NA, CA PR. NA	170. Ear Probe Inv. No. NA, GS 3 L. NA, CA PR. NA	171. Ear Probe Inv. No. NA, GS 3 L. NA, CA PR. NA
172. Ear Probe Inv. No. NA, GS 3 L. NA, CA PR. NA	173. Ear Probe Inv. No. NA, GS 3 L. NA, CA PR. NA	174. Ear Probe Inv. No. 5.101, GS 3 L. NA, CA PR. NA
175. Ear Probe Inv. No. 36.389, GS 3 L. NA, CA PR. Breite, Fig 26, Nr. 5	176. Ear Probe Inv. No. 36.39, GS 3 L. NA, CA PR. Breite, Fig 26, Nr. 5	177. Ear Probe Inv. No. 36.391, GS 3 L. NA, CA PR. Breite, Fig 26, Nr. 5
178. Ear Probe Inv. No. 36.395, GS 3 L. NA, CA PR. Breite, Fig 26, Nr. 5	179. Ear Probe Inv. No/ 36.397, GS 3 L. NA, CA PR. Breite, Fig 26, Nr. 5	180. Ear Probe Inv. No. 36.689, GS 3 L. NA, CA PR. Breite, Fig 26, Nr. 5
181. Ear Probe Inv. No. 37.3064, GS 3 L. NA, CA PR. Breite, Fig 26, Nr. 3	182. Ear Probe Inv. No. 37.3171, GS 3 L. NA, CA PR. Breite, Fig 26, Nr. 3	183. Ear Probe Inv. No. 28.1149, GS 3 L. NA, CA PR. Breite, Spillmann, Fig 26, Nr. 16
184. Ear Probe Inv. No. 27.32, GS 3 L. NA, CA PR. Breite, Spillmann, Fig 26, Nr. 17	185. Ear Probe Inv. No. 29.2583, GS 3 L. NA, CA PR. Breite, Spillmann, Fig 26, Nr. 18	186. Ear Probe Inv. No. 29.2586, GS 3 L. NA, CA PR. Breite, Spillmann, Fig 26, Nr. 18
187. Ear Probe Inv. No. 28.1829, GS 3 L. NA, CA PR. Breite, Spillmann, Fig 26, Nr. 3	188. Ear Probe Inv. No. 29.1109, GS 3 L. NA, CA PR. Breite Spillmann, Fig 26, Nr. 18	189. Ear Probe Inv. No. 29.2042, GS 3 L. NA, CA PR. Breite, Spillmann Fig 26, Nr. 18
190. Ear Probe Inv. No. 29.111O, GS 3 L. NA, CA PR. Breite, Spillmann, Fig 26, Nr. 18	191. Ear Probe Inv. No. 33.101, GS 3 L. NA, CA PR. Breite, Fig 26, Nr. 7	192. Ear Probe Inv. No. 33.289, GS 3 L. NA, CA PR. Breite, Fig 26, Nr. 7
193. Ear Probe Inv. No. 32.857, GS 3 L. NA, CA PR. Breite, Fig 26, Nr. 6	194. Ear Probe Inv. No. 31.1068, GS 3 L. NA, CA PR. Breite, Fig 26, Nr. 13	195. Ear Probe Inv. No. 31.1819, GS 3 L. NA, CA PR. Breite, Fig 26, Nr. 13
196. Ear Probe Inv. No. 31.1556, GS 3 L. NA, CA PR. Breite, Fig 26, Nr. 13	197. Ear Probe Inv. No. 33.31, GS 3 L. NA, CA PR. Breite, Fig 26, Nr. 7	198. Ear Probe Inv. No. 33.27, GS 3 L. NA, CA PR. Breite, Fig 26, Nr. 7
199. Ear Probe Inv. No. 55.138, GS 3 L. NA, Bone PR. Schutthügel, Fig 26, Nr. 1	200. Ear Probe Inv. No. 51.276, GS 3 L. NA, CA PR. NA	201. Ear Probe Inv. No. 55.137, GS 3 L. NA, CA PR. NA
202. Ear Probe Inv. No. 2183.26, GS 3 L. NA, CA PR. NA	203. Ear Probe Inv. No. 2183.42, GS 3 L. NA, CA PR. NA	204. Ear Probe Inv. No. 2183.44, GS 3 L. NA, CA PR. NA

205. Ear Probe Inv. No. 2183.5O, GS 3 L. NA, CA PR. NA	206. Ear Probe Inv. No. 2183.51, GS 3 L. NA, CA PR. NA	207. Ear Probe Inv. No. 2183.52, GS 3 L. NA, CA PR. NA
208. Ear Probe Inv. No. 2183.53, GS 3 L. NA, CA PR. NA	209. Ear Probe Inv. No. 2183.54, GS 3 L. NA, CA PR. NA	210. Ear Probe Inv. No. 2183.45, GS 3 L. NA, CA PR. NA
211. Ear Probe Inv. No. 2183.46, GS 3 L. NA, CA PR. NA	212. Ear Probe Inv. No. 2183.47, GS 3 L. NA, CA PR. NA	213. Ear Probe Inv. No. 2183.48, GS 3 L. NA, CA PR. NA
214. Ear Probe Inv. No. 2183.49, GS 3 L. NA, CA PR. NA	215. Ear Probe Inv. No. 2183.12, GS 3 L. NA, CA PR. NA	216. Ear Probe Inv. No. 2183.3, GS 3 L. NA, CA PR. NA
217. Ear Probe Inv. No. 2183.4, GS 3 L. NA, CA PR. NA	218. Ear Probe Inv. No. 2183.5, GS 3 L. NA, CA PR. NA	219. Ear Probe Inv. No. 2183.6, GS 3 L. NA, CA PR. NA
220. Ear Probe Inv. No. 2183.7, GS 3 L. NA, CA PR. NA	221. Ear Probe Inv. No. 2183.8, GS 3 L. NA, CA PR. NA	222. Ear Probe Inv. No. 2183.9, GS 3 L. NA, CA PR. NA
223. Ear Probe Inv. No. 2183.10, GS 3 L. NA, CA PR. NA	224. Ear Probe Inv. No. 2183.11, GS 3 L. NA, CA PR. NA	225. Ear Probe Inv. No. 2183.13, GS 3 L. NA, CA PR. NA
226. Ear Probe Inv. No. 5121, GS 3 L. NA, CA PR. NA	227. Ear Probe Inv. No. 5393, GS 3 L. NA, CA PR. NA	228. Ear Probe Inv. No. 4181, GS 3 L. NA, CA PR. NA
229. Ear Probe Inv. No. 5059, GS 3 L. NA, CA PR. NA	230. Ear Probe Inv. No. 5048, GS 3 L. NA, CA PR. NA	231. Ear Probe Inv. No. 2193.1, GS 3 L. NA, CA PR. NA
232. Ear Probe Inv. No. 2193.11, GS 3 L. NA, CA PR. NA	233. Ear Probe Inv. No. 2193.12, GS 3 L. NA, CA PR. NA	234. Ear Probe Inv. No. 2193.14, GS 3 L. NA, CA PR. NA
235. Ear Probe Inv. No. 2193.15, GS 3 L. NA, CA PR. NA	236. Ear Probe Inv. No. 2193.16, GS 3 L. NA, CA PR. NA	237. Ear Probe Inv. No. 2193.17, GS 3 L. NA, CA PR. NA
238. Ear Probe Inv. No. 2193.18, GS 3 L. NA, CA PR. NA	239. Ear Probe Inv. No. 2193.19, GS 3 L. NA, CA PR. NA	240. Ear Probe Inv. No. 2193.20, GS 3 L. NA, CA PR. NA
241. Ear Probe Inv. No. 1512, GS 3 L. NA, CA PR. NA	242. Ear Probe Inv. No. 1544, GS 3 L. NA, CA PR. NA	243. Ear Probe Inv. No. 1746, GS 3 L. NA, CA PR. NA
244. Ear Probe Inv. No. 2914.17, GS 3 L. NA, CA PR. NA	245. Ear Probe Inv. No. 3773, GS 3 L. NA, CA PR. NA	246. Ear Probe Inv. No. 5059, GS 3 L. NA, CA PR. NA
247. Ear Probe Inv. No. 5393, GS 3 L. NA, CA PR. NA	248. Ear Probe Inv. No. 9006, GS 3 L. NA, CA PR. NA	249. Ear Probe Inv. No. 5394, GS 3 L. NA, CA PR. Schutthügel, Fig 26, Nr. 1
250. Ear Probe Inv. No. 6876, GS 3 L. NA, CA PR. NA	251. Ear Probe Inv. No. 25 IG, GS 3 L. NA, CA PR. NA	252. Ear Probe Inv. No. 260C, GS 3 L. NA, CA PR. NA
253. Ear Probe	254. Ear Probe	255. Ear Probe

Inv. No. 2609, GS 3 L. NA, CA PR. NA	Inv. No. 263H, GS 3 L. NA, CA PR. NA	Inv. No. 569, GS 3 L. NA, CA PR. NA
256. Ear Probe Inv. No. 574, GS 3 L. NA, CA PR. NA	257. Ear Probe Inv. No. 928, GS 3 L. NA, CA PR. NA	258. Ear Probe Inv. No. 1200, GS 3 L. NA, CA PR. NA
259. Ear Probe Inv. No. 21.93, GS 3 L. NA, CA PR. Fig 26, Nr. 19	260. Ear Probe Inv. No. 3772, GS 3 L. NA, CA PR. NA	261. Ear Probe Inv. No. 4181, GS 3 L. NA, CA PR. NA
262. Ear Probe Inv. No. 5048, GS 3 L. NA, CA PR. Schutthügel, Fig 26, Nr. 1	263. Ear Probe Inv. No. 4271, GS 3 L. NA, CA PR. NA	264. Ear Probe Inv. No. 4272, GS 3 L. NA, CA PR. NA
265. Ear Probe Inv. No. 4505, GS 3 L. NA, CA PR. NA	266. Ear Probe Inv. No. 5055, GS 3 L. NA, CA PR. Schutthügel, Fig 26, Nr. 1	267. Ear Probe Inv. No. 5056, GS 3 L. NA, CA PR. Schutthügel, Fig 26, Nr. 1
268. Ear Probe Inv. No. 5057, GS 3 L. NA, CA PR. Schutthügel, Fig 26, Nr. 1	269. Ear Probe Inv. No. 5058, GS 3 L. NA, CA PR. NA	270. Ear Probe Inv. No. 5395, GS 3 L. NA, CA PR. NA
271. Ear Probe Inv. No. 5396, GS 3 L. NA, CA PR. NA	272. Ear Probe Inv. No. 5121, GS 3 L. NA, CA PR. NA	273. Ear Probe Inv. No. ST 2, GS 3 L. NA, CA PR. NA
274. Ear Probe Inv. No. ST 3, GS 3 L. NA, CA PR. NA	275. Ear Probe Inv. No. ST 4, GS 3 L. NA, CA PR. NA	276. Ear Probe Inv. No. ST 5, GS 3 L. NA, CA PR. NA
277. Ear Probe Inv. No. ST 6, GS 3 L. NA, CA PR. NA	278. Ear Probe Inv. No. ST 7, GS 3 L. NA, CA PR. NA	279. Ear Probe Inv. No. ST 8, GS 3 L. NA, CA PR. NA
280. Ear Probe Inv. No. ST 9, GS 3 L. NA, CA PR. NA	281. Ear Probe Inv. No. 13.548, GS 3 L. NA, CA PR. Dätweiler 1913, Fig 26, Nr. 2	282. Ear Probe Inv. No. 20.86, GS 3 L. NA, CA PR. NA
283. Ear Probe Inv. No. 6842, GS 3 L. NA, CA PR. NA	284. Ear Probe Inv. No. 12841, GS 3 L. NA, CA PR. NA	285. Ear Probe Inv. No. 13104, GS 3 L. NA, CA PR. NA
286. Ear Probe Inv. No. 13.548, GS 3 L. NA, CA PR. Fig 26, Nr. 3	287. Ear Probe Inv. No. 5120, GS 3 L. NA, CA PR. NA	288. Ear Probe Inv. No. 6843, GS 3 L. NA, CA PR. NA
289. Ear Probe Inv. No. 25:76, GS 3 L. NA, CA PR. Breite, Spillmann, Fig 26, Nr. 15	290. Ear Probe Inv. No. 25:218, GS 3 L. NA, CA PR. Breite, Spillmann, Fig 26, Nr. 15	291. Ear Probe Inv. No. 25:2355, GS 3 L. NA, CA PR. Breite, Spillmann, Fig 26, Nr. 15
292. Ear Probe Inv. No. 19.435, GS 3 L. NA, CA PR. NA	293. Ear Probe Inv. No. 19.669, GS 3 L. NA, CA PR. NA	294. Ear Probe Inv. No. 21.388, GS 3 L. NA, CA PR. Südtor, Fig 26, Nr. 14
295. Ear Probe Inv. No. 22.18O, GS 3 L. NA, CA PR. NA	296. Ear Probe Inv. No. 18.2OO, GS 3 L. NA, CA PR. NA	297. Ear Probe Inv. No. 23.28O, GS 3 L. NA, CA PR. NA
298. Ear Probe Inv. No. 23.33O, GS 3 L. NA, CA PR. NA	299. Ear Probe Inv. No. 23.429, GS 3 L. NA, CA PR. NA	300. Ear Probe Inv. No. 23.534, GS 3 L. NA, CA PR. NA
301. Ear Probe	302. Ear Probe	303. Ear Probe

Inv. No. 23.434, GS 3 L. NA, CA PR. NA	Inv. No. 20.86, GS 3 L. NA, CA PR. NA	Inv. No. 23.527, GS 3 L. NA, CA PR. NA
304. Ear Probe Inv. No. 23.528, GS 3 L. NA, CA PR. NA	305. Ear Probe Inv. No. 17.101, GS 3 L. NA, CA PR. NA	306. Ear Probe Inv. No. 13.1511, GS 3 L. NA, CA PR. Breite, Fig 26, Nr. 2
307. Ear Probe Inv. No. 13.1521, GS 3 L. NA, CA PR. Breite, Fig 26, Nr. 9	308. Ear Probe Inv. No. 13.1513, GS 3 L. NA, CA PR. Breite, Fig 26, Nr. 9	309. Ear Probe Inv. No. 14.96, GS 3 L. NA, CA PR. NA
310. Ear Probe Inv. No. 16.78O, GS 3 L. NA, CA PR. NA	311. Ear Probe Inv. No. 17.313, GS 3 L. NA, CA PR. NA	312. Ear Probe Inv. No. 13.803, GS 3 L. NA, CA PR. Breite, Fig 26, Nr. 9
313. Ear Probe Inv. No. 13.804, GS 3 L. NA, CA PR. Breite, Fig 26, Nr. 9	314. Ear Probe Inv. No. 13.805, GS 3 L. NA, CA PR. Breite, Fig 26, Nr. 9	315. Ear Probe Inv. No. 13.806, GS 3 L. NA, CA PR. Breite, Fig 26, Nr. 9
316. Ear Probe Inv. No. 13.807, GS 3 L. NA, CA PR. Breite, Fig 26, Nr. 9	317. Double Ended Olivary Probe Inv. No. 1414, GS 3 L. 41.0, CA PR. NA Holes were drilled through both olivary ends. The holes do not match in direction. One end also has a slit 1.3 cm long and 2.0 mm wide.	318. Double Ended Olivary Probe Inv. No. 23.4, GS 3 L. 27.4, CA PR. Schutthügel, Fig 26, Nr. 1 It has holes drilled though both olivary ends and the holes do not match in their direction.
319. Double Ended Olivary Probe Inv. No. 4275, GS 3 L. 15.4, CA PR. Schutthügel, Fig 26, Nr. 1 There are two sets of holes drilled through one of the olivary ends. The holes are not in the same direction.	320. Dipyrene Inv. No. 4273, GS 3 L. 16.3, CA PR. Schutthügel, Fig 26, Nr. 1 It is very simple without holes.	321. Needle Inv. No. 13.811, GS 3 L. 14.7, CA PR. Schutthügel, Fig 26, Nr. 1 The needle ends in a point and the cylindrical handle terminates in a slight hook.
322. Needle Inv. No. 23.353, GS 3 L. 14.8, CA PR. Schutthügel (west), Fig 26, Nr. 1 The handle terminates in an olivary end.	323. Needle Inv. No. 2193, GS 3 L. 14.8, CA PR. Schutthügel, Fig 26, Nr. 1 The cylindrical handle terminates in a point.	324. Needle Inv. No. 32:565, GS 3 L. 5.4, CA PR. Breite, Fig 26, Nr. 6 The cylindrical handle terminates in a knob.
325. Needle Inv. No. 36.495, GS 3 L. 6.7, CA PR. Breite, Fig 26, Nr. 5 The cylindrical handle is decorated above the needle, and a bit of the needle survives (1.2 cm long)	326. Oculist Stamp Inv. No. NA, GS 3 L. NA PR. NA Feugère *et al* 1985: 479, Nr. 44; V. 267	

TABLE A5.3: LADENBURG, LOPODUNUM, AUXILIARY FORT

1. Scalpel Inv. No. NA, GS 4 L. NA, CA PR. Bath von Elbe 1974: 240	2. Scalpel Inv. No. NA, GS 5 L. NA, CA PR. Grave Künzl 1983: 79 Early third century	3. Bone Scraper Inv. No. NA, GS 4 L. NA, CA PR. Bath von Elbe 1974: 240
4. Sharp Hook Inv. No. NA, GS 5 L. NA, CA, silver inlay PR. Grave Künzl 1983: 79, Early third century	5. Sharp Hook Inv. No. NA, GS 5 L. NA, CA PR. Grave Künzl 1983: 79 Early third century	6. Spoon Scoop Inv. No. NA, GS 4 L. NA, CA PR. Bath von Elbe 1974: 240

7. Spatula Probe Inv. No. NA, GS 5 L. NA, CA PR. Grave Künzl 1982: 79 Early third century	8. Spatula Probe Inv. No. NA, GS 4 L. NA, Bone PR. Bath von Elbe 1974: 240	9. Spoon Probe Inv. No. NA, GS 5 L. NA, CA PR. Grave Künzl 1983: 79 Early third century
10. Ointment Pallet Inv. No. NA, GS 4 L. NA, Stone PR. Bath von Elbe 1974: 240	11. Medical Box Inv. No. NA, GS 4 L. NA, Wood PR. Bath von Elbe 1974: 240	

TABLE A5.4: HOLZHAUSEN, AUXILIARY FORT

1. Ear Probe Inv. No. NA L. 7.0, CA PR. West Corner of the Fort Pallat 1904: 31	2. Olivary End Probe Inv. No. NA L. NA, CA PR. West Corner of the Fort Pallat 1904: 31, Nr. 21-Tab. 7 Nr. 18

TABLE A5.5: ZUGMANTEL, AUXILIARY FORT

1. Scalpel Inv. No. NA L. 10.0, CA PR. NA Fabricius 1936: 184, 17 Nr.-Tab. 26	2. Scalpel Inv. No. NA L. NA, CA PR. NA Jacobi 1909: 90, Nr. 2-Tab. 11 Nr. 44	3. Scalpel Inv. No. NA L. NA, CA PR. NA Jacobi 1909: 90, Nr. 2-Tab. 11 Nr. 64
4. Spatula Probe Inv. No. NA L. NA, CA PR. NA Jacobi 1909: 90, Nr. 5-Tab. 11 Nr. 36	5. Spatula Probe Inv. No. NA L. NA, CA PR. NA Jacobi 1909: 90, Nr. 5-Tab. 11 Nr. 37	6. Spoon Probe Inv. No. NA L. NA, CA PR. NA Jacobi 1909: 90, Nr. 6-Tab. 11 Nr. 38
7. Spoon Probe Inv. No. NA L. NA, CA PR. NA Jacobi 1909: 90, Nr. 6-Tab. 11 Nr. 39	8. Spoon Probe Inv. No. NA L. NA, CA PR. NA Jacobi 1909: 90, Nr. 6-Tab. 11 Nr. 40	9. Spoon Probe Inv. No. NA L. NA. CA PR. NA Jacobi 1909: 90, Nr. 6-Tab. 11 Nr. 42
10. Spoon Probe Inv. No. NA L. NA, CA PR. NA Jacobi 1909: 90, Nr. 6-Tab. 11 Nr. 43	11. Spoon Probe Inv. No. NA L. NA, CA PR. NA Anonymous 1930: 47, Nr. 9-Tab. 11	12. Ear Probe Inv. No. NA L. NA, CA PR. NA Jacobi 1909: 91, Nr. 9-Tab. 11 Nr. 60
13. Ear Probe Inv. No. NA L. NA, CA PR. NA Jacobi 1909: 91, Nr. 9-Tab. 11 Nr. 61	14. Ear Probe Inv. No. NA L. NA, CA PR. NA Jacobi 1909: 91, Nr. 9-Tab. 11 Nr. 62	15. Ear Probe Inv. No. NA L. NA, CA PR. NA Jacobi 1909: 91, Nr. 9-Tab. 11 Nr. 63
16. Ear Probe Inv. No. NA L. NA, Silver PR. NA Anonymous 1930: 47, Nr. 5-Tab. 11	17. Spoon Scoop Inv. No. NA L. NA, CA PR. NA Anonymous 1930: 47, Nr. 10-Tab. 11.	18. Double Ended Olivary Probe Inv. No. NA L. NA, CA PR. NA Jacobi 1909: 91, Nr. 8-Tab. 11 Nr. 35
19. Olivary End Probe Inv. No. NA L. NA, CA PR. NA Jacobi 1909: 90, Nr. 7-Tab. 11 Nr. 41		

TABLE A5.6: HEFTRICH, NUMERUS FORT

1. Spoon Probe Inv. No. NA L. NA, CA PR. NA Jacobi 1904: 8, Nr. 19	2. Olivary End Probe Inv. No. NA L. NA, CA PR. NA Jacobi 1904: 8, Nr. 20

TABLE A5.7: STADEN, NUMERUS FORT

1. Spatula Probe Inv. No. NA L. 18.7, CA PR. NA Fabricius 1936: 200, Nr. 23-Tab. 17 Nr. 20

TABLE A5.8: SAALBURG, AUXILIARY FORT

1. Scalpel Inv. No. NA, GS 6 L. NA, CA PR. NA Jacobi 1897: Nr. 2-Tab. 67	2. Forceps Inv. No. NA, GS 6 L. NA, CA PR. NA Jacobi 1897: 452, Nr. 10-Tab. 62	3. Button Probe Inv. No. NA, GS 6 L. NA, CA PR. NA von Elbe 1974: 347
4. Spoon Probe Inv. No. NA, GS 6 L. NA, CA PR. NA Jacobi 1897: 452, Nr. 1-Tab. 62	5. Spoon Probe Broken Inv. No. NA, GS 6 L. NA, CA PR. NA Jacobi 1897: 452, Nr. 6-Tab. 62	6. Spatula Probe Inv. No. NA, GS 6 L. NA, CA PR. NA Jacobi 1897: 452, Nr. 2-Tab. 62
7. Ointment Pallet Inv. No. NA, GS 6 L. NA, CA PR. NA Jacobi 1897: 453, Nr. 22-Tab. 71	8. Oculist Stamp Inv. NA L. NA PR. NA Feugère *et al* 1986: 479, Nr. 25, E. 122, V. 195	9. Oculist Stamp Inv. NA L. NA PR. NA Feugère *et al* 1986: 479, Nr. 26, E. 25, V. 224

TABLE A5.9: KAPERSBURG, AUXILIARY FORT

1. Spoon Probe Inv. No. NA L. NA, CA PR. NA Jacobi and Hofmann 1906: 27, Nr. 36	2. Forceps Inv. No. NA L. 5.8, CA PR. NA Jacobi and Hofmann 1906: 27, Nr. 38

Table A5.10: Oberflorstadt, Auxiliary Fort

Olivary End Probe Inv. No. NA L. 5.9, CA PR. NA Kofler and Jacobi 1903: 22, Nr. 12	2. Olivary End Probe Inv. No. NA L. 4.3, CA PR. N Kofler and Jacobl 1903: 22, Nr. 12

TABLE A5.11: GROß-KROTZENBURG, AUXILIARY FORT

1. Spoon Probe Inv. No. NA L. NA, CA PR. Principia Wolff and Jacobi 1903: 23, Nr. 9-Tab. 8 Nr. 18

TABLE A5.12: OKARBEN, AUXILIARY FORT

1. Spatula Probe Inv. No. NA L. 18.0, CA PR. Bath Wolff 1902: 17, Nr. 9	2. Forceps Inv. No. NA L. 9.5, CA PR. Bath Wolff 1902: 17, Nr. 10

TABLE A5.13: WIESBADEN, AUXILIARY FORT

1. Ear Probe Inv. No. 7134, GS 7 L. NA, CA PR. NA Ritterling 1909: 99, Nr. 93	2. Olivary End Probe Inv. No. 17417, GS 7 L. NA, CA PR. NA Ritterling 1909: 98. Nr. 94	3. Ointment Pallet Inv. No. NA, GS 7 L. NA, CA PR. NA von Elbe 1974: 455
4. Oculist Stamp Inv. No. NA L. NA PR. NA Feugère *et al* 1985: 479, Nr. 24, E. 123, V. 108		

TABLE A5.14: HOFHEIM, AUXILIARY FORT

1. Scalpel Inv. No. NA L. NA, CA PR. Old Baths Wolff 1897: 23, Nr. 5-Tab. 8 Nr. 12

TABLE A5.15: NECKARBURKEN, AUXILIARY FORT

1. Spatula Probe Inv. No. NA L. NA, CA PR. NA Schumacher 1898: 35, Nr. 2

TABLE A5.16: BAD WIMPFEN, AUXILIARY FORT

1. Forceps Inv. No. NA, GS 8 L. 13.3, CA PR. NA Schumacher 1900: 10	2. Forceps Inv., No. NA, GS 8 L. 11.0, CA PR. NA Schumacher 1900: 10

TABLE A5.17: STOCKSTADT AM MAIN, AUXILIARY FORT

1. Spoon Probe Inv. No. NA L. 16.3, CA PR. NA Conrady *et al.* 1910: 52, Nr. 3-Tab. 7 Nr. 77

TABLE A5.18: HÜFINGEN, AUXILIARY FORT

1. Spoon Probe Inv. No. NA L. NA, CA PR. NA Revellio 1937: 40, Nr. 64-Tab. 10

TABLE A5.19: DEGENFELD, AUXILIARY FORT

1. Scalpel Inv. No. NA L. 10.0, CA PR. NA Anthes 1936: 184

TABLE A5.20: BAD CANSTATT, AUXILIARY FORT

1. Surgical Knife Inv. No. NA L. NA, CA PR. NA Barthel 1907: 28, Nr. 45-Tab. 8 Nr. 45	2. Forceps with Olivary Probe Inv. No. NA L. NA, CA PR. Cemetery Barthel 1907: 28, Nr. 58

TABLE A5.21: KÖNGEN, GRINARIO, AUXILIARY FORT

1. Spatula Probe Inv. No. NA L. 14.2, CA PR. NA Mettler and Barthel 1907: 35, Nr. 15	2. Olivary End Probe Inv. No. NA L. 13.5, CA PR. NA Mettler and Barthel 1907: 35, Nr. 16

TABLE A5.22: LANGENHAIN, AUXILIARY FORT

1. Olivary End Probe Inv. No. NA L. NA, CA PR. NA Kofler 1897: 8, Nr. 7

TABLE A5.23: ÖHRINGEN, AUXILIARY FORT

1. Spoon Probe Broken Inv. No. NA L. NA, CA PR. NA Herzog 1897: 17, Nr. 4

TABLE A5.24: MAINHARDT, AUXILIARY FORT

1. Spatula Probe Broken Inv. No. NA L. 14.5, CA PR. East Tower Mettler and Drexel 1909: 12, Nr. 10

TABLE A5.25: BINGEN, AUXILIARY FORT

1. Cupping Vessel Inv. No. Como 1-7, GS 9 L. 12.0, CA PR. NA Como 1925: 153, Nr. 7-Fig. 1; Künzl 1983: 80, Nr. 7-Fig. 55, AD 150	2. Cupping Vessel Inv. No. Como 1-8, GS 9 L. 16.0, CA PR. NA Como 1925: 153, Nr. 8-Fig. 1; Künzl 1983: 80, Nr. 8-Fig. 55, AD 150	3. Cupping Vessel Inv. No. Como 1-9, GS 9 L. 12.0, CA PR. NA Como 1925: 153, Nr. 8-Fig. 1; Künzl 1983: 80, Nr. 8-Fig. 55, AD 150
4. Scalpel with Iron Blade Inv. No. Como 2-1, GS 9 L. 15.5, CA 32 PR. NA	5. Scalpel with Iron Blade Inv. No. Como 2-2, GS 9 L. 16.0, CA PR. NA	6. Scalpel with Iron Blade Inv. No. Como 2-3, GS 9 L. 16.0, CA PR. NA

Como 1925: 155, Nr. 1-Fig. 2; Künzl 1983: 80, Nr. 1-Fig. 56, AD 150	Como 1925: 155, Nr. 2-Fig. 2; Künzl 1983: 80, Nr. 2-Fig. 56, AD 150	Como 1925: 155, Nr. 3-Fig. 2; Künzl 1983: 80, Nr. 3-Fig. 56, AD 150
7. Scalpel with Iron Blade Inv. No. Como 2-4, GS 9 L. 16.5, CA PR. NA Como 1925: 155, Nr. 4-Fig. 2; Künzl 1983: 80, Nr. 4-Fig. 56, AD 150	8. Scalpel with Iron Blade Inv. No. Como 2-5, GS 9 L. 14.0, CA PR. NA Como 1925: 155, Nr. 5-Fig. 2; Künzl 1983: 80, Nr. 5-Fig. 56, AD 150	9. Scalpel with Iron Blade Inv. No. Como 2-6, GS 9 L. 15.0, CA PR. NA Como 1925: 155, Nr. 6-Fig. 2; Künzl 1983: 80, Nr. 6-Fig. 56, AD 150
10. Scalpel with Iron Blade Inv. No. Como 2-7, GS 9 L. 14.0, CA PR. NA Como 1925: 155, Nr. 7-Fig. 2; Künzl 1983: 80, Nr. 7-Fig. 56, AD 150	11. Scalpel Inv. No. Como 2-8, GS 9 L. 9.0, CA PR. NA Como 1925: 155, Nr. 8-Fig. 2; Künzl 1983: 80, Nr. 8-Fig. 56, AD 150	12. Scalpel Inv. No. Como 2-9, GS 9 L. 10.0, CA PR. NA Como 1925: 155, Nr. 9-Fig. 2; Künzl 1983: 80, Nr. 9-Fig. 56, AD 150
13. Bone Lever Inv. No. Como 2-10, GS 9 L. 11.0, CA PR. NA Como 1925: 155, Nr. 10-Fig. 2; Künzl 1983: 80, Nr. 10-Fig. 56, AD 150	14. Bone Lever Como 2-11, GS 9 L. 11.5, CA PR. NA Como 1925: 155, Nr. 11-Fig. 2; Künzl 1983: 80, Nr. 11-Fig. 56, AD 150	15. Bone Lever Inv. No. Como 2-12, GS 9 L. 12.5, CA PR. NA Como 1925: 155, Nr. 12-Fig. 2; Künzl 1983: 80, Nr. 12-Fig. 56, AD 150
16. Bone Lever Inv. No. Como 2-13, GS 9 L. 17.5, CA PR. NA Como 1925: 155, Nr. 13-Fig. 2; Künzl 1983: 80, Nr. 13-Fig. 56, AD 150	17. Bone Lever Inv. No. Como 2-18, GS 9 L. 15.0, CA PR. NA Como 1925: 157, Nr. 18-Fig. 2; Künzl 1983: 80, Nr. 18-Fig. 56, AD 150	18. Sharp Hook Inv. No. Como 3-15, GS 9 L. 16.8, CA PR. NA Como 1925: 159, Nr. 15-Fig. 3; Künzl 1983: 80, Nr. 15 Fig. 57, AD 150
19. Sharp Hook Inv. No. Como 3-16, GS 9 L. 14.4, CA PR. NA Como 1925: 159, Nr. 16-Fig. 3; Künzl 1983: 80, Nr. 16-Fig. 57, AD 150	20. Sharp Hook Inv. No. Como 3-17, GS 9 L. 12.2, CA PR. NA Como 1925: 159, Nr. 17-Fig. 3; Künzl 1983: 80, Nr. 17-Fig. 57, AD 150	21. Sharp Hook Inv. No. Como 3-18, GS 9 L. 16.5, CA PR. NA Como 1925 159, Nr. 18-Fig. 3; Künzl 1983: 80, Nr. 18 Fig. 57, AD 150
22. Sharp Hook Inv. No. Como 2-17, GS 9 L. 21.0, CA PR. NA Como 1925: 157, Nr. 17-Fig. 2; Künzl 1983: 80, Nr. 17-Fig. 56, AD 150	23. Needle Inv. No. Como 3-20, GS 9 L. 13.8, CA PR. NA Como 1925: 160, Nr. 20-Fig. 3; Künzl 1983: 80, Nr. 20 Fig. 57, AD 150	24. Trepanning Saw Inv. No. Como 2-19, GS 9 L. 18.5, CA PR. NA Como 1925: 157, Nr. 19-Fig. 2; Künzl 1983: 80, Nr. 19-Fig. 56, AD 150; Behrens 1939: 4-5, Figs. 1 and 2
25. Bone Borer Inv. No. Como 6-1, GS 9 L. 5.5, CA PR. NA Como 1925: 160, Nr. 1-Fig. 6; Künzl 1983: 80, Nr. 1 Fig. 58, AD 150	26. Bone Borer Inv. No. Como 6-2, GS 9 L. 4.5, CA PR. NA Como 1925 160, Nr. 2-Fig. 6; Künzl 1983: 80, Nr. 2 Fig. 58, AD 150	27. Cautery Inv. No. Como 2-16, GS 9 L. 9.0, CA PR. NA Como 1925: 157, Nr. 16-Fig. 2; Künzl 1983: 80, Nr. 16-Fig. 56; Bliquez 1981: 220. The end is missing, AD 150
28. Double Sided Spatula Inv. No. Como 3-10a, GS 9 L. 20.5, CA PR. NA Como 1925: 159, Nr. 10a-Fig. 3; Künzl 1983: 80, Nr. 10a-Fig. 57, AD 150	29. Double Sided Spatula Inv. No. Como 3-10b, GS 9 L. 19.9, CA PR. NA Como 1925: 159, Nr. 10b-Fig. 3; Künzl 1983: 80, Nr. 10b-Fig. 57, AD 150	30. Spatula Probe Inv. No. Como 3-11, GS 9 L. 16.7, CA PR. NA Como 1925: 159, Nr. 11-Fig. 3; Künzl 1983: 80, Nr. 11-Fig. 57, AD 150
31. Spoon Scoop Inv. Como 2-14, GS 9 L. 11.5, CA PR. NA Como 1925: 155, Nr. 14-Fig. 2;	32. Spoon Scoop Inv. No. Como 2-15, GS 9 L. 4.5, Iron PR. NA Como 1925: 157, Nr. 15-Fig. 2;	33. Forceps Inv. No. Como 3-12, GS 9 L. 16.3, CA PR. NA Como 1925: 159, Nr. 12-Fig. 3;

Künzl 1983 80, Nr. 14-Fig. 56, AD 150	Künzl 1983: 80, Nr. 15-Fig. 56, the handle is broken, AD 150	Künzl 1983: 80, Nr. 12-Fig. 57, AD 150
34. Forceps Inv. No. Como 3-13, GS 9 L. 15.3, CA PR. NA Como 1925: 159, Nr. 13-Fig. 3; Künzl 1983: 80, Nr. 13-Fig. 57, AD 150	35. Forceps Inv. No. Como 3-14, GS 9 L. 15.0, CA PR. NA Como 1925: 159, Nr. 14-Fig. 3; Künzl 1983: 80, Nr. 14-Fig. 57, AD 150	

TABLE A5.26: WORMS, BORBETOMAGUS, AUXILIARY FORT

1. Scalpel (S) Inv. No. R 214, GS 10 L. 12.0, Iron PR. Grave Field Maria Münster, Found in a Child's Grave Künzl 1979/81: 53, Nr. 3-Tab. 3, Künzl 1983: 78, Pl 53, The scalpel has bronze and silver inlay	2. Scalpel Inv. No. NA, GS 10 L. 10.7, CA PR. NA Künzl 1979/81: 53, Nr. 4-Tab. 3. The scalpel has bronze and silver inlay	3. Bifurcated hook Inv. No. R 208, GS 10 L. 19.9, CA PR. Grave field Maria Münster Künzl 1979/81: 59, Nr. 31-Tab. 6, The exact find spot is not known
4. Needle with a Hook Inv. No. R 4120, GS 10 L. 14.0, CA PR. Weinsheimer Zollhaus Künzl 1979/81: 60, Nr. 63-Tab. 8	5. Needle Inv. No. R 581, GS 10 L. 15.5, CA PR. Mainzer Strasse Künzl 1979/81: 60, Nr. 62-Tab. 8	6. Ear Probe Inv. No. R 213, GS 10 L. 12, CA PR. Grave field Maria Münster, 1886 Künzl 1979/81: 60, Nr. 64-Tab. 8
7. Ear Probe Inv. No. R4523, GS 10 L. 11.5, CA PR. Pfeddersheim Künzl 1979/81: 60, Nr. 65-Tab. 8	8. Ear Probe Inv. No. R 635, GS 10 L. 14.5, Silver PR. Mainzer Strasse Künzl 1979/81: 60, Nr. 66-Tab. 8	9. Ointment Pallet Inv. No. 645, GS 10 13.8x8.6, Serpentine PR. Gas Works Künzl 1979/81: 53, Nr. 2-Tab. 1-2
10. Oculist Stamp Inv. No. NA L. NA PR.NA Feugère *et al* 1985: 479, Nr. 28; E. 69; V. 88		

APPENDIX SIX

MEDICAL INSTRUMENTS FROM RAETIA

Abbreviations for Museums

R 1	Stadtmuseen, Regensburg, Germany
R 2	Heimatmuseum, Günzburg, Germany
R 3	Prähistorische Staatssammlung, Munich, Germany
R 4	Gäuboden -und Stadtmuseum, Straubing, Germany
R 5	Wurttembergischen Landesmuseum, Stuttgart, Germany
R 6	Heimatmuseum, Ehningen an der Donau, Germany

TABLE A6.1: REGENSBURG, CASTRA REGINA, LEGIONARY FORTRESS (INCLUDING THE AUXILIARY FORT)

1. Scalpel Inv. No. A 2227, R 1 L. 9.2, CA PR. NA Dietz *et al.* 1979: 152	2. Forceps Inv. No. A 1470, R 1 L. 13.0, CA PR. Auxiliary Cohort Fort, Bath Building Dietz *et al.* 1979: 152	3. Oculist Stamp Inv. No. A 1995, R 1 L. 5.66, Stone PR. Large Grave field, Grave 967 Dietz *et al.* 1979: 152
4. Spoon Probe Inv. No. A 3580, R 1 L. 10.4, CA PR. NA Dietz *et al.* 1979: 152	5. Oculist Stamp Inv. No. NA L. NA PR. NA Feugère *et al.* 1985: 479, Nr. 29; E. 152; V. 145	

TABLE A6.2: WEISSENBURG, BRICIANIS, AUXILIARY FORT

1. Spoon Probe Inv. No. NA L. NA, CA PR. NA Kohl *et al.* 1906: 38, Nr.89-Tab. 7 Nr. 39	2. Spoon Probe Inv. No. NA L. NA, CA PR. NA Kohl *et al.* 1906: 38, Nr.89-Tab. 7 Nr. 40	3. Spoon Probe Inv. No. NA L. NA, CA PR. NA Kohl *et al.* 1906: 38, Nr..89-Tab.7 Nr. 41
4. Spatula Probe Inv. No. NA L. NA, CA PR. NA Kohl *et al.* 1906: 38, Nr. 89-Tab. 7 Nr. 38	5. Ear Probe Inv. No. NA L. NA, CA PR. East Building Kohl *et al.* 1906: 38, Nr. 90-Tab. 7 Nr. 47	6. Ear Probe Inv. No. NA L. NA, CA PR. NA Kohl *et al.* 1906: 38, Nr. 90-Tab. 7 Nr. 48

TABLE A6.3: MUNNINGEN, AUXILIARY FORT

1. Spoon Probe Inv. No. NA L. 15.0, CA PR. NA Eidam 1929: 22, Nr. 28-Tab. 5

TABLE A6.4: ELLINGEN, AUXILIARY FORT

1. Sharp Hook Inv. No. 1991, 686 L. 3.6, CA PR. NA Zanier 1992: 183, Nr. 150-Tab. 19	2. Ear Probe Inv. No. 1983, 2740 L. 14.9, CA PR. Barrack Room 8 x 72/ y 67 Zanier 1992: 183, Nr. 144-Tab. 19	3. Ear Probe Inv. No. 1983, 2739 L. 12.4, CA PR. *Via Sagularis* North Building D x 35, 20/ y 89, 80 Zanier 1992: 183, Nr. 145-Tab. 19
4. Ear Probe Inv. No. 1983, 2741 L. 9.7, CA PR. Building C Middle part x 62, 40/ y 85, 10 Zanier 1992:183, Nr.146Tab. 19	5. Olivary End Probe Inv. No. 1991, 346 L. 11.6, CA PR. NA Zanier 1992: 183, Nr. 147-Tab. 19	6. Olivary End Probe Inv. No. 1991, 2426 L. 9.5, CA PR. Schacht 6, x 16.50/ y 34 Zanier 1992: 183, Nr. 148-Tab. 19

7. Olivary End Probe Inv. No. 1991, 1151 L. 6.2, CA PR. NA Zanier 1992: 183, Nr. 149-Tab. 19

Table A6.5: Günzburg, Gontia, Auxiliary Fort

1. Spoon Probe Inv. No. NA, R 2 L. NA, CA PR. Grave 496, Necropolis Künzl 1983: 121, Middle Empire	2. Needle Inv. No. NA, R. 2 L. NA, CA PR. Grave 496, Necropolis Künzl 1983: 121, Middle Empire	3. Medical box Inv. No. NA, R 2 7.2 x 5.4 x 1.8, CA PR. Grave 496, Necropolis Künzl 1983: 121; Sobel 1991: 128 Middle Empire

Table A6.6: Pfünz, Vetoniana, Auxiliary Fort

1. Spatula Probe Inv. No. NA L. NA, CA PR. NA Winkelmann and Jacobs 1901: 24, Nr. 63-Tab. 12 Nr. 7	2. Spoon Probe Inv. No. NA L. NA, CA Pr. NA Winkelmann and Jacobs 1901: 24, Nr. 63-Tab. 12 Nr.	3. Spoon Probe Inv. No. NA L. NA, CA PR. NA Winkelmann and Jacobs 1901: 24, Nr. 63-Tab. 12 Nr. 9
4. Ear Probe Inv. No. NA L. NA, CA PR. NA Winkelmann and Jacobs 1901: 24, Nr. 61-Tab. 12 Nr. 23	5. Ear Probe Inv. No. NA L. NA, CA PR. NA Winkelmann and Jacobs 1901: 24, Nr. 61-Tab. 12 Nr. 25	6. Ear Probe Inv. No. NA L. NA, CA PR. NA Winkelmann and Jacobs 1901: 24, Nr. 61-Tab. 12 Nr. 26

Table A6.7: Gnotzheim, Auxiliary Fort

1. Spatula Probe Inv. No. NA L. 9.3, CA PR. NA Obermedizininalrat and Barthel 1907: 20

Table A6.8: Dambach, Auxiliary Fort

1. Spoon Probe Inv. No. NA L. 5.5, CA PR. NA Kohl *et al* 1901: 20, Nr. 2

Table A6.9: Faimingen, Auxiliary Fort

1. Ear Probe Inv. No. 1105 L. NA, CA PR. NA Scheller and Drexel 1911: 43, Nr. 8	2. Ear Probe Inv. No. 7195 L. NA, CA PR. *Vicus* Scheller and Drexel 1911: 43, Nr. 8
3. Ear Probe Inv. No. 997 L. NA, CA PR. NA Scheller and Drexel 1911: 43, Nr. 8	4. Olivary End Probe Inv. No. NA L. 16.0, CA PR. *Vicus* Scheller and Drexel 1911: 43, Nr. 10

TABLE A6.10: HEIDENHEIM, AQUILEIA, AUXILIARY FORT

1. Spatula Probe Inv. No. NA L. 18.0, CA PR. Outside the fort Brenzstrasse Prescher and Jacobs 1900: 4, Nr. 9

TABLE A6.11: LONSEE URSPRING, AUXILIARY FORT

1. Spoon Probe Inv. No. NA L. 15.0, CA PR. Room K West Building Druck 1904: 36, Nr. 17	2. Spoon Probe Inv. No. NA L. 12.0, CA Room 5 Middle Building Druck 1904: 36, Nr. 17

TABLE A6.12: WALLHEIM, AUXILIARY FORT

1. Spoon Probe Inv. No. NA L. NA, CA PR. NA Swoboda 1967: Tab. 112- Fig. 2

TABLE A6.13: OBERSTIMM, AUXILIARY FORT (FIG. 23)

1. Double Simple Probe Inv. No. 1975, 57, R 3 L. 15.1, CA PR. NA Böhme 1978: 188, Tab. 31 B 450	2. Spatula Probe Inv. No. 1975, 314, R 3 L. 19.4, CA PR. Trench 29, Section a, Fig. 23, Nr, 1. Böhme 1978: 188, Tab. 31 B 447	3. Spatula Probe Inv. No. 1975, 189, R 3 L. 16.4, CA PR. NA Böhme 1978: 188, Tab. 31 B 448
4. Spatula Probe Inv. No. 1975, 189, R 3 L. 5.6, CA PR. Area 19, Fig. 23, Nr.2 Böhme 1978: 188, Tab. 31 B 449	5. Spatula Probe Inv. No. 1975, 289, R 3 L. 12.0, CA PR. NA Böhme 1978: 188, Tab. 31 B 452	6. Ear Probe Inv. No. 1975, 225, R 3 L. 13.9, CA PR. Area 21, Fig. 23, Nr. 4 Böhme 1978: 188, Tab. 31 B 451
7. Olivary End Probe Inv. No. 1975, 224, R 3 L. 6.6, CA PR. Area 21, Section b, Fig. 23, Nr. 4 Böhme 1978: 187, Tab. 30 B 443	8. Olivary End Probe Inv. No. 1975, 224, R 3 L. 4.5, CA PR. Area 22, section b, Fig. 23, Nr. 3 Böhme 1978: 187, Tab. 30 B 443	9. Olivary End Probe Inv. No. 1975, 185, R 3 L. 7.7, CA PR. Area 19, Fig. 23, Nr. 2 Böhme 1978: 187, Tab. 30 B 444
10. Olivary End Probe Inv. No. 1975, 207, R 3 L. 10. 8, CA PR. Area19 west section cut 1-11, Fig. 23, Nr. 2 Böhme 1978: 187, Tab. 30 445	11. Olivary End Probe Inv. No. 1975, 66, R 3 L. 12.1, CA PR. Area 4 southwest corner, Fig. 23, Nr. 5 Böhme 1978: 187, Tab. 30446	

TABLE A6.14: STRAUBING, SOVIODURUM, AUXILIARY FORT

1. Spoon Probe Inv. No. 3879, R 4 L. NA, CA PR. West *Vicus* Pl 1009/ 21-23 Walke 1965: 153, Nr. 2-Tab.109	2. Spoon Probe Inv. No. 3875, R 4 L. NA, CA PR. West *Vicus* Pl 1009/ 23-24 Walke 1965: 153, Nr. 3-Tab. 109	3. Spoon Probe Inv. No. 3878, R 4 L. NA, CA PR. South *Vicus* Pl 3602, Excavation 1896 Walke 1965: 153, Nr. 4-Tab. 109
4. Spoon Probe Inv. No. 3880, R 4 L. NA, CA Pr. NA Walke 1965: 153, Nr. 5-Tab. 109	5. Spoon Probe Inv. No. 3881, R 4 L. NA, CA PR. NA Walke 1965: 153, Nr. 6-Tab. 109	6. Spoon Probe Broken Inv. No. 3882, R 4 L. NA, CA PR. Fort West Pl. 3609/1109/0 1898 Walke 1965: 153, Nr. 8-Tab. 109

7. Spatula Probe Inv. No. 3889, R 4 L. NA, CA PR. NA Walke 1965: 153, Nr. 9-Tab. 109 Spatula has pointed end	8. Spatula Probe Inv. No. 3884, R 4 L. NA, CA PR. West *Vicus* Pl 1009/ 23, 1953 Walke 1965: 153, Nr. 10-Tab. 109	9. Spatula Probe Inv. No. 3886, R 4 L. NA, CA PR. West *Vicus* Walke 1965: 153, Nr. 11-Tab. 109
10 Spatula Probe Inv. No. 3888, R 4 L. NA, Ca PR. NA Walke 1965: 153. Nr. 12-Tab. 109	11. Small Spatula Probe Inv. No. 3890, R 4 L. NA, CA North-east *Vicus* Pl 3634/ 7. 24 1930 Walke 1965: 153, Nr. 13-Tab. 109	12. Ear Probe Inv. No. 3896, R 4 L. NA, CA PR. North-east *Vicus* Pl 3634/ 0.8 1934 Walke 1965: 153, Nr. 14-Tab. 110
13. Ear Probe Inv. No. 3911, R 4 L. NA, CA PR. NA Walke 1965: 153, Nr. 15-Tab. 110	14. Ear Probe Inv. No. 3892, R 4 L. NA, Ca PR. South *Vicus* Pl 3516/ 2, 1950 Walke 1965: 153, Nr. 16-Tab. 110	15. Ear Probe Inv. No. 3912, R 4 L. NA, CA PR. Fort South Pl 3622, 1913 Walke 1965: 153, Nr. 17-Tab. 110
16. Ear Probe Inv. No. 3903, R 4 L. NA, CA PR. NA Walke 1965: 153, Nr. 18-Tab. 110	17. Ear Probe Inv. No. 3902, R 4 L. NA, CA PR. NA Walke 1965: 153, Nr. 19-Tab. 110	18. Ear Probe Inv. No. 3913, R 4 L. NA, CA PR. NA Walke 1965: 153, Nr. 20-Tab. 110
19. Olivary End Probe Inv. No. 3883, R 4 L. NA, CA PR. North-East *Vicus* Pl 3632/ 4-6 Walke 1965:153, Nr. 7-Tab. 109	20 Olivary End Probe Inv. No. 3877, R 4 L. NA, CA PR. West *Vicus* Pl 1009/ 21-22 Walke 1965: 153, Nr. 1-Tab. 109	21. Oculist Stamp Inv. No. NA L. NA PR. NA Feugère *et al* 1985: 479, Nr. 31, V. 254

TABLE A6.15: RISSTISSEN, AUXILIARY FORT

1. Scalpel Inv. No. A 621, R 5 L. NA, CA PR. NA Ulbert 1959: 107, Nr. 6, Tab. 66	2. Sharp Hook Inv. No. A 2088, R 5 L. NA, CA PR. NA Ulbert 1959: 107, Nr 12, Tab. 66	3. Forceps Inv. No. A 787, R 5 L. NA, CA PR. NA Ulbert 1959: 107, Nr 13, Tab. 66
4. Spoon Probe Inv. No. 3953, R 6 L. NA, CA PR. NA Ulbert 1959: 107, Nr 14-Tab. 66	5. Spoon Probe Inv. No. 66/188, R 5 L. 15.3, CA PR. NA Ulbert 1970: 31, Nr 165, Tab. 11	6. Spoon Probe Inv. No. 66/77, R 5 L. 12.0, CA PR. NA Ulbert 1970: 31, Nr 166, Tab. 11
7. Spoon Probe Broken Inv. No. 66/244, R 5 L. 11.0, CA PR, NA Ulbert 1970: 31, Nr 167, Tab. 11	8. Forceps with Ear Probe Inv. No. 68/66, R 5 L. 14.0, CA PR. NA Ulbert 1970: 31, Nr 164, Tab. 11	

Appendix Seven

Medical Instruments from Noricum

Abbreviation for Museum
N 1 Museum Lauriacum, Enns, Austria

Table A7.1: Enns-Lorch, Lauriacum, Legionary Fortress

1. Scalpel Inv. No. NA, N 1 L. 11.7, CA PR. NA	2. Surgical Knife Inv. No. R VII 777, N-1 L. 11.4, CA PR. Friedhofes Lorch Deringer 1954: 149, Fig. 81, Nr. 2	3. Forceps Inv. No. R VII 913, N 1 L. 15.1, CA PR. Parz 1076/ 1KS Enns
4. Pterygotom Inv. No. R VII 692, N 1 L. 11.5, Silver PR. 1951 East end of building group one, grave Deringer 1954: 149, Nr. 1-Fig. 81; Künzl (1983) 116 Ear probe at opposite end	5. Spoon Probe Inv. No. R. VII 765, N 1 L. 13.8, CA PR. 1905 In the Camp Barrack IV Deringer 1954: 147 d, Fig. 79 Nr. 10; Groller 1907: 141, Fig. 62, Nr 55	6. Spoon Probe Inv. No. R VII 766, N 1 l. 15.6, CA PR. NA Deringer 1954: 147 e, Fig 81, Nr. 3
7. Spoon Probe Inv. No. R VII 775, N 1 L. 16.9, CA PR. 1908 Herrschaftsfeld Deringer 1954: 147 b, Fig. 79, Nr. 8	8. Spoon Probe Inv. No. RVII 768, N 1 L. 12.85, CA PR. 1894 Eichburg S-E of the schottergrube Deringer 1954: 147 g, Fig. 79, Nr. 11	9. Spoon Probe Inv. No. R VII 769, N 1 L. 9.5, CA PR. 1907 In the central area of the fortress 147 h, Fig. 79 Nr 12; Groller 1909: 99, Fig. 39, Nr. 7
10. Spoon Probe Inv. No. R VII 764, N 1 L. 16.3, CA PR. NA Deringer 1954: 147 c, Fig. 79, Nr. 9	11. Spoon Probe Inv. No. R VII 767, N 1 L. 15.6, CA PR. Sammlung Kukonnig. Found next to the train station Deringer 1954: 147 f	12. Spoon Probe Inv. No. R VII 776, N 1 L. 17.5, CA PR. Deringer 1954: 147a, Fig. 79, Nr. 7
13. Spatula Probe Inv. No. R VII 765/1, N 1 L. 13.85, CA 1905 Barrack II Deringer 1954: 149a, Fig. 79 Nr. 13a; Groller 1907: 141, Fig. 62, Nr. 4	14. Spatula Probe Inv. No. R VII 772, N 1 L. 9.5, CA PR. NA Deringer 1954: 149c, Fig. 79, Nr. 15	15. Spatula Probe Inv. No. R VII 774, N 1 L. 10.0, CA PR. 1919 *Limes* excavation Deringer 1954: 149e, Fig. 79, Nr. 16
16. Spatula Probe Inv. No. R VII 585, N 1 L. 11.0, CA PR. 1930 Civil settlement Deringer 1954: 149g, Fig. 79, Nr. 18	17. Spatula Probe Inv. No. R VII 771, N 1 L. 13.7, CA PR. 1916 Friedhoff soldier's grave Deringer 1954: 149 b, Fig. 79, Nr. 14	18. Spatula Probe Broken Inv. No. R VII 773, N 1 L. 7.4, CA PR. NA Deringer 1954: 149d, Fig. 79, Nr. 17
19. Ear Probe Inv. No. R VII 756, N 1 L. 13.4, CA PR. 1906 By the *limes* Deringer 1954: 146 c	20. Ear Probe Inv. No. R VII 733, N 1 L. 11.6, CA PR. 1905 Camp excavations Deringer 1954: 146, Fig 79, Nr. 4 d; Groller 1907: 141	21. Ear Probe Inv. No. R VII 734, N 1 L. 11.6, CA PR. Found in a hypocaust in the fort
22. Ear Probe (S/T) Inv. No. R VII 251, N 1 L. NA, CA PR. Dedrahntsfeld by Habdschuhmacher House Sammlung Bukong	23. Ear Probe (S/T) Inv. No. R VII 474, N 1 L. 13.4, CA PR. 1914 Limes excavation Deringer 1954: 146 a; Groller 1924: 11-12, Fig. 8	24. Ear Probe (S/T) Inv. No. R VII 739, N 1 L. 8.0, CA PR. 1911 *Limes* excavation Deringer 1954: 146 f
25. Ear Probe (S/T) Inv. No. R VII 471, N 1 L. 15.6, CA PR. 1914 Limes Excavation Deringer 1954: 146 b; Groller 1924: 11-12, Fig. 8	26. Olivary End Probe (S/T) Inv. No. R VII 770 N 1 L. 11.2, CA PR. 1900 The bath of the camp Deringer 1954: 148 k, Fig. 79, Nr. 13	27. Olivary End Probe (S/T) Inv. No. R V 130, N 1 L. 11.15, CA PR. NA Deringer 1954: 149 a, Fig. 79, Nr. 19
28. Olivary End Probe (S/T)	29. Ointment Pallet (S/T)	30. Oculist Stamp

Inv. No. R V 131, N 1 L. 10.4, CA PR. NA Deringer 1954: 150b, Fig. 79, Nr. 20	Inv. No. R V 169, N 1 L. 21.5, CA PR. Water canal in the *retentura* Deringer 1954: 150 b, Fig. 83, Nr. 2	Inv. No. NA L. NA PR. NA Feugère *et al* 1985: 479, Nr. 31, E. 51, V. 216

Appendix Eight

Medical Instruments from Pannonia Superior

Abbreviations for Museums
PS 1 Carnuntum Museum, Bad Deutsch Altenburg, Austria
PS 2 Museum der Stadt, Wien, Vienna, Austria

Table A.8.1: Bad-Deutsch Altenburg, Carnuntum, Legionary Fortress and Auxiliary Fort

1. Scalpel Inv. No. 21872, PS 1 L. 6.5, CA PR. *Canabae* Hauff 1993/94: 116, Nr.1-Tab. 1, 1-2 century	2. Scalpel Inv. No. 21392A, PS 1 L. 11.5, CA PR. *Canabae* Hauff 1993/94: 116, Nr. 2 Tab. 1, 3rd Century	3. Scalpel Inv. No. 14610, PS 1 L. NA, CA PR. Carnuntum Hauff 1993/94: 116, Nr. 3-Tab. 1 Copper and Silver Inlay, Blunt dissector broken, 1-2 century
4. Scalpel Inv. No. 13228, PS 1 L. 5.6, CA PR, Carnuntum Hauff 1993/94: 116, Nr. 4-Tab. 1, 1-2 century	5. Scalpel Inv. No. 19863, PS 1 L. 6.5, CA PR. Civil Settlement Hauff 1993/94: 116, Nr. 5-Tab. 1. It has a small handle with a knob at the top, 1-2 century	6. Scalpel Inv. No, NA, PS 1 L. 6.8, CA PR. Carnuntum Hauff 1993/94: 118, Nr. 6-Tab. 1, 1-4 century
7. Sharp Hook Inv. No. 15053, PS 1 L. 15.4, CA PR. Carnuntum Hauff 1993/94: 124, Nr. 23- Tab. 5	8. Sharp Hook Inv. No. 15597, PS 1 L. 13.9, CA PR. North Section of the *Retentura* Right Side, Map 66 Hauff 1993/94: 124, Nr. 24- Tab. 5, Appears to be a Ligula with a diagonal handle, 1-4 century	9. Sharp Hook Inv. No. 13176, PS 1 L. 15.0, CA PR. *Valetudinarium* West of the *Quaestorium* Hauff 1993/94: 124, Nr. 25- Tab. 5, Baluster formation at the top, 1-4 century
10. Sharp Hook Inv. No. 13081, PS 1 L. 16.5, CA PR. *Valetudinarium* West of the *Quaestorium* Hauff 1993/94: 124, Nr. 26- Tab. 5, Baluster formation at the top of the instrument, 1-4 century	11. Sharp Hook Inv. No. 12324, PS 1 L. 15.3, CA PR. Area Between the *Via Secunda* and *via Quintana* Hauff 1993/94: 124, Nr. 27- Tab. 6, Silver inlay on the handle, curved neck, Blunt hook, 1 century	12. Hook with Spatula Inv. No. 15570, PS 1 L. 13.5, CA PR. Carnuntum Hauff 1993/94: 126, Nr. 28- Tab. 6. The hook is broken and the other end has a spatula, 1 century.
13. Needle handle Inv. No. 13230, PS 1 L. 4.8, CA PR. Carnuntum Hauff 1993/94: 126, Nr. 29- Tab. 6, Handle Decorated with an acanthus formation and the other end has a hole for an iron needle, 3 century	14. Needle handle Inv. No. 14578, PS 1 L. 5.6, CA PR. Carnuntum Hauff 1993/94: 126, Nr. 30 -Tab. 6, Decorated cylindrical handle with a hole on the bottom for a needle, 3 century	15. Dental Forceps Inv. No. 15445, PS 1 L. 18.0, Iron PR. Carnuntum Hauff 1993/94: 126, Nr. 31 -Tab. 7, Silver inlay, a bolt in the centre holds the forceps together, 1-2 century
16. Bone Knife Inv. No. 15039, PS 1 L. 11.4, CA PR. Carnuntum Hauff 1993/94: 126, Nr. 32 -Tab. 7, a knife for cutting bone, 1-2 century	17. Female Catheter Inv. No. 15446, PS 1 L. 14.4, CA PR. Carnuntum Hauff 1993/94: 126, Tab. 7, Nr. 33, the top opening is 0.9 cm and the bottom end is circular, 1 century	18. Male Catheter Inv. No. NA, PS 1 L. 22.3, CA PR. Carnuntum Hauff 1993/94: 128, Tab, 7. Nr. 34, the opening is 0.5 cm l, the utility end is rounded with an opening to its side, and the bottom end is circular, 1 century
19. Forceps Inv. No. 15623, PS 1 L. 12.0, CA PR. Civil Settlement *Insula* VI 1952 Hauff 1993/94: 118, Nr. 7- Tab. 2, Clamp and Jagged teeth 2-3 century	20. Forceps Inv. No. 15461, PS 1 L. 16.6, CA PR. Carnuntum Hauff 1993/94: 118, Nr. 8- Tab. 2, Jagged teeth 3rd Century	21. Forceps Inv. No. 16026, PS 1 L. 11.7, CA PR. NA Hauff 1993/94: 118, Nr. 9- Tab. 2, 2-3 century
22. Forceps	23. Spatula Probe	24. Spatula Probe

Inv. No. 167/90, PS 1 L. 9.8, CA PR. Civil Settlement 1989-90 Hauff 1993/94: 118, Nr. 10- Tab. 2, Ball Formation at the top, ends turn inwards, 2-3 century	Inv. No. 15052, PS 1 L. 18.5, CA PR. Carnuntum Hauff 1993/94: 128, Nr. 36 -Tab. 8, 1-4 century	Inv. No. 15067, PS 1 L. 15.3, CA PR. Carnuntum Hauff 1993/94: 128, Nr. 37 -Tab. 8, 1-4 century
25. Spatula Probe Inv. No. 15605, PS 1 L. 19.4, CA PR. Civil Settlement *Insula* VI 1949 Hauff 1993/94: 128, Nr. 38 -Tab. 8	26. Spatula Probe Inv. No. 15065, PS 1 L. 18.1, CA PR. Civil Settlement *Insula* VI 1952 Hauff 1993/94: 128, Nr. 39 -Tab. 8, 1-4 century	27. Spatula Probe Inv. No. VI 2612 KhM/AS Wien, PS 1 L. 18.8, CA PR. Carnuntum Hauff 1993/94: 128-130, Nr. 40 - Tab. 9, 1-4 century
28. Spatula Probe Inv. No. VI. 4121 KhM/AS Wien, PS 1 L. 15.5, CA PR. Carnuntum Hauff 1993/94: 130, Nr. 41 -Tab. 9, 1-4 century	29. Spatula Probe Inv. No. 15469, PS 1 L. 11.2, CA PR. Carnuntum Hauff 1993/94: 130, Nr. 42 -Tab. 9, 1-4 century	30. Spatula Probe Inv. No. 16071, PS 1 L. 15.4, CA PR. Carnuntum Hauff 1993/94: 130, Nr. 43 -Tab. 9, 1-4 century
31. Spatula Probe Inv. No. 15599, PS 1 L. 14.3, CA PR. Carnuntum Hauff 1993/94: 130, Nr. 44 -Tab 9, 1-4 century	32. Spatula Probe Inv. No. NA, PS 1 L. 15.2, CA PR. Bad Deutsch-Altenburg Hauff 1993/94: 130, Nr. 45 -Tab. 10, 1-4 century	33. Spatula Probe Inv. No. 3915 NO LM, PS 1 L. 8.4, CA PR NA Hauff 1993/94: 132, Nr. 46-Tab. 10, 1-4 century
34. Spatula Probe Inv. No. 5860 NO LM, PS 1 L. 17.0, CA PR. Carnuntum Hauff 1993/94: 134, Nr. 55-Tab. 11, 1-4 century	35. Spatula Probe Inv. No. 15468, PS 1 L. 15.3, CA PR. Between *Via Secunda* and *Via Quintana* Hauff 1993/94: 134, Nr. 56-Tab. 11, 1-4 century	36. Spatula Probe Inv. No. 15070, PS 1 L. 17.7, CA PR. Carnuntum Hauff 1993/94: 134, Nr. 57-Tab. 11
37. Spatula Probe Broken Inv. No. 15598, PS 1 L. 15.3, CA PR. Carnuntum Hauff 1993/94: 128, Nr. 35 -Tab. 8, 1-4 Century	38. Spatula Probe Broken Inv. No. 15613, PS 1 L. 7.3, CA PR. East and South-east of Camp Hauff 1993/94: 132, Nr. 47 -Tab. 10, 1-4 century	39. Spatula Probe Broken Inv. No. 21909, PS 1 L. 5.2, CA PR. Carnuntum Hauff 1993/94: 132, Nr. 48 -Tab. 10, 1-4 century
40. Spatula Probe Broken Inv. No. 21997a, PS 1 L. 6.0, CA PR. Carnuntum Hauff 1993/94: 132, Nr. 49 -Tab. 10, 1-4 century	41. Spatula Probe Broken Inv. No. 21997b, PS 1 L. 8.5, CA PR. Carnuntum Hauff 1993/94: 132, Nr. 50 -Tab. 10, 1-4 century	42. Spatula Probe Broken Inv. No. 22014, PS 1 L. 4.1, CA PR. Carnuntum Hauff 1993/94: 132, Nr. 51 -Tab. 10, 1-4 century
43. Spatula Probe Broken Inv. No. NA, PS 1 L. 4.6, CA PR. *Canabae* (west) Hauff 1993/94: 134, Nr. 52 -Tab. 10, 1-4 century	44. Spatula Probe Broken Inv. No. NA, PS 1 L. 3.3, CA PR. Carnuntum Hauff 1993/94: 134, Nr. 53 -Tab. 10, 1-4 century	45. Spatula Probe Broken Inv. No. NA, PS 1 L. 4.5, CA PR. *Canabae* 1986 Hauff 1993/94: 134, Nr. 54 -Tab. 10, 1-4 century
46. Spatula Probe (Small Blade) Inv. No. 15609, PS 1 L. 14.2, CA PR. Carnuntum Hauff 1993/94: 152, Nr. 104-Tab. 20, 1-4 Century	47 Spatula Probe (Small Blade) Inv. No. 15517, PS 1 L. 7.2, CA PR. Carnuntum Hauff 1993/94: 154, Nr. 105-Tab. 20, 1-4 century	48. Spoon Probe Inv. No. 16056, PS 1 L. 18.2, CA PR. Carnuntum Hauff 1993/94: 136, Nr. 58-Tab. 12, 1-4 century
49. Spoon Probe Inv. No. 15058, PS 1 L. 14.8, CA PR. Carnuntum Hauff 1993/94: 136, Nr. 59-Tab. 12, 1-4 century	50. Spoon Probe Inv. No. NA, PS 1 L. 14.5, CA PR. Civil Settlement 1952 Hauff 1993/94: 136, Nr. 60-Tab. 12, 1-4 century	51. Spoon Probe Inv. No. 15607, PS 1 L. 12.1, CA PR. Carnuntum Hauff 1993/94: 136, Nr. 61-Tab. 12, 1-4 century
52. Spoon Probe Inv. No. 22347, PS 1 L. 10.9, CA	53. Spoon Probe Inv. No. 15854,PS 1 L. 12.6, CA	54. Spoon Probe Inv. No. 15060, PS 1 L. 11.8, CA

PR. Carnuntum Hauff 1993/94: 136, Nr. 62-Tab. 12, 1-4 century	PR. Bad Deutsch-Altenburg 1963 Hauff 1993/94: 136-140, Nr. 63-Tab. 12, 1-4 century	PR. Carnuntum Hauff 1993/94: 140, Nr. 64-Tab. 13, 1-4 century
55. Spoon Probe Inv. No. 15606,PS 1 L. 13.7, CA PR. Carnuntum Hauff 1993/94: 140, Nr. 65-Tab. 13, 1-4 century	56. Spoon Probe Inv. No. 4 89, PS 1 L. 10.2, CA PR. Civil Settlement 1989-90 Hauff 1993/94: 140, Nr. 66-Tab. 13, 1-4 century	57. Spoon Probe Inv. No. 15057, PS 1 L. 16.8, CA PR. Carnuntum Hauff 1993/94: 140, Nr. 67-Tab. 13, 1-4 century
58. Spoon Probe Inv. No. 15601, PS 1 L. 17.1, CA PR. Carnuntum Hauff 1993/94: 140, Nr. 68 Tab. 14, 1-4 century	59. Spoon Probe Inv. No. 15602, PS 1 L. 14.7, CA PR. Carnuntum Hauff 1993/94: 140, Nr. 69 Tab. 14, 1-4 century	60. Spoon Probe Inv. No. 15055, PS 1 L. 15.7, CA PR. Carnuntum Hauff 1993/94: 142, Nr. 70- Tab. 14, 1-4 century
61. Spoon Probe Inv. No. 15059, PS 1 L. 11.6, CA PR. Carnuntum Hauff 1993/94: 142, Nr. 71-Tab. 14, 1-4 century	62 Spoon Probe Inv. No. 15066, PS 1 L. 18.7, CA PR. Carnuntum Hauff 1993/94: 142, Nr. 72-Tab. 15, 1-4 century	63. Spoon Probe Inv. No. 3914 NO LM, PS 1 L. 13.4, CA PR. Carnuntum Hauff 1993/94: 142, Nr. 73-Tab. 15, 1-4 century
64. Spoon Probe Inv. No. 15620, PS 1 L. 13.8, CA PR. *Valetudinarium* West of *Quaestorium* Hauff 1993/94: 142, Nr. 74-Tab. 15, 1-4 century	65. Spoon Probe Inv. No. 15608, PS 1 L. 10.0, CA PR. Carnuntum Hauff 1993/94: 144, Nr. 75-Tab. 15, 1-4 century	66. Spoon Probe Inv. No. 15611, PS 1 l. 11.0, CA PR. Carnuntum Hauff 1993/94: 144, Nr. 76-Tab. 15, 1-4 century
67. Spoon Probe Inv. No. 21909, PS 1 L. 8.9, CA PR. Carnuntum Hauff 1993/94: 144, Nr. 77-Tab. 16, 1-4 century	68. Spoon Probe Broken Inv. No. 15603, PS 1 L. 4.7, CA PR. Carnuntum Hauff 1993/94: 144, Nr. 78-Tab. 16, 1-4 century	69. Spoon Probe Broken Inv. No. 15612, PS 1 L. 4.0, CA PR. Carnuntum Hauff 1993/94: 144, Nr. 79-Tab. 16, 1-4 century
70. Spoon Probe Broken Inv. No. 21842, PS 1 L. 4.4, CA PR. Carnuntum Hauff 1993/94: 144, Nr. 80-Tab. 16, 1-4 century	71. Spoon Probe Broken Inv. No. 21909a, PS 1 L. 3.0, CA PR. Carnuntum Hauff 1993/94: 146, Nr. 81-Tab. 16, 1-4 century	72. Spoon Probe Broken Inv. No. 21909b, PS 1 L. 5.5, CA PR. Carnuntum Hauff 1993/94: 146, Nr. 82-Tab. 16, 1-4 century
73. Spoon Probe Broken Inv. No. 22152, PS 1 L. 6.0, CA PR. Carnuntum Hauff 1993/94: 146, Nr. 83-Tab. 16, 1-4 century	74. Spoon Probe Broken Inv. No. 22151, PS 1 L. 5.5, CA PR. Carnuntum Hauff 1993/94: 146, Nr. 84-Tab. 16, 1-4 century	75. Ear Probe Inv. No. 13172, PS 1 L. 8.2, CA PR. Carnuntum Hauff 1993/94: 150, Nr. 95-Tab. 19, 1-4 century
76. Ear Probe Inv. No. 13158, PS 1 L. 11.2, CA PR. Civil Settlement 1963 Hauff 1993/94: 150, Nr. 96-Tab. 19, 1-4 century	77. Ear Probe Inv. No. 13157, PS 1 L. 11.4, CA PR. Carnuntum Hauff 1993/94: 150, Nr. 97-Tab. 19, 1-4 century	78. Ear Probe Inv. No. 13153, PS 1 L. 12.7, CA PR. Carnuntum Hauff 1993/94: 152, Nr. 98-Tab. 19, 1-4 century
79. Ear Probe Inv. No. 13152, PS 1 L. 13.3, CA PR. Carnuntum Hauff 1993/94: 152, Nr. 99-Tab. 19, 1-4 century	80. Ear Probe Inv. No. 13151, PS 1 L. 15.2, CA PR. Carnuntum Hauff 1993/94: 152, Nr. 100-Tab. 20, 1-4 century	81. Ear Probe Inv. No. 12329, PS 1 L. 13.8, CA PR. Carnuntum Hauff 1993/94: 152, Nr. 101-Tab. 20, 1-4 century
82. Ear Probe Inv. No. 13107, PS 1 L. 8.3, CA PR. Carnuntum Hauff 1993/94: 152, Nr. 102-Tab. 20, 1-4 century	83. Ear Probe Inv. No. 13080, PS 1 L. 12.3, CA PR. Carnuntum Hauff 1993/94: 152, Nr. 103-Tab. 20, 1-4 century	84. Ear Probe Inv. No. 13032, PS 1 L. 11.9, CA PR. Civil Settlement *Insula* VI 1953 Hauff 1993/94: 154, Nr. 106-Tab. 21
85. Ear Probe	86. Ear Probe	87. Ear Probe

Inv. No. 13046, PS 1 L. 10.3, CA PR. Carnuntum Hauff 1993/94: 154, Nr. 107-Tab. 21	Inv. No. 13079, PS 1 L. 12.6, CA PR. Carnuntum Hauff 1993/94: 154, Nr. 108-Tab. 21	Inv. No. 13081, PS 1 L. 12.0, CA PR. *Valetudinarium* west of the *Quaestorium*, Map 66 Hauff 1993/94: 154, Nr. 109-Tab. 21
88. Ear Probe Inv. No. 13078, PS 1 L. 12.5, CA PR. Carnuntum Hauff 1993/94: 154, Nr. 110-Tab. 21	89. Ear Probe Inv. No. 13084, PS 1 L. 11.5, CA PR. Carnuntum Hauff 1993/94: 156, Nr. 111-Tab. 22	90. Ear Probe Inv. No. 13083, PS 1 L. 11.5, CA PR. Carnuntum Hauff 1993/94: 156, Nr. 112-Tab. 22
91. Ear Probe Inv. No. 13085, PS 1 L. 10.9, CA PR. Grave lined street west of the camp Hauff 1993/94: 156, Nr. 113-Tab. 22	92. Ear Probe Inv. No. 13087, PS 1 L. 10.9, CA PR. Carnuntum Hauff 1993/94: 156, Nr. 114-Tab. 22	93. Ear Probe Inv. No. 13088, PS 1 L. 10.5, CA PR. Carnuntum Hauff 1993/94: 156, Nr. 115-Tab. 22
94. Ear Probe Inv. No. 13089, PS 1 L. 10.4, CA PR. Carnuntum Hauff 1993/94: 156, Nr. 116-Tab. 22	95. Ear Probe Inv. No. 13091, PS 1 L. 9.5, CA PR. Carnuntum Hauff 1993/94: 156, Nr. 117-Tab. 23	96. Ear Probe Inv. No. 13090, PS 1 L. 10.1, CA PR. Carnuntum Hauff 1993/94: 158, Nr. 118-Tab. 23
97. Ear Probe Inv. No. 13093, PS 1 L. 9.5, CA PR. Carnuntum Hauff 1993/94: 158, Nr. 119-Tab. 23	98. Ear Probe Inv. No. 13094, PS 1 L. 9.0, CA PR. Legionary Camp Hauff 1993/94: 158, Nr. 120-Tab. 23	99. Ear Probe PR. 13095, PS 1 L. 9.2, CA PR. Carnuntum Hauff 1993/94: 158, Nr. 121-Tab. 23
100. Ear Probe Inv. No. 13096, PS 1 L. 8.9, CA PR. Carnuntum Hauff 1993/94: 158, Nr. 122-Tab. 23	101. Ear Probe Inv. No. 13097, PS 1 L. 8.6, CA PR. Carnuntum Hauff 1993/94: 158, Nr. 123-Tab. 24	102. Ear Probe Inv. No. 13098, PS 1 L. 8.5, CA PR. Carnuntum Hauff 1993/94: 158, Nr. 124-Tab. 24
103. Ear Probe Inv. No. 13099, PS 1 L. 8.3, CA PR. *Praetentura* left half, barracks, *scamnum tribunorum* Hauff 1993/94: 160, Nr. 125-Tab. 24	104 Ear Probe Inv. No. 13100, PS 1 L. 9.5, CA PR. Civil Settlement 1958 Hauff 1993/94: 160, Nr. 126-Tab. 24	105. Ear Probe Inv. No. 13101, PS 1 L. 8.1, CA PR. Carnuntum Hauff 1993/94: 160, Nr. 127-Tab. 24
106. Ear Probe Inv. No. 13102, PS 1 L. 7.9, CA PR. Carnuntum Hauff 1993/94: 160, Nr. 128-Tab. 24	107. Ear Probe Inv. No. 13104, PS 1 L. 7.8, CA PR. *Retentura* North section, Map 66 Hauff 1993/94: 160, Nr. 129-Tab. 25	108. Ear Probe Inv. No 13104, PS 1 L. 8.0, CA PR. *Praetentura* left half, barracks *scamnum tribunarum*, Map 66 Hauff 1993/94: 160, Nr. 130-Tab. 25
109. Ear Probe Inv. No. 13106, PS 1 L. 8.0, CA PR. Carnuntum Hauff 1993/94: 162, Nr. 131-Tab. 25	110. Ear Probe Inv. No. 13108, PS 1 L. 7.8, CA PR. Carnuntum Hauff 1993/94: 162, Nr. 132-Tab. 25	111. Ear Probe Inv. No. 13109, PS 1 L. 7.7, CA PR. Carnuntum Hauff 1993/94: 162, Nr. 133-Tab. 25
112. Ear Probe Inv. No. 13110, PS 1 L. 7.5, CA PR. *Praetentura* left half, *scamnum tribunorum*, barracks. Hauff 1993/94: 162, Nr. 134-Tab. 25	113. Ear Probe Inv. No. 13113, PS 1 L. 7.2, CA PR. *Praetentura* left half, *scamnum tribunorum*, barracks. Hauff 1993/94: 162, Nr. 135-Tab. 26	114. Ear Probe Inv. No. 13116, PS 1 L. 7.0, CA PR. Carnuntum Hauff 1993/94: 162, Nr. 136-Tab. 26
115. Ear Probe Inv. No. 13117, PS 1	116. Ear Probe Inv. No. 13118, PS 1	117. Ear Probe Inv. No. 13119, PS 1

L. 7.0, CA PR. Between *Via Secunda* and *Via Quintana* Hauff 1993/94: 162, Nr. 137-Tab. 26	L. 7.1, CA PR. Carnuntum Hauff 1993/94: 164, Nr. 138-Tab. 26	L. 7.6, CA PR. Carnuntum Hauff 1993/94: 164, Nr. 139-Tab. 26
118. Ear Probe Inv. No. 13120, PS 1 L. 6.7, CA PR. *Praetentura* left half, *scamnum tribunorum*, barracks. Hauff 1993/94: 164, Nr. 140-Tab. 26	119. Ear Probe Inv. No. 13121, PS 1 L. 6.9, CA PR. Carnuntum Hauff 1993/94: 164, NR 141 Tab 27	120. Ear Probe Inv. No. 13122, PS 1 L. 6.7, CA PR. Carnuntum Hauff 1993/94: 164, Nr. 142-Tab. 27
121. Ear Probe Inv. No. 13123, PS 1 L. 7.6, CA PR. Carnuntum Hauff 1993/94: 164, Nr. 143-Tab. 27	122. Ear Probe Inv. No. 13124, PS 1 L. 5.9, CA PR. Carnuntum Hauff 1993/94: 164, Nr. 144-Tab. 27	123. Ear Probe Inv. No. 13125, PS 1 L. 4.4, CA PR. *Praetentura* left half, *scamnum tribunorum*, barrack. Hauff 1993/94: 166, Nr. 145-Tab. 27
124. Ear Probe Inv. No. 13126, PS 1 L. 3.7, CA PR. Carnuntum Hauff 1993/94: 166, Nr. 146-Tab. 27	125. Ear Probe Inv. No. 13127 (PS 1) L. 3.5, CA PR. Carnuntum Hauff 1993/94: 166, Nr. 147-Tab. 28	126. Ear Probe Inv. No. 13128, PS 1 L. 9.1, CA PR. Legionary Camp 1912 Hauff 1993/94: 166, Nr. 148-Tab. 28
127. Ear Probe Inv. No. 13129, PS 1 L. 7.2, CA PR. Carnuntum Hauff 1993/94: 166, Nr. 149-Tab. 28	128. Ear Probe Inv. No. 13130, PS 1 L. 7.8, CA PR. Carnuntum Hauff 1993/94: 166, Nr. 150-Tab. 28	129. Ear Probe Inv. No. 13131, PS 1 L. 6.0, CA PR. Carnuntum Hauff 1993/94: 168, Nr. 151-Tab. 28
130. Ear Probe Inv. No. 13134, PS 1 L. 12.6, CA PR. Civil Settlement *Insula* VI 1949 Hauff 1993/94: 168, Nr. 152-Tab. 28	131. Ear Probe Inv. No. 13135, PS 1 L. 5.1, CA PR. Civil Settlement *Insula* III 1950 Hauff 1993/94: 168, Nr. 153-Tab. 29	132. Ear Probe Inv. No. 13136, PS 1 L. 6.4, CA PR. Carnuntum Hauff 1993/94: 168, Nr. 154-Tab. 29
133. Ear Probe Inv. No. 13137, PS 1 L. 8.0, CA PR. Carnuntum Hauff 1993/94: 168, Nr. 155-Tab. 29	134. Ear Probe Inv. No. 13138, PS 1 L. 9.1, CA PR. Civil Settlement *Insula* VI 1953 Hauff 1993/94: 168, Nr. 156-Tab. 29	135. Ear Probe Inv. No. 13139, PS 1 L. 7.7, CA PR, Carnuntum Hauff 1993/94: 168, Nr. 157-Tab. 29
136. Ear Probe Inv. No. 13139a, PS 1 Il. 17.1, CA PR. Civil Settlement *Insula* VI 1949 Hauff 1993/94: 172, Nr. 158-Tab. 29	137. Ear Probe Inv. No. 21320, PS 1 L. 10.8, CA PR. Carnuntum Hauff 1993/94: 172, Nr. 159-Tab. 30	138. Ear Probe Inv. No. 21993, PS 1 L. 8.0, CA PR. Carnuntum Hauff 1993/94: 172, Nr. 160-Tab. 30
139. Ear Probe Inv. No. 21994, PS 1 L. 5.6, CA PR. Carnuntum Hauff 1993/94: 172, Nr. 161-Tab. 30	140. Ear Probe Inv. No. 21995, PS 1 L. 4.3, CA PR. Carnuntum Hauff 1993/94: 172, Nr. 162-Tab. 30	141. Ear Probe Inv. No. 21996, PS 1 L. 7.0, CA PR. Carnuntum Hauff 1993/94: 172, Nr. 163-Tab. 30
142. Ear Probe Inv. No. 21997, PS 1 L. 7.7, CA PR. Carnuntum Hauff 1993/94: 172, Nr. 164-Tab. 30	143. Ear Probe Inv. No. NA, PS 1 L. 4.8, CA PR. *Canabae* 1986 Hauff 1993/94: 174, Nr. 165-Tab. 31	144. Ear Probe Inv. No. NA, PS 1 L. 7.8, CA PR. Carnuntum Hauff 1993/94: 174, Nr. 166-Tab. 31
145. Ear Probe Inv. No. NA, PS 1 L. 9.6, CA PR. Carnuntum Hauff 1993/94: 174, Nr. 167-Tab.	146. Ear Probe Inv. No. NA, PS 1 L. 3.0, CA PR. Carnuntum Hauff 1993/94: 174, Nr. 168-Tab.	147. Ear Probe Inv. No. 13915, PS 1 L. 6.9, CA PR. Carnuntum Hauff 1993/94: 174, Nr. 169-Tab.

31	31	31
148. Ear Probe Inv. No. 13114, PS 1 L. 7.3, CA PR. Carnuntum Hauff 1993/94: 174, Nr. 170-Tab. 31	149. Ear Probe Inv. No. 13112, PS 1 L. 7.3, CA PR. Carnuntum Hauff 1993/94: 176, Nr. 171-Tab. 32	150. Ear Probe Inv. No. 13103, PS 1 L. 7.5, CA PR. South Part of the right principal side of the *Retentura*. Hauff 1993/94: 176, Nr. 172-Tab. 32
151. Ear Probe Inv. No. 13111, PS 1 L. 9.0, CA PR. Carnuntum Hauff 1993/94: 176, Nr. 173-Tab. 32	152. Ear Probe Inv. No. 13132, PS 1 L. 12.4, CA PR. Carnuntum Hauff 1993/94: 176, Nr. 174-Tab. 32	153. Ear Probe Inv. No. 13077, PS 1 L. 14.7, CA PR. *Praetentura* left half, *scamnum tribunorum*, Barracks. Hauff 1993/94: 176, Nr. 175-Tab. 32
154. Ear Probe Inv. No. 13076, PS 1 L. 17.9, CA PR. *Valetudinarium* west of the *Quaestorium*. Hauff 1993/94: 176, Nr. 176-Tab. 33	155. Ear Probe Inv. No. NA, PS 1 L. 8.2, CA PR. Civil Settlement 1993 Hauff 1993/94: 176, Nr. 177-Tab. 33	156. Ear Probe Inv. No. NA, PS 1 L. 7.4, CA PR. Civil Settlement 1993 Hauff 1993/94: 176, Nr. 178-Tab. 33
157. Ear Probe Inv. No. NA, PS 1 L. 4.85, CA PR. Civil Settlement 1986 Hauff 1993/94: 178, Nr. 179-Tab. 33	158. Ear Probe Inv. No. NA, PS 1 L. 8.0, CA PR. Civil Settlement 1986 Hauff 1993/94: 178, Nr. 180-Tab. 33	159. Ear Probe Inv. No. 21788, PS 1 L. 10.9, Silver PR. *Canabae* 1987 Hauff 1993/94: 178, Nr. 181-Tab. 34
160. Ear Probe Inv. No. 13730, PS 1 L. 11.3, Silver PR. Carnuntum Hauff 1993/94: 178, Nr. 182-Tab. 34	161. Ear Probe Inv. No. 13174, PS 1 L. 9.4, Silver PR. Bad Deutsch-Altenburg Hauff 1993/94: 178, Nr. 183-Tab. 34	162. Ear Probe Inv. No. 13156, PS 1 L. 11.9, Silver Pr. *Valetudinarium* west of the *Quaestorium*. Hauff 1993/94: 178, Nr. 184-Tab. 34
163. Ear Probe (S/T) Inv. No. NA, PS 1 L. 16.1, CA PR. Carnuntum Hauff 1993/94: 180, Nr. 185-Tab. 34	164. Ear Probe Inv. No. 13154, PS 1 L. 12.5, CA PR. Carnuntum Hauff 1993/94: 180, Nr. 186-Tab. 35	165. Ear Probe Inv. No. 13159, PS 1 L. 11.0, CA PR. Carnuntum Hauff 1993/94: 180, Nr. 187-Tab. 35
166. Ear Probe Inv. No. 13160, PS 1 L. 11.2, CA PR. Carnuntum Hauff 1993/94: 180, Nr. 188-Tab. 35	167. Ear Probe Inv. No. 13161, PS 1 L. 11.0, CA PR. Carnuntum Hauff 1993/94: 180, Nr. 189-Tab. 35	168. Ear Probe Inv. No. 13162, PS 1 L. 10.0, CA PR. Carnuntum Hauff 1993/94: 180, Nr. 190-Tab. 35
169. Ear Probe Inv. No. 13163, PS 1 L. 9.9, CA PR. Carnuntum Hauff 1993/94: 182, Nr. 191-Tab. 36	170. Ear Probe Inv. No. 13164, PS 1 L. 9.5, CA PR. Carnuntum Hauff 1993/94: 182, Nr. 192-Tab. 36	171. Ear Probe Inv. No. 13165, PS 1 L. 8.2, CA PR. Carnuntum Hauff 1993/94: 182, Nr. 193-Tab. 36
172. Ear Probe Inv. No. 13166, PS 1 L. 7.5, CA PR. Carnuntum Hauff 1993/94: 182, Nr. 194-Tab. 36	173. Ear Probe Inv. No. 13167, PS 1 L. 7.4, CA PR. Legionary Camp 1912 Hauff 1993/94: 182, Nr. 195-Tab. 36	174. Ear Probe Inv. No. 13168, PS 1 L. 4.5, CA PR. Carnuntum Hauff 1993/94: 182, Nr. 196-Tab. 36
175. Ear Probe Inv. No. 13169, PS 1 L. 4.4, CA PR. Carnuntum Hauff 1993/94: 184, Nr. 197-Tab. 36	176. Ear Probe Inv. No. 13171, PS 1 L. 6.0, CA PR. Carnuntum Hauff 1993/94: 184, Nr. 198-Tab. 37	177. Ear Probe Inv. No. 13170, PS 1 L. 6.6, CA PR. Carnuntum Hauff 1993/94: 184, Nr. 199-Tab. 37
178. Ear Probe	179. Ear Probe	180. Ear Probe

Inv. No. 13173, PS 1 L. 4.9, CA PR. South side of the *Raetentura*. Hauff 1993/94: 184, Nr. 200-Tab. 37	Inv. No. NA, PS 1 L. 8.2, CA PR. Carnuntum Hauff 1993/94: 184, Nr. 201-Tab. 37	Inv. No. 13174, PS 1 L. 11.2, CA PR. Carnuntum Hauff 1993/94: 184, Nr. 202-Tab. 37
181. Ear Probe Inv. No. 13277, PS 1 L. 14, CA PR. Carnuntum Hauff 1993/94: 184, Nr. 203-Tab. 37	182. Ear Probe Inv. No. 13283, PS 1 L. 9.2, CA PR. Carnuntum Hauff 1993/94: 186, Nr. 204-Tab. 38	183. Ear Probe Inv. No. 13092, PS 1 L. 9.9, CA PR. Carnuntum Hauff 1993/94: 186, Nr. 205-Tab. 38
184. Ear Probe Inv. No. 13285, PS 1 L. 7.5, CA PR. Carnuntum Hauff 1993/94: 186, Nr. 206-Tab. 38	185. Ear Probe Inv. No. 13287, PS 1 L.6.4, CA PR. Carnuntum Hauff 1993/94: 186, Nr. 207-Tab. 38	186. Ear Probe Inv. No. 13178, PS 1 L. 10.1, CA PR. *Canabae* 1987 Hauff 1993/94: 186, Nr. 208-Tab. 38
187. Olivary End Probe Inv. No. 15610, PS 1 L. 13.5, CA PR. Carnuntum Hauff 1993/94: 146, Nr. 85-Tab. 17, 1-4 century	188. Olivary End Probe Inv. No. 15614, PS 1 L. 8.0, CA PR. Carnuntum Hauff 1993/94: 148, Nr. 86-Tab. 17, 1-4 century	189. Olivary End Probe Inv. No. 15615, PS 1 L. 9.0, CA PR. Carnuntum Hauff 1993/94: 148, Nr. 87 Tab. 17, 1-4 century
190. Olivary End Probe Inv. No. 15616, PS 1 L. 8.0, CA PR. East and South east of the camp Hauff 1993/94: 148, Nr. 88-Tab. 17, 1-4 century	191. Olivary End Probe Inv. No. 21320, PS 1 L. 5.3, CA PR. Carnuntum Hauff 1993/94: 148, Nr. 89-Tab. 17, 1-4 century	192. Olivary End Probe Inv. No. 21909, PS 1 L. 10.9, CA PR. Carnuntum Hauff 1993/94: 148, Nr. 90-Tab. 18, 1-4 century
193. Olivary End Probe Inv. No. 21909, PS 1 L. 10.0, CA PR. Carnuntum Hauff 1993/94: 148, Nr. 91, Tab. 18, 1-4 century	194. Olivary End Probe Inv. No. 21639, PS 1 L. 8.9, CA PR. Carnuntum Hauff 1993/94: 150, Nr. 92, Tab. 18, 1-4 century	195. Olivary End Probe Inv. No. 22001, PS 1 L. 9.3, CA PR. Carnuntum Hauff 1993/94: 150, Nr. 93, Tab. 18, 1-4 century
196. Olivary End Probe Inv. No. NA, PS 1 L. 10.5, CA PR. Carnuntum Hauff 1993/94: 150, Nr. 94-Tab. 18, 1-4 century		

TABLE A8.2: VIENNA, VINDOBONA, LEGIONARY FORTRESS AND AUXILIARY FORT

1. Scalpel Inv. No. MV 9496, PS 2 L. 9.0, CA PR. Neuer Markt 1943 Gschwantler and Ubls 1978: 260, Nr. 81	2. Spoon Probe Inv. No. MV 1561, PS 2 L. 12.5, CA PR. Rudolph Spital 1909/10 (Auxiliary Fort) Gschwantler and Ubls 1978: 260, Nr. 80

TABLE A8.3: SZÓNY, BRIGETIO, LEGIONARY FORTRESS

1. Spoon Probe Inv. No. NA, PS 3 L. 17.5, CA PR. Necropolis Bonis 1968: 29	2. Ear Probe Inv. No. NA, PS 3 L. NA, CA PR. Necropolis Bonis 1968: 30	3. Cylindrical Instrument Case Inv. No. NA, PS 3 L. 20.3, CA PR. Necropolis Bonis 1968: 29
4. Oculist Stamp Inv. No. NA L. NA PR. NA Feugère *et al.* 1985: 479, Nr. 56, E. 52, V. 204		

APPENDIX NINE

MEDICAL INSTRUMENTS FROM PANNONIA INFERIOR

Abbreviations for Museums

PI 1 Aquincum Museum, Budapest, Hungary
PI 2 Historical Museum, Budapest, Hungary
PI 3 National Museum, Budapest, Hungary
PI 4 Museum Intercisa, Dunaújváros, Hungary

TABLE A9.1: BUDAPEST, AQUINCUM, LEGIONARY FORTRESS

1. Cupping Vessel Inv. No. 50305, PI 1 4.0 x 2.8, CA PR. Obuda Korbuly 1934: 22, Nr. 17-Tab. 9	2. Bifurcated Hook Inv. No. 3024, PI 1 L. 22.5, CA PR. Aquincum Anonymous 1986: 174, Nr. 157, 2nd century.	3. Scalpel Inv. No. 50303, PI 1 L. 11.9, CA PR. Aquincum Korbuly 1934: 23-24, Nr. 2-Tab. 9, 2nd century.
4. Iron Knife Blade Inv. No. NA, PI 1 L. NA, CA Grave 216, Aranyheger Bach Necropolis Künzl 1983: 116, 2nd century	5. Needle Inv. No. NA, PI 1 L. NA, CA PR. Grave 86, Aranyheger Bach Necropolis Künzl 1983:116, 2nd century	6. Needle Handle Inv. No. 40309, PI 1 L. 9.5, CA PR. Aquincum Anonymous 1986: 174, Nr. 158, 2nd century.
7. Needle Handle Inv. No. 40307, PI 1 L. 9.0, CA PR. Aquincum Anonymous 1986: 174, Nr. 158, 2nd century	8. Forceps with Ear Probe Inv. No. NA, PI 1 L. NA, CA PR. Grave 216, Aranyheger Bach Necropolis Künzl 1983: 116, 2nd century	9. Forceps Inv. No. 50302, PI 1 L. 11.8, CA PR. Aquincum Korbuly 1934: 12, Nr. 4-Tab. 12, 2nd century.
10. Spoon Probe Inv. No. 50310, PI 1 L. 11.8, CA PR. Obuda (Gas Factory) Civil Settlement Nágy 1942: 529, Pl. C1; Anonymous 1986: 174, Nr. 160, 2nd century	11. Spoon Probe Inv. No. 50299, PI 1 L. 16.0, CA PR. Aquincum Korbuly 1934: 25, Nr. 7-Tab. 10	12. Ear Probe Inv. No. NA, PI 1 L. NA, CA PR. Grave 216, Aranyheger Bach Necropolis Künzl 1983: 116, 2nd century
13. Ear Probe Inv. No. NA, PI 1 L. NA, CA PR. Grave 86, Aranyheger Bach Necropolis Künzl 1983: 116, 2nd century	14. Scale Inv. No. NA, PI 1 L. NA, CA PR. Grave 86, Aranyheger Bach Necropolis Künzl 1983: 116, 2nd century	15. Medical Box Inv. No. 50312, PI 1 12.8 x 7.0 x 2.2, CA PR. Grave 219, Aranyheger Bach Necropolis Sobel 1991: 135

TABLE A9.2: DUNAÚJVÁROS, INTERCISA, AUXILIARY FORT

1. Scalpel Inv. No. 194/1910-45, PI 3 L. 12.0, CA PR. Grave 26 Part 18 of the Necropolis Künzl 1983: 117; Radnóti1957: 237, Nr. 132-Tab. 47 Nr. 14, 2nd/3rd century	2. Scalpel Inv. No. Szfv 1153, PI 4 L. 7.3, CA PR. NA Radnóti 1957: 239, Nr. 173	3. Broken Spoon Probe Inv. No. 14/ 1907-113, PI 3 L. 5.4, CA PR. NA Radnóti 1957: 233, Nr. 42 Tab. 46 Nr. 18
4. Spoon Probe Inv. No. 28/1908-123, PI 3 L. 15.0, CA PR. Building 3 Radnóti 1957: 239, Nr. 173	5. Spoon Probe Inv. No. 43/1902-14, PI 3 L. 14.5, CA PR. NA Radnóti 1957: 235, Nr. 94-Tab. 47 Nr. 12	6. Spoon Probe Inv. No. 46/1910-98, CA L. 17.1, CA PR. Building Nr 6 Radnóti 1957: 236, Nr. 111-Tab. 47 Nr. 19
7. Spoon Probe Inv. No. 23/ 1927-11, PI 3 L. 14.0, CA PR. NA Radnóti 1957: 238, Nr. 160	8. Spoon Probe Inv. No. Szfv 2408, PI 4 L. 16.6, CA PR. NA Radnóti 1957: 239, Nr. 179	9. Spoon Probe Inv. No. Szfv 2428, PI 4 L. 14.0, CA PR. NA Radnóti 1957: 239, Nr. 180

10. Spoon Probe Inv. No. Szfv 9752, PI 4 L. 7.8, CA PR. NA Radnóti 1957: 240, Nr. 202	12. Ear Probe Inv. No. 8/1908-32, PI 3 L. 10.0, CA PR. NA Radnóti 1957: 234, Nr. 59	12. Ear Probe Inv. No. 8/1908-32, PI 3 L. 10.0, CA PR. NA Radnóti 1957: 234, Nr. 59
13. Ear Probe Inv. No. Szfv 2771, PI 4 L. 7.2, CA PR. NA Radnóti 1957: 239, Nr. 181	14. Ear Probe Inv. No. Szfv 3605, PI 4 L. 11.4, CA PR. NA Radnóti 1957: 239, Nr. 183	15. Medical Box Inv. No. 82.4.27, PI 4 10.0 x 5.3 x 2.9, CA PR. Camp 22 Sobel 1991: 135, 3rd century

Appendix Ten

Medical Instruments from Britain

Abbreviations for Museums

BR 1	Yorkshire Museum, York, England
BR 2	Roman Legionary Museum, Caerleon, Wales
BR 3	Newport Museum and Art Gallery, Newport, Wales
BR 4	Grosvenor Museum, Chester, England
BR 5	Corbridge Museum, England
BR 6	Arbeia Museum, South Shields, England
BR 7	Museum of Antiquities, Newcastle upon Tyne, England
BR 8	Chesters Museum, England
BR 9	Tulley House Museum, Carlisle, England

Table A10.1: York, Eboracum, Legionary Fortress

1. Oculist Stamp Inv. No. NA L. NA PR. NA Feugère et al. 1985: 480, Nr. 78; V. 247	2. Oculist Stamp Inv. No. NA L. NA PR. NA Feugère et al. 1985: 480, Nr. 79; V. 147

Table A10.2: Caerleon, Isca Silurum, Legionary Fortress (Fig. 21)

1. Scalpel Inv. No. 84.119 H, BR 2 L. 8.5, CA PR. Isca Grange 3, Rubbish Pits, Fig. 21, Nr. 8 The scalpel bent at 90 degrees.	2. Needle Inv. No. 55T, BR 2 L. 6.2, CA PR. Jenkins Field II (Workshops), Fig. 21, Nr. 6 Cylindrical handle with a hole in the bottom centre, possibly for a needle.	3. Needle Inv. No, NA, BR 3 L. 8.5, CA PR. NA Cylindrical handle with needle coming from the bottom centre. Boon, in his unpublished work, refers to this as a cataract needle.
4. Dental Tool Inv. No. 31.78, BR 2 L. 14.6, CA PR. NA Lee 1862: 67, Nr. 9-Pl. 34	5. Forceps Inv. No. 81.79 H, BR 2 L. 12.6, CA PR. Fortress Baths, Fig. 21, Nr. 5 Zienkiewicz 1986: 189, Nr. 188-Fig. 64	6. Forceps Inv. No. 54.389A, BR 2 L. 13.4. CA PR. *Vicus* Main Lateral Drain Boon (draft copy) 104, 130-230 AD. The forceps have an olivary probe on its end
7. Forceps Inv. No. 31.78, BR 2 L. 13.7, CA PR. Castle Baths, Outside fortress Lee 1862: 67, Nr. 6-Pl. 34 The arms terminate in sharp points.	8. Forceps Inv. No. 82.112/267, BR 3 L. 9.0, CA PR. NA	9. Spoon Probe Inv. No. NA, BR 2 L. 17.0, CA PR. Castle Baths, Outside fortress Lee 1862: 68, Nr. 9-Pl. 35
10. Spoon Probe Inv. No. 54.389 A, BR 2 L. 15.8, CA PR. *Vicus*, Main Lateral Drain Boon (draft copy) Nr. 101, 130-230 AD	11. Spoon Probe Inv. No. 344.90(966), BR 2 L. NA, CA PR. Roman Gates Block B, Fig. 21, Nr. 1	12. Spoon Probe Broken Inv. No. 513/79/161/001 UCC, BR 3 L. 9.0, CA PR. NA
13. Spoon Probe Broken Inv. No. NA, BR 2 L. 9.0, CA PR. Amphitheatre, Fig. 21, Nr. 2 Wheeler 1928: 166, Nr 36- Fig. 14. 90-120 AD found with a coin of Titus.	14. Spoon Probe Broken Inv. No. 35.119, BR 2 L. 8.1, Bone PR. Amphitheatre, Fig. 21, Nr. 2 Wheeler 1928: 169, Nr. 19-Pl. 33.1	15. Spoon Probe Broken Inv. No. 69.326, BR 2 L. 10.2, CA PR. Vicarage Garden (Headquarters Building), Fig. 21, Nr. 7 Boon 1970: 57, Nr. 4-Fig. 57
16. Spoon Probe Broken Inv. No. 56.214 B F4, Br 2 L. 6.0, CA Pr. *Vicus*, Under building VIII Boon (unpublished draft) Nr. 103	17. Spoon Probe Broken Inv. No. 58.330 F 13, BR 2 L. 8.6, CA PR. *Vicus*, Main Lateral Drain Boon (unpublished draft) Nr. 102,	18. Spatula Probe Inv. No. 277, BR 2 L. 8.7, CA PR. Post Hole Centurion 1st Cohort, Fig. 21, Nr. 3

	130-230 AD	The spatula is flat and triangular, possibly a cautery.
19. Spatula Probe Broken Inv. No. NA, BR 2 L. NA, CA PR. Prysg Field Trench 1, Fig. 21, Nr. 4 Fox 1940: 127, Nr. 1-Fig. 5. Has Inscription (CIL VII, 1144)	20. Spatula Probe Broken Inv. No. CBT 138/396 781, BR 2 L. 6.5, CA PR. British Telecom, (Workshop), Fig. 21, nr. 6	21. Ear Probe Inv. No. NA, BR 2 L. 14.5, CA PR. NA
22. Ear Probe L. 32.6, BR 2 L. 9.8, CA PR. Barrack C room 11, Prysg Field, Fig. 21, Nr. 4 Nash-Williams 1932: 90, Nr. 5-Fig. 38	23. Ear Probe Inv. No. 39.386, BR 2 L. 12.5, CA PR. Barrack IV, Trench I Layer 2, Fig. 21, Nr. 4 Fox 1940: 32, Nr. 7-Fig. 5, Late 3rd or early 4th	24. Ear Probe Inv. No. 35.119, BR 2 L. NA, CA PR. Amphitheatre A-H Section, Bank, Fig. 21, Nr. 2
25. Ear Probe Inv. No. 54.389 A F 45, BR 2 L. 9.8, CA Il. 39 PR. *Vicus* Main Lateral Drain Boon (unpublished draft) 112	26. Ear Probe Inv. No. CBT 138/409 814, BR 2 L. 13.6, CA Il. 39 PR. British Telecom, Bath Drain? Fig. 21, Nr. 5	27. Ear Probe Inv. No. NA, BR 2 L. 12.4, CA Il. 39 PR. *Vicus*
28. Ear Probe Inv. No. 32.6, BR 2 L. 9.8, CA PR. Prysg Field Trench 1 Barrack V, Fig. 21, Nr. 4 Nash-Williams 1932: 90, Nr. 5-Fig. 38	29. Ear Probe Inv. No. 35.119, BR 2 L. 12.2, CA PR. Amphitheatre, Fig. 21, Nr. 2 Wheeler 1928: 169, Nr. 4-Fig. 33.1.	30. Ear Probe Inv. No. 2392 (1632), BR 2 L. NA, CA PR. Roman Gates Block B, Fig. 21, Nr. 1
31. Ear Probe Inv. No. 82/389, BR 3 L. NA, CA PR, NA	32. Ear Probe Bent Inv. No. 88.165 H, BR 2 L. 8.6, CA PR. Roman gates Rampart Area, Fig. 21, Nr. 1	33. Olivary End Probe Inv. No. NA, BR 2 L 9.6, CA PR. NA
34. Olivary End Probe Inv. No. 84.43 H, BR 2 L. 10.5, CA PR. Museum Basement Area Zienkiewicz Forthcoming Report 39	35. Olivary End Probe Inv. No. 242/ 354, BR 2 L. 11.2, CA PR. Museum Gardens Zienkiewicz Forthcoming Report 29	36. Olivary End Probe Inv. No. 31/548 778/1636, BR 2 L. 12.0, CA PR. Roman Gates Rampart Area, Fig. 21, Nr. 1
37. Olivary End Probe Inv. No. 35.119, BR 2 L. 5.9, CA PR. Amphitheatre, Fig. 21, Nr. 2	38. Olivary End Probe Inv. No. 1684 (1301), BR 2 L. NA, CA PR. Roman Gates, Rampart Area, Fig. 21, Nr. 1	

TABLE A10.3: CHESTER, DEVA, LEGIONARY FORTRESS (FIG. 20)

1. Double Ended Olivary Probe Inv. No. NA, BR 4 L. 18.0, CA PR. Antonine Deposit Room 18, N-E Corner Barracks, Dearney Field, Fig. 20, Nr. 1 Hole in one end of the probe	2. Forceps Inv. No. 250. R. 176 28 A67/3, BR 4 L. 10.3, CA PR. Amphitheatre East Entrance Antonine Deposit	3. Forceps Inv. No. CHE NSM 88 306, BR 4 L. 8.0, CA PR. Extra Mural, Fig. 20, Nr. 6 There is an ear scoop attached to the top and an incised vine decoration on the arms.
4. Spoon Probe Broken Inv. No. CRS 1973-74 524 5, BR 4 L. NA, CA PR. First cohort Barracks, Fig. 20, Nr. 5	5. Spoon Probe Broken Inv. No. CHE/HSS 79 201, BR 4 L. 4.8, CA PR. Courtyard Building Hunter Street, Fig. 20, Nr. 3	6. Ear Probe Inv. No. CHE/NSM 88 271, BR 4 L. 3.2, CA PR. Extra Mural West St. Nicholas Mews, Fig. 20, Nr. 6
7. Ear Probe Inv. No. CHE/HSS 79 258, BR 4 L. 10.4, CA PR. Courtyard Hunter Street, Fig. 20, Nr. 2	8. Ear Probe Inv. No. CHE/PP 89 136, BR 4 L. NA, CA PR. Priory Place Extra Mural East, Fig. 20, Nr. 7	9. Ear Probe Inv. No. CHE/PP 89 84, BR 4 L. 5.5, CA PR. Priory Place Extra Mural East, Fig. 20, Nr. 7

10. Ear Probe Inv. No. CHE/CRS 63-64 187, BR 4 L. 15.6, Bone PR. First Cohort's Barrack, Fig. 20, Nr. 4	11. Olivary End Probe Inv. No. NA, BR 4 L. 3.36, CA PR. *Vicus* Love Street East of Fort	12. Olivary End Probe Inv. No. CHE/OMH 67-9 600, BR 4 L. 2.1, CA PR. Pit 17, Fig. 20, Nr. 3
13. Olivary End Probe Inv. No. CHE/CRS 73-4 148, BR 4 L. 7.4, CA PR. First Cohort Centurion's Quarters, Fig. 20, Nr. 5	14. Oculist Stamp Inv. No. NA L. NA Il. 32 Feugère *et al.* 1985: 480, Nr. 72; V. 271	

TABLE A10.4: CORBRIDGE, CORSTOPITUM, AUXILIARY FORT

1. Scalpel Inv. No. CO 11311 75.897, BR 5 L. 7.7, CA PR. Forum Site Gilson 1981: Nr.1-Fig. 1, Possible Forum Site because it is in a photograph Archaeologia Aeliana 1911	2. Scalpel Inv. No. CO 11322 75. 896, BR 5 L. 5.8, CA PR. NA Gilson 1981: Nr.2-Fig. 1	3. Scalpel Inv. No. CO11323 75. 899, BR 5 L. 10.6, CA PR. NA Gilson 1981: Nr.3-Fig. 1
4. Surgical Knife Inv. No. CO11312 75.1449, BR 5 L. 8.2, CA PR. NA Gilson 1981: Nr.1-Fig. 2	5. Surgical Knife Inv. No. CO11311 75. 897, BR 5 L. 5.0, CA PR. NA Gilson 1981: Nr.2-Fig. 2	6. Arm of Forceps Inv. No. CO11325 75.911, BR 5 L. 9.0, CA PR. NA Gilson 1981: Nr.1-Fig. 3
7. Double Simple Probe Inv. No. CO10294 75. 906, BR 5 L. 13.0, CA PR. NA Gilson 1981: Nr.1-Fig. 4	8. Spatula Probe Inv. No. CO10293 75.903, BR 5 L. 17.3, CA PR. NA Gilson 1981: Nr.5-Fig. 4	9. Spatula Probe bent Inv. No. CO10295 75. 909, BR 5 L. 16.0, CA PR. NA Gilson 1981: Nr.4-Fig. 4
10. Spoon Probe Inv. No. CO11306 75.459, BR 5 L. 10.5, CA PR. NA Gilson 1981: Nr.7-Fig. 4	11. Spoon Probe Inv. No. CO11285 75.463, BR 5 L. 6.5, CA PR. NA Gilson 1981: Nr.8-Fig. 4	12. Spoon Scoop Inv. No. CO11306 75.461, BR 5 L. 15.0, CA Pr. NA Gilson 1981: Nr.6-Fig. 4
13. Ear Probe Bent Inv. No. CO11321 75.904, BR 5 L. 8.0, CA PR. NA Gilson 1981: Nr. 3-Fig. 3 Bent in the centre, suggesting a possible use as a tongue depressor	14. Ear Probe Inv. No. CO10286 75. 457, BR 5 L. 5.1, CA PR. NA Gilson 1981: Nr.1-Fig. 5	15. Ear Probe Inv. No. CO10288 75. 460, BR 5 L. 9.9, CA PR. Forum Site Gilson 1981: Nr.4-Fig. 5, Possibly found in Forum due to Photograph in Archaeologia Aeliana 1911
16. Ear Probe Inv. No. CO10287 75. 458, BR 5 L. 9.4, CA PR. NA Gilson 1981: Nr.3-Fig. 5	17. Ear Probe Inv. No. CO10290 75. 910, BR 5 L. 13.5, CA PR. NA Gilson 1981: Nr.5-Fig. 5	18. Ear Probe Broken Inv. No. CO6729 R 236/452, BR 5 L. 8.1, CA PR. NA
19. Ear Probe Bent Inv. No. CO8515 75. 137, BR 5 L. 13.5, Ca PR. NA Bent at 45 degrees, suggesting use as a tongue depressor	20. Ear Probe Bent and Broken Inv. No. CO584 68 150 IP 68, BR 5 L. 6.1, CA PR. Temple III B6	21. Probe With Diamond Shaped Head Inv. No. CO10291 75.905, BR 5 L. 12.5, CA PR. NA Gilson 1981: Nr. 6-Fig. 5 the spatula is 0.7 cm at its widest point
22. Olivary End Probe Inv. No. CO10296 75. 908, BR 5 L. 7.5, CA PR. NA Gilson 1981: Nr 2-Fig. 4	23. Olivary End Probe Inv. No. CO1297 75. 907, BR 5 L. 9.5, CA PR. NA Gilson 1981: Nr 3 Fig. 4	24. Ointment Pallet Inv. No. CO1582 75. 3754, BR 5 5.4 x 3.0 x 0.7, Schist PR. NA Bishop and Dore 1988: 214, Nr. 1

TABLE A10.5: SOUTH SHIELDS, ARBEIA, AUXILIARY FORT

1. Spoon Probe Inv. No. SS 1900 8 (2), BR 6	2. Spoon Probe Inv. No. SS 1900 8 (1), BR 6	3. Ear Probe Inv. No. MA 1956. 128. 66 A (2).

L. 11.3, CA PR. NA Allason-Jones and Miket 1984: 170, Nr. 451-Fig. 3	L. 14.7, CA PR. NA Allason-Jones and Miket 1984: 170, Nr. 453-Fig. 3	BR 7 L. 4.3, CA PR. NA Allason-Jones and Miket 1984: 170, Nr. 458-Fig. 3
4. Ear Probe Inv. No. MA 1956. 128. 66 A (1), BR 7 L. 11.7, CA PR. NA Allason-Jones and Miket 1984: 172, Nr.459-Fig. 3	5. Ear Probe Inv. No. MA 1925. 35+37 (28), BR 7 L. 5.4 , CA PR. NA Allason-Jones and Miket 1984: 172, Nr. 460-Fig. 3	6. Ear Probe Inv. No. SS 1900.7 (3), BR 6 L. 13.7, CA PR. NA Allason-Jones and Miket 1984: 172, Nr. 461-Fig. 3
7. Ear Probe Inv. No. SS 1900.7 (1), BR 6 L. 15.1, CA PR. NA Allason-Jones and Miket 1984: 172, Nr. 462-Fig. 3	8. Ear Probe Inv. No. MA 1929.120 (1), BR 7 L. 6.0, CA PR. NA Allason-Jones and Miket 1984: 172, Nr. 463-Fig. 3	9. Ear Probe Inv. No. MA 1929. 119, BR 7 L. 11.4, CA PR. NA Allason-Jones and Miket 1984: 172, Nr. 464-Fig. 3
10. Ear Probe Inv. No. MA 1929. 119, BR 7 L. 12.0, CA PR. NA Allason-Jones and Miket 1984: 172, Nr. 465-Fig. 3		

TABLE A10.6: WALLSEND, SEGEDUNUM, AUXILIARY FORT

1. Spatula Probe Broken Inv. No. C11 4 (1196) L. 5.1, CA PR. NA Allason-Jones (Unpublished Draft)	2. Spatula Probe Broken Inv. No. C1332 (886) L. 2.6, CA PR. NA Allason-Jones (Unpublished Draft)	3. Olivary End Probe Inv. No. C11 4 (1199) L. 12.5, CA PR. NA Allason-Jones (Unpublished Draft)

TABLE A10.7: HALTON CHESTERS, HUNNUM, AUXILIARY FORT

1. Spoon Probe Inv. No. H60 IR L. 17.0, CA PR. NA Allason-Jones (Unpublished Draft)	2. Spoon Probe Inv. No. H61 QO 333 L. 5.8, CA PR. NA Allason-Jones (Unpublished Draft)

TABLE A10.8: CHESTERS, CILURNUM, AUXILIARY FORT

1. Spoon Probe Inv. No. CH 1043, BR 8 L. 7.8, CA PR. NA Both ends are broken	2. Spoon Probe Inv. No. CH 1045, BR 8 L. 10.0, CA PR. NA The handle is slightly bent	3. Spoon Probe Broken Inv. No. CH 744, BR 8 L. 4.5, CA PR. NA Most of the spoon is broken.
4. Ear Probe Inv. No. 1512, 74014 EER/50, BR 5 L. 11.5, CA PR. NA	5. Ear Probe Inv. No. 818 (1072), BR 5 L. 11.0, CA PR. 37 Below the scoop is a rectangular decoration with a hole through the centre	6. Ear Probe Inv. No. CH2432, 1083, BR 5 L. 7.4, CA PR. NA
7. Ear Probe Inv. No. CH1044, BR 8 L. 11.0, CA PR. NA There is a circular design below the spoon with a hole through its centre.	8. Ear Probe Bent Inv. No. CH2431, 1041,1516, BR 5 L. 5.5, CA PR. NA The handle is bent in the middle at a right angle.	9. Ear Probe Bent Inv. No. CH 2439, BR 5 L. 8.0, CA PR. NA
10. Ear Probe Broken Inv. No. CH 695, BR 8 L. 7.2, CA	11. Shears Inv. No. CH 1041, BR 8 L. 8.9, CA	12. Ointment Pallet Inv. No. CH 1210, BR 8 7.0 x 7.3, Stone

PR. NA The end is broken.	PR. NA One arm is broken	PR. NA
13. Ointment Pallet Inv. No. CH1209, BR 8 7.6 x 7.9, Stone PR. NA		

TABLE A10.9: HOUSESTEADS, BORCOVICIUM, AUXILIARY FORT

1. Sharp Hook Inv. No. NA, BR 7 L. NA, CA PR. Trial Trench, South of Fort, Fig. 25 Bosanquet 1904: 289	2. Spoon Scoop Inv. No. 81072056, BR 5 L. 14.5, CA PR. *Valetudinarium*, Fig. 25 The handle is hollow and opens onto the spoon.	3. Spoon Probe Inv. No. 79208631(75. 4879), BR 5 L. 12.5, CA PR. NA
4. Ear Probe Inv. No. H13. 1075. 444, BR 5 L. 12.0, CA PR. Outside the Commandant's Quarters, Fig. 25	5. Ear Probe Inv. No. 79208511, BR 5 L. 12.5, CA PR. NA	6. Ointment Pallet Inv. No. HSE1 23 (9254), BR 5 6.4 x 8.0, Stone PR. NA

TABLE A10.10: BIRDOSWALD, BANNA, AUXILIARY FORT

1. Ear Probe Inv. No. 575 127, BR 9 L. 10.6, CA PR. Building 197 (Granary) Period 5 Floor Layer, Fig. 24 Wilmott and Hird 1997: 287, Nr. 102 Period 5	2. Ear Probe Inv. No. 712 235, BR 9 L. 12.0, CA PR. Building 198 (Granary) Dump Period 5. Fig. 24 Wilmott and Hird 1997: 287, Nr. 103 Period 5	3. Ear Probe Inv. No. 923 1505, BR 9 L. 12.7, CA PR. Via Praetoria Period 4 B, Fig. 7o Wilmott and Hird 1997: 287, Nr. 103 Period 4b
4. Ointment Pallet Inv. No. 903 1403, BR 9 6.4 x 3.7, Sandstone PR. Building 198 Dump, Fig. 24 Wilmott and Hird 1997: 288, Nr. 108 Phase Five	5. Ointment Pallet Inv. No. 581 1, BR 9 6.3 x 3.0, Slate PR. Area A Topsoil, Fig. 24 Wilmott and Hird 1997: 288, Nr. 109	

TABLE A10.11: CARLISLE, AUXILIARY FORT

1. Sharp Hook Inv. No. Ae 219, BR 9 L. 12.5, CA PR. Building One Period 4 McCarthy 1990: 137-8, Nr. 123, Fig. 122, mid second century	2. Scalpel Inv. No. A1237 Ae 656, BR 9 L. 9.0, CA PR. Annetwell St. Excavations McCarthy 1990: 137-8, Nr. 123, Fig 123, mid second century	3. Cataract Needle Inv. No. A3550 Ae 881. 4 B, BR 9 L. 11.0, CA PR. Annetwell St. Excavations McCarthy 1990: 137-8, Nr. 123-Fig. 124, mid second century

TABLE A10.12: BOWNESS ON SOLWAY, MAIA, AUXILIARY FORT

1. Ear Probe Inv. No. 15-1939-1, BR 9 L. 19.0, CA PR. Sewer Trench

Appendix Eleven

Chi-Squared Test One

Q. Is there an association between province and fortification with or without instruments?

Province	Instruments	Without Instruments	Total
GI	9	23	32
GS	26	59	85
R	15	25	40
N	1	16	17
PS	4	7	11
PI	2	17	19
B	12	10	22
Total	**69**	**157**	**226**

		O	E	(O-E)	(O-E)2	(O-E)2/E
GI	W	9	9.76	-0.76	0.57	0.059
	W/O	23	22.2	0.8	0.64	0.028
GS	W	26	25.95	0.05	0.0025	0.000
	W/O	59	59.09	0.04	0.0016	0.000
R	W	15	12.2	2.8	7.85	0.64
	W/O	25	27.7	-2.7	7.29	0.26
N	W	1	5.19	-4.19	17.55	3.3
	W/O	16	11.8	4.2	17.64	1.49
PS	W	4	3.35	0.65	0.42	0.12
	W/O	7	7.6	-0.6	0.36	0.05
PI	W	2	5.80	-3.8	14.44	2.48
	W/O	17	13.1	3.9	15.21	1.16
B	W	12	6.71	5.29	27.98	4.17
	W/O	10	15.8	-5.8	33.64	2.12
					Total	**15.87=$\chi 2$**

d.f.= (7-1)(2-1)
= (6)(1)
= 6

For 6 d.f. the 0.1% level is 22.5. The $\chi 2$ value is 15.87, allowing for the null hypothesis to be rejected just above the 1% level which has a $\chi 2$ value of 16.8. Thus for the number of fortifications with instruments compared to those fortifications without there is a significant number of fortifications to have a mathematically significant association.

Appendix Twelve

Chi-Squared Test Two

Q. Is there an association between province and the types of fortifications with instruments?

Province	**Legion**	**Auxiliary**	**Numerus**	**Total**
GI	4	5	0	9
GS	2	22	2	26
R	1	14	0	15
N	1	0	0	1
PS	3	1	0	4
PI	1	1	0	2
B	3	9	0	12
Total	**14**	**52**	**2**	**69**

		O	**E**	**(O-E)**	**(O-E)2**	**(O-E)2/E**
GI	Leg	4	1.9	2.1	4.41	2.32
	Aux	5	6.78	-1.78	3.16	0.46
	Num	0	0.26	-0.26	0.067	0.26
GS	Leg	2	5.6	-3.6	12.96	2.31
	Aux	22	19.59	2.41	5.8	0.296
	Num	2	0.75	1.25	1.56	2.08
R	Leg	1	3.2	2.2	4.84	1.51
	Aux	14	11.3	2.7	7.29	0.645
	Num	0	0.43	-0.43	0.18	0.43
N	Leg	1	0.21	0.79	0.62	2.95
	Aux	0	0.75	-0.75	0.56	0.75
	Num	0	0.028	-0.028	0.0007	0.028
PS	Leg	3	0.86	2.14	4.57	5.3
	Aux	1	3.01	-2.01	4.04	1.34
	Num	0	0.115	-0.115	0.013	0.115
PI	Leg	1	0.43	0.57	0.32	0.74
	Aux	1	1.5	-0.5	0.25	0.16
	Num	0	0.05	-0.05	0.0.0025	0.05
B	Leg	3	2.6	0.4	0.16	0.06
	Aux	9	0.04	-.04	0.005	0.0005
	Num	0	0.34	-0.34	0.115	0.34
					Total	**22.144=χ2**

d.f. = (7-1)(3-1)
= (6)(2)
= 12

For 12 d.f. the 0.1% value is 32.9. The χ2 value is 22.144, allowing for a null hypothesis to be rejected at the 5% level which has a d.f. value of 21.0 and the 1% value is 26.2. There is just a significant association between provinces and the types of fortifications with instruments.

APPENDIX THIRTEEN

CHI-SQUARED TEST THREE

Q. Is there an association between instrument numbers per unit type and province?

Province	Legion	Auxiliary	Numerus	Total
GI	118	25	0	143
GS	360	111	3	474
R	5	73	0	78
N	30	0	0	30
PS	201	1	0	202
PI	15	15	0	30
B	54	67	0	121
Total	**783**	**292**	**3**	**1078**

	O	E	(O-E)	(O-E)2	(O-E)2/E
GI					
Leg	118	103.86	14.14	199.9	1.92
Aux	25	38.7	-13.7	187.69	4.84
Num	0	0.39	-0.39	0.1521	0.39
GS					
Leg	360	344.2	15.8	246.64	0.72
Aux	111	128.3	-17.3	299.29	2.3
Num	3	1.31	1.69	2.85	2.18
R					
Leg	5	56.6	-51.6	2662.56	47.0
Aux	73	21.12	51.88	2691.53 1	27.4
Num	0	0.21	-0.21	0.044	0.21
N					
Leg	30	21.8	8.2	67.24	3.08
Aux	0	8.12	-8.12	65.9	8.12
Num	0	0.08	-0.08	0.0064	0.08
PS					
Leg	201	146.7	54.3	2948	20.08
Aux	1	54.7	-53.7	2883.6	52.7
Num	0	0.56	-0.56	0.313	0.56
PI					
Leg	15	21.8	-6.8	47.3	5.82
Aux	15	8.12	6.88	47.3	5.82
Num	0	0.08	-0.08	0.0064	0.08
B					
Leg	54	87.8	-33.8	1142.4	13.01
Aux	67	32.7	34.3	1176.49	35.9
Num	0	0.33	-0.33	0.108	0.33
				Total	**328.88=χ2**

d.f. = (7-1)(3-1)
(6)(2)
12

For 12 d.f the 0.1% value is 32.9. The χ2 value is 328.88, allowing the null hypothesis to be rejected at the 0.1% level. There is a significant association between the numbers of instruments per unit type in comparison with the provinces.

BIBLIOGRAPHY

ABBREVIATIONS FOR INSCRIPTIONS AND PAPYROLOGY

AE=*L'Annee Epigraphique: Revue des Publications Epigraphiques Relatives a l'antique Romaine.* 1888- Paris.

BGU= *Berliner Griechische Urkunden Ägyptische Urkunden aus den Königlichen Museen zu Berlin.* 1895 - Berlin.

CIL=*Corpus Inscriptorum Latinorum. Consilio et Ductoritate Academie Litterarum Regiae Borussical Edition.* Berlin: Academieder Wissenschaften1862-.

E= e Espérandieu, *Signacula medicorum oculariorum. Corpus Inscriptionum Latinarum* vol. 13, pars 3, fasc 2. Berlin: Academieder Wissenschaften 1906.

IGRR= Cagnet, R. L. V. and J. F. Toutain 1964. *Inscriptiones Graecae ad Res Romanas Pertinentes: Auctoritate et Impensis Academiae Inscriptionum et litterarum humaniarum.* Rome: L'Erma Bretschneider.

ILS= Dessau, H. 1892-1916. *Inscriptiones Latinae Selectae.* Berlin: Apud Weidmannos.

P.Mich.= *Papyri in the University of Michigan Collection.* Ann Arbour: University of Michigan Press

P.Oxy=B. Grenfell, A. S. Hunter et al. (eds). *The Oxyrhynchus Papyri.* 1898- London.

P. Rainer=*Papyrus Erzherzog Rainer der Papyrussammlung der Österreichischen Nationalbibliothek.* Vienna: Verlag Brüder Hollinek 1883-

RIB=Collingwood, R. G. and R. P. Wright 1995. *The Roman Inscriptions of Britain.* Stroud: Alan Sutton.

V=Voinot, J. 1984. *Inventaire des cachets d'oculistes gallo-romains. Conférences Lyonnaises d'Optalmologie* Nr. 150, 1981/2.

PRIMARY SOURCES

Albucasis. *Albucasis on Surgery and Instruments.* M. S. Spink,. and G. L. Lewis (Trans.) 1973.London: Wellcome Institute of the History of Medicine

Caesar, C. Iulii Caesaris. *Commentarius de Bello Africo.* E. Wölfflin (ed.) 1896. Leipzig: B. G. Teubner.

Caesar. C. Iulii Caesaris. *Commentariorum Libri III De Bello Civili.* R. du Pontèt (ed.) 1900-1908. Oxford: Clarendon Press.

Caesar. C. Iulii Caesaris. *Commentariorum Libri VII De Bello Gallico.* R. du Pontèt (ed.) 1900-1908. Oxford: Clarendon Press.

Cato. Caton. *De L'Agriculture.* R. Goujard (ed.) 1975.Paris: Société d'Édition les Belles Lettres.

Celsus. A. Cornelii Celsi. *Corpus Medicorum Latinorum.* F. Marx (ed.) 1915. Leipzig: B. G. Teubner.

Celsus. *De Medicina.* W. G. Spencer (Trans.) 1971. (Loeb). Cambridge MA and London: Harvard University Press and William Heinemann Ltd.

Codex Iustiniaunus Corpus Iuris Civilis. P. Kruger, Th. Mommsen, R. Scholl and J. W. Kroll(eds.) 1954. Berlin: Apud Weidmann.

Codex Theodosianus. C. Pharr (Trans.) 1952. New York: Greenwood Press.

Digest of Justinian. A. Watson (Trans.) 1985. Th. Mommsen and P. Krueger (eds.) Philadelphia: University of Pennsylvania Press.

Dio Cassius. Dionis Cassii Cocceiani. *Historia Romana* (vol. 4). L. Dindorf (ed.) 1864. Leipzig: B. G. Teubner.

Dio Cassius. *Roman History* (Book 58). E. Cary (Trans.) 1968. (Loeb). Cambridge, MA and London: Harvard University Press and William Heinemann Ltd.

Dionysus of Halicarnassus. E. Carey (Trans.). 1947 Cambridge, MA and London: William Heinemann Ltd and Harvard University Press

Frontinus. Iuli Frontini. *Strategematon.* G. Gundermann (ed.) 1888. Leipzig: B. G. Teubner.

Galen. *Claudii Galeni opera omnia.* C. G. Kühn (ed) 20 vols. in 22 1821-1833. Leipzig: Cnobloch.

Galen. *On the Parts of Medicine.* M.E. Lyons (Trans. and ed.) 1969. Berlin: Akademie-Verlag.

Herodian. 2 vols. C. R. Whittaker (Trans.) 1969-70 (Loeb). London and Cambridge, MA:

William Heinemann LtD and Harvard University Press.
Heron of Alexandria. *Pneumatica et Automata.* W. Schmidt (Trans.) 1899. Leipzig: Druck and Verlag B. G. Teubner.
Herophilus. H. von Staden (Trans. and ed.) 1989. *The Art of Medicine in Early Alexandria.* Cambridge: Cambridge University Press.
Hippocrates. *Decorum.* W. H. S. Jones (Trans.) 1953 (Loeb). London and Cambridge, MA: William Heinemann LtD and Harvard University Press.
Hippocrates. Hippocratis. *De Medico.* I. L. Heiberg (ed.) 1927. Leipzig and Berlin: B. G. Teubner.
Hippocrates. *In the Surgery.* W. H. S. Jones (Trans.) 1953. (Loeb). London and Cambridge, MA: William Heinemann LtD and Harvard University Press.
Hippocrates. *On the Physician.* W. H. S. Jones (Trans.) 1953. (Loeb). London and Cambridge, MA: William Heinemann LtD and Harvard University Press.
Hyginus Gromaticus. Hygini Gromatici. *Liber de Munitionibus Castrorum.* W. Gemoll (ed.) 1897. Leipzig: B. G. Teubner.
Livy. Titi Livi. *Ab Urbe Condita* (vols. I and II). C. F. Walters and R. S. Conway (eds.) 1974 (I); 1919 (II). Oxford: Clarendon Press.
Lucian. *The Ignorant Book Collector.* A. M. Harmon (Trans.) 1921. (Loeb). London and New York William Heinemann Press LtD and G. P. Putnam's and Sons.
Martial. M. Val. Martialis. *Epigrammata.* W. M. Linday (ed.) 1929. Oxford: Clarendon Press.
Martial. *Epigrams.* D. R. Shackleton Bailey (Trans) 1993. (Loeb). Cambridge, MA and London: Harvard University Press.
Onasander. *The General.* The Illinois Greek Club (Trans.) 1977. (Loeb). Cambridge, MA and London: Harvard University Press and William Heinemann LtD.
Oribasius. *Collectionum Medicarum Reliquiae* (vols. I and II). I. Raeder (ed.) 1928-31. Leipzig: B. G. Teubner.
Paul of Aegina. *Paulus Aegineta.* I. L. Heiberg (ed.) 1921-24. Leipzig and Berlin: B. G. Teubner.
Pliny. C. Plini Secundi. *Naturalis Historiae* (vol. IIII Lib. XXIII-XXXII). L. Ianus (ed.) 1880. Leipzig: B. G. Teubner.
Qur'an. Abdullah Yusuf Ali (Trans.) 2000. Ware: Wordsworth.
Res Gestae Divi Augusti. P. A. Brunt and J. M. Moore (eds.) 1967. Oxford: Oxford University Press.
Scriptores Historia Augusta. D. Magie (Trans.) 1922. (Loeb). London and New York: William Heinemann Ltd.
Soranus. *Gynecology.* O. Temkin (Trans.) 1956. Baltimore: The Johns Hopkins University Press.
Soranus. Sorani. *Gynaecia.* J. Ilberg (ed) 1927. Leipzig: B. G. Teubner.
Suetonius. Suétone. *Vies des douze Césars* (vols. I and II). H. Ailloud (ed.) 1931-31. Paris: Société d'Édition les Belles Lettres.
Tacitus. Cornelii Taciti. *Annalium.* C. D. Fischer (ed.) 1967. Oxford: Clarendon Press.
Tacitus. Cornelii Taciti. *Historiarum Libri.* C. D. Fischer (ed.) 1967. Oxford: Clarendon Press.
Tibullus. Albii Tibulli. *Aliurum Carminum Libri Tres.* F. W. Lenz (ed.) 1937. Leipzig: B. G. Teubner.
Vegetius. *Epitome of Military Science.* N. P. Milner (Trans.) 1993. Liverpool: Liverpool University Press.
Vegetius. Flavi Vegeti Renati. *Epitoma rei Militaris.* C. Lang (ed.) 1967. Leipzig: Aedibus B. G. Teubner.
Velleius Paterculus. Velleii Paterculi. Second edition. C. S. de Pritzwald (ed.) 1933. Stuttgart: B. G. Teubner.
Virgil. P. Virgili Maronis. *Aeneidos Liber Primus.* R. G. Austin (ed.) 1971. Oxford: Clarendon Press.
Vitruvius. Vitruvii. *De Architectura.* V. Rose (ed.) 1899. Leipzig: B. G. Teubner.
Xenophon. Xénophon. *Helléniques* (Vol. I) J. Hatzfeld (ed.) 1949. Paris: Société d'Édition les Belles Lettres.

SECONDARY SOURCES

Alföldy, G. 1974. *Noricum.* A. Birley (Trans.). London and Boston: Routledge and Kegan Paul.
Allason-Jones, L. Unpublished Draft. *List of Small Finds from Roman Sites in Britain.*
Allason-Jones, L. and R. Miket 1984. *The Catalogue of Small Finds from South Shields Roman Fort.* Newcastle upon Tyne: The Society of Antiquaries.
Allason-Jones, L. and B. McKay 1985. *Coventina's Well: A Shrine on Hadrian's Wall.* Chollerford, Hexam: Trustees of the Clayton Collection, Chesters Museum.
Allason-Jones, L. 1993. Health care in the Roman North. In D. Gardner-Medwin, A. Hargreaves and E. Lazenby (eds.) *Medicine in Northumbria: Essays on the History of Medicine in the North East of*

England. Newcastle upon Tyne: The Pybus society for the history and bibliography of medicine, pp. 24-39.

Allason-Jones, L. and Dungworth, D. B. 1997. Metalworking on Hadrian's Wall. In W. Groenman-van Waateringe, B. L. van Beek, W. J. H. Willems and S. L. Wynia (eds.) *Roman FrontierStudies 1995.* Oxbow Monograph 91. Oxford: Oxbow Books, pp. 317-22.

Allason-Jones, L. 1999. Health Care in the Roman North. *Britannia* 31: 131-46.

Allison, P. 1997. Why do Excavation Reports Have Finds' Catalogues? In C. G. Cumberpatch and P. W. Blinkhorn (eds.) *Not so Much a Pot, More a Way of Life.* Oxbow Monograph 83. Oxford: Oxbow Books, pp. 77-84.

Anonymous 1750. *The Manners and Customs of the Romans.* London.

Anonymous 1930. Kastell Zugmantel die Ausgraben 1925. *Saalburg Jahrbuch* 7: 35-78.

Anonymous 1970-71. Das römische Legionslager von Vindonissa. *Helvetia Archaeologica* 2: 33-7.

Anonymous 1986. *Das römische Budapest.* Münster: Austellungskatalog.

Anonymous 2000. More Evidence of Roman PoW Camps on Hadrian's Wall. *British Archaeology.* August 2000: 6.

Anthes, E. 1936. Die Wetteraulinie vom Köpperner Tal bei der Saalburg bis zum Main bei Gross-Krotzenburg. *Der Obergermanisch-Raetische Limes des Roemerreiches.* Berlin and Leipzig: Verlag von Otto Petters.

Argyle, M. 1988. *Bodily Ccommunication.* New York and London: Routledge.

Baader, G. 1967. Spezialärzte in der Spätantike. *Medizinhistorisches Journal* 2: 231-8.

Baatz, D. 1970. Krankenhauser bei den Römern. *Kurz und Gut* 2: 8-10.

Baatz, D. 1975. *Das Kastell am kleinen Feldberg.* Führungsblatt des Saalburgmuseums.

Baatz, D. and F. R. Herrmann 1982. *Die Römer in Hessen.* Stuttgart: Konrad Theiss Verlag.

Baker, P. 1995. Unpublished Master's Dissertation, University of Newcastle upon Tyne. *Valentinean's supply system on the Rhine and Danube: an examination of secured granaries.*

Baker, P., C. Forcey, S. Jundi and R. Witcher (eds) 1999.*TRAC 98: Proceedings of the Eighth Annual Theoretical Roman Archaeology Conference, Leicester 1998.* Oxford: Oxbow Books.

Baker, P. 2001. Medicine, Culture and Military Identity. In G. Davies, A. Gardner, K. Lockyear (eds.). *TRAC 2000, Theoretical Roman Archaeology Conference Proceedings: London 2000. Oxford:* Oxbow Press, pp. 51-70

Baker, P. 2002a. Diagnosing Some Ills: the Archaeology, Literature and History of Roman Medicine. In P. Baker and G. Carr (eds.) *Practitioners, Practices and Patients: New Approaches to Medical Archaeology and Anthropology.* Oxford: Oxbow Press, pp. 16-29.

Baker, P. 2002b. The Roman Military *Valetudinaria*: Fact or Fiction? In R. Arnott (ed.) *The Archaeology of Medicine* BAR International Series 1064. Oxford: British Archaeological Reports, pp 69-79.

Baker, P. 2004. Roman Medical Instruments: Archaeological Interpretations of their Possible 'Non-functional' Uses. *Social History of Medicine* 17 (1): 3-21.

Barker, G. and T. Rasmussen 1998. *The Etruscans.* Oxford: Blackwell Publishers.

Barrett, J. C. 1989. Afterwards: Render unto Caesar. In J. C. Barrett, A. P. Fitzpatrick and L. Macinnes (eds.) *Barbarians and Romans in north-west Europe from the Later Republic to Late Antiquity.* Oxford: BAR International Series, 471, pp. 235-41.

Barrett, J. C. and A. P. Fitzpatrick 1989. Introduction. In J. C. Barrett, A. P. Fitzpatrick and L. Macinnes (eds.) *Barbarians and Romans in north-west Europe from the Later Republic to Late Antiquity.* Oxford: BAR International Series, 471, pp. 9-13.

Barthel, W. 1907. Das Kastell Cannstatt. *Der Obergermanisch-Raetische Limes des Roemerreiches.* Heildelberg: Verlag von Otto Petters.

Bartlett, A. 1994. Spatial Order and Psychiatric Disorder. In M. Parker Pearson and C. Richards (eds.) *Architecture and Order: Approaches to Social Space.* New York and London: Routledge, pp. 178-95.

Becker, M. J. 1999. Etruscan Gold Dental Appliances: Three Newly "Discovered" Examples. *American Journal of Archaeology* 103 (1): 103-11.

Becker, M. J. 2002. Etruscan Female Tooth Evulsion: Gold Dental Appliances as Ornaments. In P. Baker and G. Carr (eds.) *Practitioners, Practices and Patients: New Approaches to Medical Archaeology and Anthropology.* Oxford: Oxbow Press, pp. 238-59.

Beckmann, B. 1975. *Das Kastell Kapersburg im Taunus.* Föhrschungsblatt des Saalburgmuseums.

Behrens, G. and E. Brenner 1911. Ausgrabungen im Legionskastell zu Mainz während des

Jahres 1910. *Mainzer Zeitschrift* 6: 53-120.
Behrens, G. 1939. Schädeltrepanation im römischen Bingen. *Saalburg Jahrbuch* 9: 4-5.
Bidwell, P. 1997. *Book of Roman Forts in Britain.* London: B. T. Batsford/ English Heritage.
Birley, A. 1997. Supplying the Batavians at Vindolanda. In W. Groenman-van Waateringe, B. L. van Beek, W. J. H. Willems and S. L. Wynia (eds.) *Roman Frontier Studies 1995.* Oxbow Monograph 91. Oxford: Oxbow Books, pp. 273-80.
Birley, E. (ed.) 1952. *The Congress of Roman Frontier Studies 1949.* Durham: Durham University Registrar.
Bishop, M. C. and J. Dore 1988. *Corbridge. Excavations at the Roman Fort and Town 1947-80.* London: English Heritage.
Bishop, M. and J. Coulston 1993. *Roman Military Equipment from the Punic Wars to the Fall of Rome.* London: B. T. Batsford.
Bliquez, L. 1981a. An Unidentified Roman Surgical Instrument in Bingen. *Journal of History of Medicine* 36 (2): 219-20.
Bliquez, L. 1981b. Greek and Roman Medicine. *Archaeology* 34 (2): 10-17.
Bliquez, L. 1985. Λιθουλκός, Κιρσουλκός *American Journal of Philology* 106: 119-21.
Bliquez, L. 1988. *Roman Surgical Instruments and Minor Objects Found in the University of Mississippi.* Göteborg: Paul Åstroms Fõrlag.
Bliquez, L. and J. P. Oleson 1994. The Origins, Early History and Applications of the *Pyoulkos* (syringe). In G. Argoud (ed.) *Science et Vie Intellectuelle a Alexandrie.* Saint-Étienne: Publications de l'Universitéde Saint-Étienne, pp. 83-103.
Böcking, W. 1987. *Der Niederrhein zur römischen Zeit Archäologische Ausgrabungen in Xanten.* Kleve: Verlag für Kultur und Technik.
Bogaers , J. E. and H. Rüger 1974. *Der niedergermanische Limes.* Cologne: Rhineland Verlag.
Böhme, A. 1978. Metallfünde in H. Schönberger (ed.) *Kastell Oberstimm: Die Grabungen von 1968 bis 1971. Limesforschungen* 18. Berlin: Mann Verlag, pp. 64-226.
Bonis, E. 1968. Emaillierte Palästra-Geräte aus Brigetio. *Folia Archaeologica* 19: 25-58.
Boon, G. C. Unpublished Draft. *Civil Settlement Report for Caerleon.*
Boon, G. C. 1970. Excavations at the Site of the Basilica Principiorum at Caerleon, 1968-69. *Archaeologia Cambriensis* 119: 10-63.
Boon, G. C. 1972. *Isca: The Roman Legionary Fortress at Caerleon, Monmouthshire.* Cardiff: National Museum of Wales.
Boon, G. C. 1987: *The Legionary Fortress of Caerleon-Isca.* Cardiff: National Museum of Wales.
Boon, G. C. and C. Williams 1967. *Plan of Caerleon Isca: Legio II Augusta. Discoveries to December 1966.* Cardiff: National Museum of Wales.
Bormann, E. 1906. *Der Römische Limes in Österreich* 7: 133-6.
Bosanquet, R. C. 1904. Excavations on the Line of the Roman Wall in Northumberland. *Archaeologia Aeliana* 25 (Series 3): 193-300.
Bosman, A. V. A. J. 1995. Velserbroek B6 Velsen 1-Velsen 2: Is there a Relationship between the Military Equipment from the Ritual Site and the Fortress of Velsen? *Journal of Roman Military Equipment Studies* 6: 89-98.
Bounegru, O. 1997. Considérations concernant le transport des merchandises et le ravitaillement de l'armee sur le limes du Bas-Danube. In W. Groenman-van Waateringe, B. L. van Beek, W. J. H. Willems and S. L. Wynia. (eds.) *Roman Frontier Studies 1995.* Oxbow Monograph 91. Oxford: Oxbow Books, pp. 311-16.
Bowman, A. K. and J. D. Thomas 1991. A Military Strength Report from Vindolanda. *Journal of Roman Studies* 81: 62-73.
Bowman, A. K. and J. D. Thomas 1994. *The Vindolanda Writing Tablets (Tabulae Vindolandenses II).* London: British Museum Press.
Braadbaart, S. 1994a. Medical and Cosmetic Instruments in the Collection of the 'Rijksmuseum van Oudheden te Leiden', The Netherlands. *Oudheidkundige Mededelingen uit het Rijksmuseum van Oudheden te Leiden* 74: 163-75.
Braadbaart, S. 1994b. Romeinse medische instrumenten. *Geschiedenis der Geneeskunde* 1 (5): 51-5.
Brat, L. 1966. *Die Geschichte des Peter Friedrich Ludwigs Hospitals (1841-1966).* Oldenburg: Oldenburg.
Breeze, D. J. 2002 (3rd edition). Britain. In J. Wacher. (ed), *The Roman World.* London Routledge and Kegan Paul, pp. 198-221.
Breeze, D. J. and B. Dobson 1991. *Hadrian's Wall.* London: Penguin Press.
Breitwieser, R. 1998. *Medizin im römischen Österreich.* Linz: Linzer Archäologische Forschungen.
Britton, F. 1987. *London Delftware.* London:

Jonathon Horne.
Bult, E. J. and D. P. Hallewas 1986. *Graven bij Valkenburg: Het archeologisch onderzoek in 1985.* Delft: Eburon.
Burkert, W. 1979. *Structure and History in Greek Mythology and Ritual.* Berkeley: University of California Press.
Callies, H. 1968. Zur Stellung der *Medici* im römischen Herr. *Medizinhistorisches Journal* 3: 18-27.
Campbell, J. B. 1994. *The Roman Army 31 BC-AD 337: A Sourcebook.* London and New York: Routledge.
Carlin, M. 1989. Medieval English hospitals. In L. Granshaw and R. Porter (eds.) *The Hospital in History.* New York and London: Routledge, pp. 21-40.
Carr, G., E. Swift and J. Weekes (eds.) 2003. *TRAC 2002: Proceedings of the Twelfth Annual Theoretical Roman Archaeology Conference, Canterbury 2002.* Oxford: Oxbow Books.
Caton, R. 1914. Notes on A Group of Medical and Surgical Instruments Found near Kolophon. *Journal of Hellenic Studies* 34: 114-18.
Charlesworth, D. 1976. The Hospital: Housesteads. *Archaeologica Aeliana* (Series 5) 4: 17-30.
Clarke, S. and R. Jones. 1994. The Newstead Pits. *Journal of Roman Military Equipment Studies* 5: 109-24.
Clarke, S. 1999. Contact, Architectural Symbolism and the Negotiation of Cultural Identity in the Military Zone. In P. Baker, C. Forcey, S. Jundi. and R. Witcher (eds.) *TRAC 98: Proceedings of the Eighth Annual Theoretical Roman Archaeology Conference, Leicester 1998.* Oxford: Oxbow Books, pp. 36-45.
Cleal, R. Walker, K. Montigue, R. 1995. *Stonehenge in its Landscape: Twentieth Century Excavations.* London: English Heritage.
Comelles, J. M. 1997. The Fear of (One's Own) History. On the Relations Between Medical Anthropology, Medicine and History. *Dynamis* 17: 37-68.
Como, J. 1925. Das Grab eines römische Arztes in Bingen. *Germania* 9: 152-62.
Conrad, L. 1995. The Arab-Islamic Medical Tradition. In Conrad, L., M. Neve, V. Nutton, R. Porter and A. Wear (eds.) *The Western Medical Tradition.* Cambridge: Cambridge University Press, pp. 94-138.
Conrad, L., M. Neve, V. Nutton, R. Porter and A. Wear (eds.) 1995. *The Western Medical Tradition.* Cambridge: Cambridge University Press.
Conrady, W., C. Wirth and F. Drexel 1910. Das Kastell Stockstadt. *Der Obergermanisch-Raetische Limes des Roemerreiches.* Heildelberg: Verlag von Otto Petters.
Cook, S. A. et al. (eds.) 1979. *Cambridge Ancient History 1979. Volume X: The Augustan Empire.* Cambridge: Cambridge University Press.
Cornell, T. and K. Lomas (eds.) 1997. *Gender and Ethnicity in Ancient Italy.* London: Accordia Research Institute, University of London.
Cottam, S., D. Dungworth, S. Scott and J. Taylor (eds.) 1994. *TRAC 94: Proceedings of the Fourth Annual Theoretical Roman Archaeology Conference, Durham 1994.* Oxford: Oxbow Books.
Counihan, C. 1999. *The Anthropology of Food and the Body: Gender, Meaning and Power.* New York and London: Routledge.
Creighton, J. D. and R. Wilson. (eds.) 1999. *Roman Germany Studies in Cultural Interaction.* Portsmouth, Rhode Island: Journal of Roman Archaeology Supplementary Series, no. 32.
Crow, J. 1995. *Housesteads.* Bath: B. T. Batsford/ English Heritage.
Crummy, P. 2002. A Preliminary Account of the Doctor's Grave at Stanway, Colchester, England. In P. Baker and G. Carr (eds.) *Practitioners, Practices and Patients: New Approaches to Medical Archaeology and Anthropology.* Oxford: Oxbow Books, pp. 47-57.
Cunliffe, B. 1988: *Greeks, Romans and Barbarians: Spheres of Interaction.* London: Guild Publishing.
Cuppers, H. and H. Bernhard 1990. *Die Römer in Rheinland-Pfalz.* Stuttgart: Konrad Theiss Verlag.
Curchin, L. A. 1991. *Roman Spain Conquest and Assimilation.* New York and London: Routledge.
Czysz, W. et al. 1995. *Die Römer in Bayern.* Stuttgart: Konrad Theiss Verlag.
Daniels, C. 1969. Corbridge. *Current Archaeology* 15: 97-101.
Daniels, C. 2002 (3rd edition). Africa. In J. Wacher (ed.) *The Roman World.* London and New York: Routledge Press, pp. 223-65.
Davies, R. 1969a. Joining the Roman Army. *Bonner Jahrbücher* 169: 208-32.
Davies, R. 1969b. The *Medici* of the Roman Armed Forces. *Epigraphische Studien* 8: 83-99.
Davies, R. W. 1969/70. A Note on the Hoard of Roman Equipment Buried at Corbridge. *Durham University Journal* 62: 177.
Davies, R. 1970. Some Roman Medicine. *Medical*

History 14 (1): 101-6.
Davies, R. 1972. Some More Military *Medici. Epigraphische Studien* 9: 3-11.
Davies, R. 1974. The Daily Life of the Roman Soldier under the Principate. *Aufstieg und Niedergang das Römischen Welt.* II, I 299-338.
Davies, R. 1989 (original 1970). The Roman Military Medical Service. In D. Breeze and V. Maxfield (eds.) *Service in the Roman Army.* Edinburgh: Edinburgh University Press: pp, 209-36.
Deetz, J. 1977. *In Small Things Forgotten.* New York: Anchor Press/ Doubleday.
Deringer, H. 1954. Die Medizinischen Instrumente des Ennser Museum. *Forschungen in Lauriacum* 2: 1952: Linz, pp. 144-55.
Dietler, M. 1995. The Cup of Gyptis: Rethinking the Colonial Encounter in Early-Iron-Age Western Europe and the Relevance of the World-Systems Model. *Journal of European Archaeology* 3 (2): 89-112.
Dietz, K., U. Osterhaus, S. Rieckhoff-Pauli and K. Spindler 1979. *Regensburg zurRömerzeit.* Regensburg: Verlag Friedrich Pustet.
Döderlein, G, 1973. Medizinische Instrumente aus Vindonissa und Aquae Helveticae. *Medizinische Monatschrift* 27: 409-12.
Dolmans, M. Th. R. M. 1992. De medische verzorging van de Romeinse soldaat. *Hermeneus* 64: 1-11.
Domaszewski, A. von 1908. Die Rangordung des römischen Heeres. *Bonner Jahrbücher* 108: 1-278.
Doppler, H. W. 1970-71. Baden in römischer Zeit. *Helvatia Archaeologica* 2: 26-32.
Dore, J. 1989. *Corbridge Roman Site.* London: English Heritage.
Drabkin, I. E. 1944. On Medical Education in Greece and Rome. *Bulletin of the HistoryofMedicine*, 15 (4): 333-51.
Drack, W. and R. Fellmann 1988. *Die Römer in der Schweiz.* Stuttgart: Konrad Theiss Verlag.
Drinkwater, J. F. 1983. *Roman Gaul.* London and Canberra: Croom Helm.
Drück, T. 1904. Das Kastell Urspring. *Der Obergermanisch-Raetische Limes des Roemerreiches.* Heildelberg: Verlag von Otto Petters.
Drummond, S. K. and L. H. Nelson 1994. *The Western Frontiers of Imperial Rome.* New York and London: M. E. Sharpe.
Dyczek, P. 1995. The *Valetudinarium* at Novae: New Components. In *Acts of the 12th International Congress on Ancient Bronzes (NAR).* Amersfoort, pp. 365-72.
Dyson, S. L. 1985. *The Creation of the Roman Frontier.* Princeton: Princeton University Press.
Edelstein, L. 1952. The Relation of Ancient Philosophy to Medicine. *The Bulletin of the History of Medicine* 24 (4): 298-316.
Eidam, Dr. 1929. Das Kastell Munningen. *Der Obergermanisch-Raetische Limes des Roemerreiches.* Berlin and Leipzig: Verlag von Otto Petters.
Elton, H. 1996. *Frontiers of the Roman Empire.* London: BT. Batsford.
Elgood, C. 1951. *A Medical History of Persia and the Eastern Caliphate from the Earliest Times until the Year AD 1932.* Cambridge: Cambridge University Press.
Evans, C. 1990. 'Power on Silt': Towards an Archaeology of the East India Company. *Antiquity* 64 (244 Sept.): 643-61.
Fabricius, E. 1936. Die Wetterau Limie von Köpperrner Tal bei der Saalburg bis zum Main bei Gross-Krotzenburg. *Der Obergermanisch-Raetische Limes des Roemerreiches.* Heildelberg: Verlag von Otto Petters.
Feugère, M., E. Künzl, U. Weisser 1985. Die Starnalden von Montbellet (Saône-et-Loire). Ein Beitrag zur antiken und islamischen Augenheilkunde. *Jahrbuch des Römisch-Germanischen Zentral museums.* 32: 436-508.
Filtzinger, P., D. Planck and B. Cämmerer 1986. *Die Römer in Baden Wurttemberg.* Stuttgart: Konrad Theiss Verlag.
Fletcher, M. and G. R. Lock 1991. *Digging Numbers: Elementary Statistics for Archaeologists.* Oxford: University Committee for Archaeology Monograph 33.
Forcey, C., J. Hawthorne and R. Witcher (eds.) *TRAC 97: Proceedings of the Seventh Annual Theoretical Roman Archaeology Conference, Nottingham 1997.* Oxford: Oxbow Books.
Fox, A. 1940. The Legionary Fortress at Caerleon in Monmouthshire: Excavations at Myrtle Cottage Orchard 1939. *Archaeologia Cambriensis* 95: 101-52.
Frere, S. S. 1983. Sites Explored 1982. *Britannia* 14: 279-335.
Frere, S. S. 1984. Sites Explored 1983. *Britannia* 15: 265-332.
Fröhlich, L. 1910. Bericht über die Grabungen am Schutthügel im Jahre 1909. *Anzeiger für Schweizer Altertumskunde* 12: 126-29.
Furniss, D. A. 1970. Mediaeval Hospitals. *History of Medicine* 2 (1): 2-4.
Gaitzsch, W. 1983. Die römische Schraube aus dem Kastell von Niederbieber. *Bonner Jahrbücher* 183: 595-602.
Gautier, E. F. 1952. *Le passé de l'Afrique du Nord.* Paris: Payot.
Geertz, C. 1984. Anti Anti-Relativism. *American*

Anthropologist. 86: 263-78.
Genser, K. 1986. *Der römische Limes in Österreich.* Vienna: Verlag von der Österreichischen Akademie der Wissenschaften.
Giddens, A. 1984. *The Constitution of Society.* Cambridge: Polity Press.
Gillam, J. P. and J. Tate 1971. The Investigation of the Commander's House Area, on site XI, Corbridge, 1958 to 1970. The Structures. *Archaeologia Aeliana* (series 4) 49: 1-28.
Gilson, A. 1978. A Doctor at Housesteads. *Archaeologia Aeliana* 6 (series 5): 162-165.
Gilson, A. 1981. A Group of Roman Surgical and Medical Instruments from Corbridge. *Saalburg Jahrbuch* 37: 5-9.
Gladigow, B. 1995. *Anatomia sacra* Religiös motivierte Eingriffe in menschliche oder tierische Körper. In Ph. J. van der Eijk, H. F. J. Horstmannshoff and P. H. Schrijvers (eds). *Ancient Medicine in its Socio-Cultural Context.* Amsterdam and Atlanta: Rodopi Press, pp. 345-61.
Gordon, R. 1995. The Healing Event in Graeco-Roman Folk-Medicine. In Ph. J. van der Eijk, H. F. J. Horstmannshoff and P. H. Schrijvers (eds). *Ancient Medicine in its Socio-cultural Context.* Amsterdam: and Atlanta: Rodopi Press, pp. 363-76.
Gosden, C. 1999. *Anthropology and Archaeology a Changing Relationship.* New York and London: Routledge.
Gostenčnik, K. 1997. Zwei Pinzetten mit Agathangelus-Stempel vom Magdalensberg. *Sonderdruck aus Carinthia* I, 187: 141-68.
Groenman-van Waateringe, W., B. L. van Beek, W. J. H. Willems and S. L. Wynia (eds.) *Roman Frontier Studies 1995.* Oxbow Monograph 91. Oxford: Oxbow Books.
Groller, M. 1906. Bericht des Vereins Carnuntum in Wien für die Jahr 1904 und 1905. *Der römische Limes in Österreich* 7.
Groller, M. V. 1907. Die Grabung in Lager Lauriacum. *Der römische Limes in Österreich* 8: 119-56.
Groller, M. V. 1909. Die Grabungen im Lager Lauriacum. *Der römische Limes in Österreich* 10: 79-114.
Groller, M. V. 1924. Die Grabungen im Lager Lauriacum in Jahre 1914 und 1915. *Der römische Limes in Österreich* 14: 1-54.
Gschwantler, K. and H. von Ubls 1978. *Catalogue in Vindobona - die Römer in Wiener Raum.* Vienna: Historisches Museums der Stadt Wien.
Gummerus, H. 1932. *Der Ärztesstand im römischen Reiche nach dem Inschriften.* Helsinki: Akademische Buchhandlung.
Haalebos, J. K. 1995. *Castra und Canabae Ausgrabungen auf dem Hunerberg in Nijmegen 1987-1994.* Nijmegen: Katholieke Universiteit.
Haberling, W. 1909. Die Militärlazarette im alten Rom. *Deutsche Militärärztliche Zeitschrift* 11 (5 June): 441-67.
Haberling, W. 1910. *Die altrömischen Militärärzte.* Verlag von August Hirschwald: Berlin.
Hanson, W. S, C. M. Daniels, J. N. Dore and J. P. Gillam 1979. The Agricolan Supply Base at Red House, Corbridge. *Archaeologia Aeliana* (series 5), 7: 1.
Hanson, W. S. 1989. The Nature and Function of Roman Frontiers. In J. C. Barrett, A. P. Fitzpatrick and L. Macinnes (eds.) *Barbarians and Romans in North-west Europe from theLater Republic to Late Antiquity.* Oxford: BAR International Series, 471, pp. 55-63.
Harig, G. 1971. Zum Problem „Krankenhaus" in der Antike. *Klio* 53: 179-95.
Hassall, M. 1983. *The Internal Planning of Roman Auxiliary Forts in Rome and her Northern Provinces.* London: Alan Sutton.
Hauff, E. 1993/94. Die Medizinische Versorgung von Carnuntum. *Carnuntum Jahrbuch* 10: 89-196.
Haynes, I. 1999. Military Service and Cultural Identity in the *Auxilia.* In A. Goldsworthy and I. Hayens (eds.) *The Roman Army as a Community.* Portsmouth, Rhode Island: Journal of Roman Archaeology Supplementary Series 34, pp. 165-74.
Healy, J. F. 1978. *Mining and Metallurgy in the Greek and Roman world.* London: Thames and Hudson:.
Henderson, J. 1989. The Hospitals of Late-Medieval and Renaissance Florence: A Preliminary Survey. In L. Granshaw and R. Porter (eds.) *The Hospital in History.* New York and London: Routledge, pp. 63-92.
Herzog, E. 1897. Das Kastelle bei Öhringen. *Der Obergermanisch-Raetische Limes des Roemerreiches.* Heildelberg: Verlag von Otto Petters.
Hill, J. D. 1995. *Ritual and Rubbish in the Iron Age of Wessex.* Oxford: BAR British Series 242.
Hill. J. D. and Jundi, S. 1998. Brooches and identities in first century Britain: More than Meets the Eye? In. Forcey, C., J. Hawthorne and R. Witcher (eds.) *TRAC 97: Proceedings of the Seventh Annual Theoretical Roman Archaeology Conference, Nottingham.* Oxford: Oxbow Books, pp. 125-37.
Hingley, R. 1999. The Imperial Context for

Romano-British Studies and Proposals for a New Understanding of Social Change. In P. Paulo, A. Funari, M. Hall and S. Jones (eds.) *Historical Archaeology Back from the Edge*. New York and London: Routledge, pp. 137-50.

Hodder, I. 1982. *Symbols in Action*. Cambridge: Cambridge University Press.

Hodder, I. 1989. Post-modernism, Post-structuralism and Post-processual Archaeology. In. I. Hodder (ed.) *The Meaning of Things: Material Culture and Symbolic Expression*. London: Harper Collins Academic, pp. 64-78.

Hogg, A. H. A. 1968. Pen Llystyn: a Roman Fort and Other Remains. *Archaeological Journal* 125: 101-92.

Horn, H. G. 1987. *Die Römer in Nordrhein-Westfalen*. Stuttgart: Konrad Theiss Verlag.

Horstmanshoff, H. F. J. 1995. Galen and his Patients. In Ph. J. van der Eijk, H. F. J. Horstmanshoff and P. H. Schrijvers (eds.) *Ancient Medicine in its Socio-cultural Context*. Amsterdam and Atlanta: Rodopi Press, pp. 83-99.

Houdas, Y. 2003. *La Médicine Arabe aux Siècles d'Or VIIIème – VIIème Siecles*. Paris, Budapest and Toranto: L'Harmattan.

Isaac, B. 2004. *The Inverntion of Racism in Classical Antiquity*. Princeton: Princeton University Press.

Jackson, R. 1988. *Doctors and Diseases in the Roman Empire*. University of Oklahoma Press: Norman and London.

Jackson, R. 1990. Roman Doctors and their Instruments: Recent Research into Ancient Practice. *Journal of Roman Archaeology*. 3: 5-27.

Jackson, R. 1993. Roman Medicine: Practitioners and their Practices. *Aufstieg und Niedergang der Romischen Welt* II 37. 1, 79-100.

Jackson, R 1994a. *Styphylagra, Staphylocaustes*, Uvulectomy and Haemorrhoidectomy: The Roman Instruments and Operations. In A. Krug (ed.) *From Epidauros to Salerno: Symposium Held at the European University Centre for Cultural Heritage, Ravello, April 1990*. Rixensart: Pact Belgium, pp. 167-85.

Jackson, R. 1994b. The Surgical Instruments, Appliances and Equipment in Celsus' *De Medicina*. In G. Sabbah and J. Mundry (eds.) *La Médecine de Celse*. Saint-Étienne: Publications de l'Université Saint-Étienne, pp. 167-209.

Jackson, R. 1995. The Composition of Roman Medical Instrumentaria as an Indicator of Medical Practice: a Provisional Assessment. In Ph. J. van der Eijk, H. F. J, Horstmannshoff and P. H. Schrijvers (eds.) *Ancient Medicine in its Socio-cultural Context*. Amsterdam and Atlanta: Rodopi Press, pp. 189-208.

Jackson, R. 1996. Eye Medicine in the Roman Empire. *Aufstieg und Niedergang der romischen Welt*. II. 37. 3. Berlin and New York: Walter de Gruyter, pp. 2,228-51.

Jackson, R. 1997. An Ancient British Medical Kit from Stanway, Essex. *The Lancet* 350 (9089): 1471-3.

Jackson, R. 2002. Roman Surgery: The Evidence of the Instruments. In R. Arnott (ed.) *The Archaeology of Medicine*. Oxford: BAR International Series 1064, pp. 87-94.

Jackson, R. and P. T. Craddock 1998. The Ribchester Hoard: A Descriptive and Technological Study. In B. Raftery, V. Megaw and V. Rigby (eds.) *Sites and Sights of the Iron Age*. Oxford: Oxbow Books, pp. 75-102.

Jacobi, L. 1897. *Das Rômerkastell Saalburg bei Homburg vor der Hôhe*. Homburg vor der Höhe: Selbsteverlagedes Verfussers.

Jacobi, L. 1904. Das Kastell Alteburg-Heftrich. *Der Obergermanisch-Raetische Limes des Roemerreiches*. Heildelberg: Verlag von Otto Petters.

Jacobi, L. and H. Hofmann 1906. Das Kastell Kapersburg. *Der Obergermanisch-Raetische Limes des Roemerreiches*. Heildelberg: Verlag von Otto Petters.

Jacobi, L. 1909. Das Kastell Zugmantel. *Der Obergermanisch-Raetische Limes des Roemerreiches*. Heildelberg: Verlag von Otto Petters.

James, S. 1999. The Community of the Soldiers: A Major Identity and Centre of Power in the Roman Empire. In P. Baker, C. Forcey, S. Jundi and R. Witcher (eds) *TRAC 98: Proceedings of the Eighth Annual Theoretical Roman Archaeology Conference, Leicester 1998*. Oxford: Oxbow Books, pp. 14-25.

James, S. 2002. Writing the Legions: The Development and Future of Roman Military Studies in Britain. *Archaeological Journal* 159: 1-58.

Jarrett, M. J. 1969. *The Roman Frontier in Wales* (2nd edition). Cardiff: University of Wales Press.

Jettner, D. 1966. Geschichte des Hospitals. *Sudhoffs Archive für Geschichte der Medizin und der Naturwissenschaften* 11. Wiesbaden: Franz Steiner Verlag GMBh.

Johnson, A. 1983. *Roman Forts*. London: Adam and Charles Black.

Johnson, M. 1999. *Archaeological Theory: An*

Introduction. Oxford: Blackwell Publishers.
Jones, B. W. 1973. The Dating of Domitian's War against the Chatti. *Historia* 22: 79-90.
Jones, S. 1997. *The Archaeology of Ethnicity*. London and New York: Routledge.
Kent, S. 1990. Activity Areas and Architecture: An Interdisciplinary View of the Relationship between Use of Space and Domestic Built Environment. In S. Kent (ed.) *Domestic Architecture and the Use of Space: An Interdisciplinary Cross-Cultural Study*. Cambridge: Cambridge University Press, pp. 1-8.
Khan, A. H. 1983. Early Hospitals in Muslim World. *Studies in History of Medicine* 7 (3-4): 196-208.
King, A. 1990. *Roman Gaul and Germany*. London: British Museum Press.
King, H. 1991. Using the Past: Nursing and the Medical Profession in Ancient Greece. In P. Holden and J. Littlewood (eds.) *Anthropology and Nursing*. New York and London: Routledge, pp. 7-24.
Kleinman, A. 1980. *Patients and Healers in the Context of Culture*. Berkeley: University of California Press.
Knorzer, K. H. 1963. Römerzeitliche Heilkräuter aus Novaesium. *Sudhoffs Archiv für Geschichte der Medizin und Naturwissenschaften* 47: 311-16.
Koenen, C. 1904. Beschreibung von Novaesium. *Bonner Jahrbucher* 111/112: 97-242.
Kofler, F. 1897. Das Kastell Langenhain. *Der Obergermanisch-Raetische Limes des Roemerreiches*. Heildelberg: Verlag von Otto Petters.
Kofler, F. and J. Jacobi 1903. Das Kastell Okarben. *Der Obergermanisch-Raetische Limes des Roemerreiches*. Heildelberg: Verlag von Otto Petters.
Kohl, W., A. D. Popp and J. Jacobs 1901. Das Kastell Dambach. *Der Obergermanisch-Raetische Limes des Roemerreiches*. Heildelberg: Verlag von Otto Petters.
Kohl, W. J. Tröltsch, J. Jacobs, W. Barthel and E. Fabricius 1906. Das Kastell Weissenburg. *DerObergermanisch-Raetische Limes des Roemerreiches*. Heidelberg: Verlag von Otto Petters.
Korbuly, G. 1934. *Die ärztlichen Denkmäler von Aquincum*. Budapest: Dissertationes Pannonia I, 3.
Krausse, D. 1999. Romanization in the Middle Rhine and Moselle Region: New Evidence from Recent Excavations in Luxembourg, Rhineland-Pfalz and Saarland. In J. D. Creighton and R. Wilson (eds.) *Roman Germany Studies in Cultural Interaction*. Portsmouth, Rhode Island: Journal of Roman Archaeology Supplementary Series, no. 32, pp. 54-70.
Krug, A. 1984. *Heilkunst und Heilkult: Medizin in der Antike*. Munich: Verlag C. H. Beck.
Künzl, E. 1979/81. Medizinische Instrumente aus dem römischen Altertum in Städtischen Museum Worms. *Der Wormsgau* 13: 49-63.
Künzl, E. 1982. Römische Medizin im Spiegel archäologischer Funde. *Archäologie in Deutschland* 1 (Jan-März) 14.
Künzl, E. 1983. *Medizinische Instrumente aus Sepulkralfunden der römischen Kaiserzeit*. Cologne: Rheinland Verlag GmbH.
Künzl, E. 1984. Einige Bemerkungen zu den Herstellern der romischen medizinischen Instrumente. *Alba Regia* 21: 59-65.
Künzl, E. 1984/85. Der Schropfkopf vom Limeskastell Zugmantel. *Saalburg Jahrbuch* 40/41: 30-33.
Künzl, E. 1986a. Archaeology and the History of Medicine: Basic Questions of Methodology. *Proceedings of the Third Congress of the European Association of Museums of the history of medicine*, pp. 27-34.
Künzl, E. 1986b. Operationsräume in römischen Thermen. *Bonner Jahrbücher* 186: 491-509.
Künzl, E. 1989/90. Römisches Thermen als Spitäler. *Römisches Österreich* 17/18: 147-52.
Künzl, E. 1991. Die medizinische Versorgung der römischen Armee zur Zeit des Kaisers Augustus und die Reaktion der Römer auf die Situation bei den Kelten und Germanen. In B. Trier (ed.) *Die römische Okkupation nordlich der Alpen zur Zeit des Augustus*. Münster: Aschendorff Verlagsbuchhandlung, pp. 185-202.
Künzl, E. 1996. Forschungsbericht zu den antiken medizinischen Instrumenten. *Aufstieg und Niedergang der romischen Welt* II, 37. 3: 2433-639.
Künzl, E. 2002. *Medizin in der Antike: aus einer Welt ohne Narkose und Aspirin*. Stuttgart: Konrad Theiss Verlag GmBh.
Kuzsinszky, V. 1934. *Aquincum: Ausgrabungen und Funde*. Budapest: Herausgegeben von der Haupstadt.
Landy, D. 1977. Role Adaptation: Traditional Curers under the Impact of Western Medicine. In D. Landy (ed.) *Culture, Disease and Healing: Studies in Medical Anthropology*. New York: Macmillan Publishing Co., pp. 468-81.
Langeveld, A. P. M. 1989. The Development of the Military Hospitals in the Netherlands' Army Medical Service. In Y. Kawakita, S. Sakaig and Y. Otuska (eds.) *History of*

Hospitals the Evolution of Health Care Facilities. Proceedings of the 11th International Symposium on the Comparative History of Medicine East and West 1986. Japan: The Taniguchi Foundation, pp. 89-126.

Lawrence, A. E. 1972. *Greek and Roman Sculpture*. London: Jonathon Cape.

Lee, E. J. 1862. *Isca Silurum or an Illustrated Catalogue of the Museum of Antiquities at Caerleon*. London: Longman, Green, Longmans and Roberts.

Lehner, H. 1904. Die Einzelfunden von Novaesium. *Bonner Jahrbucher* 111/112: 243-418.

Lehner, H. 1929. Ausgrabung in Vetera 1928. *Germania* 13: 126-32.

Lehner, H. 1930. Die Ausgrabung von Vetera bei Xanten. In G. Rodenwaldt (ed.) *Neue Deutsche Ausgrabungen*. Münster: Aschendorffsche Verlagsbuchhandlung, pp. 177-89.

Lévi-Strauss, C 1963. *Structural Anthropology*. Garden City, NY: Doubleday.

Lévi-Strauss, C. 1969. *The Raw and the Cooked: Introduction to a Science of Mythology*. New York: Harper and Row.

Lindenschmitt, L. 1889. *Das Römisch-Germanische Central-Museum in Bildlichen Darstellung aus Seinen Sammlungen*. Mainz: Verlag von Victor Zabern.

Lloyd, G. E. R. 1983. *Science Folklore and Ideology*. Cambridge: Cambridge University Press.

Longfield-Jones, G. M. 1986. A Graeco-Roman Speculum in the Wellcome Museum. *Medical History* 30: 81-9.

Longrigg, J. 1993. *Greek Rational Medicine: Philosophy and Medicine from Alcmaeon to the Alexandrians*. London and New York: Routledge.

Longrigg, J. 1998. *Greek Medicine from the Heroic to the Hellenistic Age: A Sourcebook*. London: Duckworth.

Lorgar, F. 1919. Vorläufiger über Ausgrabungen nächst. Lotschitz bei Cilli. *Jahreshefte des Österreich Archäologischen Institutes* 19-20: 107-34.

Lupton, D. 1994. *Medicine as Culture*. London: Sage.

Luttrell, A. 1994. The Hospitaler's Medical Tradition. In M. Barber (ed.) *The Military Orders Fighting for the Faith and Caring for the Sick*. Hampshire: Variorum, pp. 64-78.

MacMahon, A. 2003. The Realm of Janus: Doorways in the Roman World. In G. Carr, E. Swift and J. Weekes (eds.) *TRAC 2002: Proceedings of the Twelfth Annual Theoretical Roman Archaeology Conference, Canterbury 2002*. Oxford: Oxbow books, pp. 58-73.

Majno, G. 1975. *The Healing Hand*. Cambridge, MA and London: Harvard University Press.

Mann, J. C. 1974. The Frontiers of the Principate. *Aufstieg und Niedergang der romischen Welt, II, Principate (i)*, pp. 508-33.

Manning, W. 1997. Ptolemy and the pre-Flavian sites of Britain. In W. Groenman-van Waateringe, B. L. van Beek, W. J. H. Willems and S. L. Wynia (eds.) *Roman Frontier Studies 1995*. Oxbow Monograph 91. Oxford: Oxbow Books, pp. 33-40.

Mason, D. 2000. Chester the Elliptical Building. *Current Archaeology* 167: 404-16.

Matthäus, H. 1989. *Der Arzt in römischer Zeit*. Aalen: Limesmuseum.

Matthews, K. 1994. An Archaeology of Homosexuality? Perspectives from the Classical World. In S. Cottam, D. Dungworth, S. Scott, and J. Taylor (eds.) *TRAC 94: Proceedings of the Fourth Annual Theoretical Roman Archaeology Conference, Durham 1994*. Oxford: Oxbow Books, pp. 118-32.

Maxfield, V. A. 2002 (3rd Edition). Mainland Europe. In J. Wacher (ed.) *The Roman Empire*. London: Routledge. pp. 139-97.

McCarthy, M. R. 1990. *The Roman, Anglican and Medieval Site At Blackfriers Street*. Carlisle: Cumberland and Westmorland Antiquarian and Archaeological Society Research Series 4.

Meadows, K, C. Lemke J. and Heron (eds.) 1997. *TRAC 96: Proceedings of the Sixth annual Theoretical Roman Archaeology Conference, Sheffield 1996*. Oxford: Oxbow Books.

Mettler, A. and W, Barthel 1907. Das Kastell Köngen. *Der Obergermanisch-Raetische Limes des Roemerreiches*. Heildelberg: Verlag von Otto Petters.

Mettler, A. and F. Drexel 1909. Das Kastell Mainhardt. *Der ObergermanischRaetische Limes des Roemerreiches*. Heildelberg: Verlag von Otto Petters.

Meyer-Steineg, Th. 1921. *Geschichte der Medizin im Überblick mit Abbildungen*. Jena: Verlag von Gustav Fischer.

Millar, F. 1967. *The Roman Empire and its Neighbours*. London: Duckworth.

Miller, D. 1994. Artefacts and the Meaning of Things. In T. Ingold (ed.) *Companion Encyclopaedia of Anthropology*. New York and London: Routledge, pp. 396-419.

Miller, T. 1985. *The Birth of the Hospital in the Byzantine Empire.* Baltimore and London: The Johns Hopkins University Press.

Millett, M. 1990. *The Romanisation of Britain an Essay on Archaeological Interpretaion.* Cambridge: Cambridge University Press.

Milne, J. 1907. *Surgical Instruments in Greek and Roman Times.* Oxford: Clarendon Press.

Mócsy, A. 1974. *Pannonia and Upper Moesia.* London and Boston: Routledge and Kegan Paul.

Moore, H. L. 1982. The Interpretation of Spatial Patterning in Settlement Residues. In I. Hodder (ed.) *Symbolic and Structural Archaeology.* Cambridge: Cambridge University Press, pp. 74-9.

Moore, H. L. 1999a. Anthropology at the Turn of the Century. In H. L. Moore (ed.) *Anthropological Theory Today.* Cambridge: Polity Press, pp. 1-23.

Moore, H. L. 1999b. Whatever Happened to Women and Men? Gender and Other Crises in Anthropology. In H. L. Moore (ed.) *Anthropological Theory Today.* Cambridge: Polity Press, pp. 151-171.

Morford, M. and R. Lenardon 1985. *Classical Mythology.* New York and London: Longman.

Morley, P. 1978. Culture and the Cognitive World of Traditional Medical Beliefs: Some Preliminary Considerations. In P. Morley and R. Wallis (eds.) *Culture and Curing: Anthropological Perspectives on Traditional Medical Beliefs and Practices.* London: Peter Owen.

Morsy, S. A. 1993. *Gender, Sickness and Healing in Rural Egypt: Ethnography in Historical Context.* Boulder: Westview press.

Murray-Threipland, L. 1969. The Hall Caerleon Excavations on the Site of the Legionary Hospital. *Archaeologia Cambriensis* 118: 86-123.

Nágy, L. 1942. *Budapest az Ókorban.* (With a German Summary). Budapest: Története.

Nash-Williams, V. E. 1932. The Roman Legionary Fortress at Caerleon in Monmouthshire: Report on the Excavations Carried out at Prysg Field 1927-9, Part II: The Finds. *Archaeologia Cambriensis* 87: 48-104.

Navarro, J. M. de 1955. A Doctor's Grave of the Middle La Tène Period from Bavaria. *Proceedings of the Prehistoric Society.* 21: 231-49.

Németh, M. 1994. Roman Military Camps in Aquincum. In Gábor Hajnóczi (ed) *La Pannonia e l' Impero Romano Accedemia d' Ungheria e l' Istituto Austriaco di Cultura (Roma 13-16 gennaio).* Rome: Annuario Dell' Accademia d' Ungheria in Roma, 139-52.

Neumann, A. 1965. Spital und Bad des Legionslagers Vindobona. *Jahrbuch des Römisch-Germanischen Zentral Museums, Mainz* 12: 99-117.

Neumann, A. 1967. *Forschungen in Vindobona 1948 bis 1967. I Teil Lager und Lagerterritorium.* Vienna: Der römische Limes in Österreich 23.

Neumann, A. 1980. *Vindobona.* Vienna: Hermann Böhhlaus Nachf.

Nijhuis, K. 1995. Greek Doctors and Roman Patients: a Medical Anthropological Approach. In Ph. J. van der Eijk, H. F. J. Horstmannshoff and P. H. Schrijvers (eds). *Ancient Medicine in its Socio-cultural Context.* Amsterdam and Atlanta: Rodopi Press, pp. 49-66.

Nutton, V. 1969. Medicine and the Roman Army: A Further Reconsideration. *Medical History* 13: 260-70.

Nutton, V. 1970. A Greek Doctor at Chester. *Journal of Chester Archaeological Society* 55: 7-13.

Nutton, V. 1995a. Medicine in Medieval Western Europe. In L. Conrad, M. Neve, V. Nutton, R. Porter and A. Wear (eds.) *The Western Medical Tradition.* Cambridge: Cambridge University Press, pp. 139-206.

Nutton, V. 1995b. Roman Medicine, 250 BC to AD 200. In L. I. Conrad, M. Neve, V. Nutton, R. Porter and A. Wear (eds.) *The Western Medical Tradition.* Cambridge: Cambridge University Press, pp. 39-70.

Nutton, V. 1995c. Medicine in Late Antiquity and the Early Middle Ages. In L. I. Conrad, M. Neve, V. Nutton, R. Porter and A. Wear (eds.) *The Western Medical Tradition.* Cambridge: Cambridge University Press, pp. 71-88.

Nutton, V. 2004. *Ancient Medicine.* London and New York: Routledge.

Obermedizinalrat, E. and W. Barthel 1907. Das Kastell Gnotzheim. *Der Obergermanisch-Raetische Limes des Roemerreiches.* Heildelberg: Verlag von Otto Petters.

Oelmann, F. 1931. Ausgrabung in 1930. *Germania* 15: 221-29.

Okun, M. 1989. *The Early Roman Frontier in the Upper Rhine Area.* Oxford: British Archaeological Reports International Series 547.

Ottaway, P. Recent Excavations of the Late Roman Signal Station at Filey, North Yorkshire. In W. Groenman-van Waateringe, B. L. van Beek., W. J. H. Willems and S. L. Wynia (eds.). *Roman*

Frontier Studies 1995. Oxbow Monograph 91. Oxford: Oxbow Books, pp. 135-42.
Pallat, L. 1904. Das Kastell Holzhausen. *Der Obergermanisch-Raetische Limes des Roemerreiches*. Heildelberg: Verlag von Otto Petters.
Parker-Pearson, M. 1999. *The Archaeology of Death and Burial*. Somerset: Sutton Publishing.
Penn, R. G. 1964. Medical Service in the Roman Army. *Journal of the Royal Army Medical Corps* 110: 253-58.
Pitts, L. and J. K. St. Joseph 1985. *Inchtuthil, The Roman Legionary Fortress. Britannia Monograph Series no.* 6. London: The Society for the Promotion of Roman Studies.
Pollitt, J. J. 1972. *Art and Experience in Classical Greece*. Cambridge: Cambridge University Press.
Prescher, F. and J. Jacobs 1900. Das Kastell Heidenheim. *Der Obergermanisch-Raetische Limes des Roemerreiches*. Heildelberg: Verlag von Otto Petters.
Press, L. 1988. Valetudinarium at Novae and Other Roman Danubian Hospitals. *Archeologia* 39: 69-89.
Radnóti, A. 1957. *Intercisa II (Dunapentelle) Geschichte der Stadt in der Römerzeit*. Budapest: Akadémiai Kiadó.
Ramage, N. H. and A. Ramage 2000. *Roman Art* (3rd Edition). London: Laurence King.
Rapaport, A. 1990. Systems of Activities and Systems of Settings. In S. Kent (ed.) *Domestic Architecture and the Use of Space: An Interdisciplinary Cross-Cultural Study*. Cambridge: Cambridge University Press, pp. 9-20.
Raven, S. 1993. *Rome in Africa*. New York and London: Routledge.
RCHME 1959. *City of Cambridge*. London: HMSO.
Revellio, P. 1937. Das Kastell Hüfingen. *Der Obergermanisch-Raetische Limes des Roemerreiches*. Berlin and Leipzig: Verlag von Otto Petters.
Richmond, I. A. 1952. The Roman Army Medical Service. *University Medical Gazette* June 1952: 2-7.
Richmond, I. A. 1968. *Hod Hill vol 2, Excavations Carried out Between 1951 and 1958*. London: The Trustees of the British Museum.
Richmond, I. A. and J. McIntyre 1938-39. The Agricolan Fort at Fendoch. *Proceedings of the Society of Antiquaries of Scotland* 73: 110-54.
Rickman, G. 1971. *Roman Granaries and Storebuildings*. Cambridge: Cambridge University Press.
Riha, E. 1986. Römische *Toilettgerät und Medizinische Instrumente aus Augst und Kaiser Augst*. Augst: Forschungen in Augst 6.
Ritterling, E. 1909. Das Kastell Wiesbaden. *Der Obergermanisch-Raetische Limes des Roemerreiches*. Heildelberg: Verlag von Otto Petters.
Rowland, R. 1977. Some New *Medici* in the Roman Empire. *Epigraphica* 39 (1-2): 174-79.
Roxan, M. 1997. Settlement of Veterans of the Auxilia - A Preliminary Study. In W. Groenman-van Waateringe, B. L. van Beek, W. J. H. Willems S. L. and Wynia (eds.) *Roman Frontier Studies 1995*. Oxbow Monograph 91. Oxford: Oxbow Books, pp. 483-92.
Saddington, D. B. 1997. The 'Politics' of the Auxilia and the Forging of Auxiliary Regimental Identity. In W. Groenman-van Waateringe, B. L. van Beek, W. J. H. Willems S. L. and Wynia (eds.) *Roman Frontier Studies 1995*. Oxbow Monograph 91. Oxford: Oxbow Books, pp. 493-96.
Sahlins, M. 1985. *Islands of History*. Chicago: Chicago University Press.
Salazar, C. 2000. *The Treatment of War Wounds in Graeco-Roman Antiquity*. Leiden: Brill.
Sayili, A. 1980. The Emergence of the Prototype of the Modern Hospital in Medieval Islam. *Studies in History of Medicine* 4: 112-18.
Scarborough, J. 1968. Roman Medicine and the Legions: A Reconsideration. *Medical History* 12: 254-61.
Scarborough. J. 1976. *Roman Medicine*. Ithaca: Cornell University Press.
Scheller, M. and F. Drexel 1911. Das Kastell Faimingen. *Der Obergermanisch-Raetische Limes des Roemerreiches*. Heildelberg: Verlag von Otto Petters.
Schiffer, M. B. 1987. *Formation Processes of the Archaeological Record*. Alberquerque: University of New Mexico Press.
Schönberger, H. 1952. *The Roman Camp at the Saalburg*. Bad Homburg: C. Zeuner & Co.
Schönberger, H. 1969. The Roman Frontier in Germany: An Archaeological Survey. *Journal of Roman Studies* 59: 144-97.
Schönberger, H. 1972. *Kastell Oberstimm: Die Grabung von 1968 bis 1971*. Gebr. Mann Verlag: Berlin.
Schönberger, H. 1975. Kastell Künzing-Quintana die Grabungen von 1958 bis 1966. *Limesforschungen* 13. Berlin: Gebr. Mann Verlag.
Schönberger, H. 1979. Praetorium oder Fabrica. *Germania* 57: 135-41.

Schumacher, K. 1898. Das Kastelle bei Neckarburken. *Der Obergermanisch-Raetische Limes des Roemerreiches.* Heildelberg: Verlag von Otto Petters.
Schumacher, K. 1900. Das Kastell Wimpfen. *Der Obergermanisch-Raetische Limes des Roemerreiches.* Heildelberg: Verlag von Otto Petters.
Schultze, R. 1934. Die römischen Legionslazarette in Vetera und anderen Legionslagern. *Bonner Jahrbücher.* 139: 54-63.
Scott, E. 1991. Animal and Infant Burials in Romano-British Villas: A Revitalization Monument. In P. Garwood, D. Jennings, R. Skeates and J. Toms (eds.) *Sacred and Profane: Proceedings of a Conference in Archaeology, Ritual and Religion.* Oxford: Oxford University Committee for Archaeology monograph 32, pp. 115-21.
Scott, E. 1997. Introduction: on the Incompleteness of Archaeological Narratives. In J. Moore and E. Scott (eds.) *Invisible People and Processes.* Leicester: Leicester University Press, pp. 1-12.
Scullard, H. H. 1979. *Roman Britain: Outpost of the Empire.* London: Thames and Hudson.
Shanks, M. and Tilley, C. 1987. *Social Theory and Archaeology.* Cambridge: Polity Press.
Shanks, M. 1996. *Classical Archaeology of Greece: Experiences of the Discipline.* New York and London: Routledge.
Shanks, M. 1999. *Art and the Early Greek State: An Interpretive Archaeology.* Cambridge: Cambridge University Press.
Shennan, S. 1996. Cultural Transmission and Cultural Change. In R. W. Preucel and I. Hodder (eds.) *Contemporary Archaeology in Theory.* Oxford: Blackwell Publishers, pp. 282-96.
Siller, W. 1996. The Dead and the Drying: Techniques for Transforming People and Things in the Andes. *Journal of Material Culture* 1 (November): 259-90.
Simonett, C. 1937. Grabung Gesellschaft Pro Vindonissa in den Jahren 1935 und 1936 auf der Breite. *Anzeiger für Schweiz Altertums Kunde* 39: 201-17.
Simpson, F. G. and I. A. Richmond 1941. The Roman Fort on Hadrian's Wall at Benwell. *Archaeologia Aeliana* (series 4) 19: 1-43.
Simpson, J. Y. 1856. *Was the Roman Army Provided with Medical Officers?* Sutherland and Knox: Edinburgh.
Small, D. B. 1999. The Tyranny of the Text: Lost Social Strategies in Current Historical Period Archaeology in the Classical Mediterranean. In P. Paulo, A. Funari, M. Hall and S. Jones (eds.) *Historical Archaeology Back from the Edge.* New York and London: Routledge, pp. 122-36.
Sobel, H. 1991. Römische Arzneikästchen. *Saalburg Jahrbucher* 46: 121-47.
Sommer, C. S. 1999. From Conquered Territory to Roman Province: Recent Discoveries and Debate on the Roman Occupation of SW Germany. In J. D. Creighton and R. Wilson (eds.) *Roman Germany Studies in Cultural Interaction.* Portsmouth, Rhode Island: Journal of Roman Archaeology Supplementary Series, no. 32, pp. 160-98.
Stather, H. 1997. Zur Frage eines spätromischen Kastells in Konstanz und einer Burgi-Kette entlang des sudlichen Bodensees. In W. Groenman-van Waateringe, B. L. van Beek, W. J. H. Willems and S. L. Wynia (eds.) *Roman Frontier Studies 1995.* Oxbow Monograph 91. Oxford: Oxbow Books, pp. 159-64.
Stieren, A. 1928. Die neuen Grabungen in Haltern. *Germania* 12: 70-6.
Stieren, A. 1930. Die römischen Lager bei Haltern. In G. Rodenwaldt (ed.) *Neue Deutsche Ausgrabungen.* Munster:Aschendorffsche Verlagsbuchhandlung, pp. 170-98.
Swoboda, E. 1937. Lauriacum: Grabungen in Enns im Jahre 1936. *Jahreshefte des Österreichischen Archäologischen Institutes in Wien* 30: 252-307.
Swoboda, J. 1967. Wallheim. *Fundberichte aus Schwaben* 18 (2): 111-13.
Szirmai, K. 1997. Excavations on the Military *Vicus* of Budapest/Albertfalva 1994. In W. Groenman-van Waateringe, B. L. van Beek, W. J. H. Willems and S. L. Wynia (eds.) *Roman Frontier Studies 1995.* Oxbow Monograph 91. Oxford: Oxbow Books, pp. 527-30.
Tabanelli, M. 1958. *Lo Strumento Chirurgico e la Sua Storia.* Milan: University of Milan.
Thomas, J. C. 1990. Some other Analogy. In F. Baker and J. Thomas (eds.) *Writing in the Past.* Lampeter: St. David's University Press, pp. 18-24.
Thomas, J. 1991. Reading the Body: Beaker Funerary Practice in Britain. In P. Garwood, D. Jennings, R. Skeates and J. Toms (eds.) *Sacred and Profane: Proceedings of a Conference in Archaeology, Ritual and Religion.* Oxford: Oxford University Committee for Archaeology monograph 32, pp.33-42.
Topping, 1988. Early Cultivation in Northumberland and the Borders. *Proceedings of the Prehistoric Society* 55: 161-80.
Turner, F. J. 1893. The Significance of the Frontier in American History. *Annual report of the*

American Historical Association. 199-207.
Turner, V. W. 1974. *The Ritual Process.* Middlesex: Penguin Books.
Ulbert, G. 1959. *Die römischen Donau-Kastelle Aislingen und Burghöfe.* Berlin: Verlag Gebr. Mann.
Ulbert, G. 1970. *Das römische Donau-Kastell Risstissen Teil I. Die Funde aus Metall, Horn und Knochen.* Stuttgart: Verlag Müller and Graff Kommissionsverlag.
Unz, C. and E. Deschler-Erb 1997. *Katalog der Militaria aus Vindonissa: Militärische Funde, Pferdegeschirr und Jochteile bis 1976.* Brugg: Veröffentlichungen der Gesellschaft pro Vindonissa.
van der Veen, M. 1992. *Crop Husbandry Regimes: An Archaeological Study of Farming in Northern England 1000 BC-AD 500.* Sheffield Archaeological Monograph, 3. Sheffield: Sheffield Academic Press.
van Driel-Murray, C. and M. Gechter 1984. Funde aus der Fabrica der legio I Minerva am Bonner Berg. *Beiträge zur Archäologie des Romischen Rheinlands* 4. Cologne: Rheinland-Verlag GMBh.
van Driel-Murray, C. 1999. And did those Feet in Ancient Times...Feet and Shoes as a Material Projection of the Self. In P. Baker, C. Forcey, S. Jundi. and R. Witcher (eds.) *TRAC 98: Proceedings of the Eighth Annual Theoretical Roman Archaeology Conference, Leicester 1998.* Oxford: Oxbow Books, pp 131-40.
van Enckevort, H. and W. J. H. Willems 1994. Roman Cavalry Helmets in Ritual Hoards from the Kops Plateau at Nijmegen, The Netherlands. *Journal of Roman Military Equipment Studies* 5: 125-37.
Vermeulen, W. G. J. R. 1932. *Een Romeinsch Grafveld op den Hunnerberg Te Nijmegen.* Amsterdam: H. J. Paris.
Visy, Z. 1988. *Der Pannonische Limes in Ungarn.* Stuttgart: Konrad Theiss Verlag.
von Elbe, J. 1974. *Roman Germany: A Guide to the Sites.* Mainz: Verlag Philipp von Zabern.
von Petrikovitz, H. 1975. *Die Innenbauten römischer Legionslager während der Prinzipatzeit.* Berlin: Westdeutscher Verlag.
von Schnurbein, S. 1974. *Die römischen Militäranlagen bei Haltern.* Münster: Aschendorf.
von Uslar, R. 1934. Die germanische Keramik in den Kastellen Zugmantel und Saalburg. *Saalburg Jahrbuch* 8: 61-96.
von Uslar, R. 1980. Germanische Keramik aus Steinkastell und vicus in Heddernheim und aus dem Osthafen in Frankfurt: Zur Entstehung der rhein-wesergermanischen Keramik. *Fundberichte aus Hessen* 19/20: 697-724.
Walke, N. 1965. Das römischen Donaukastell Straubing-Sorviodurum. *Limes Forschungen 3.* Berlin: Verlag Gebr. Mann.
Watermann, R. A. 1970. *Ärztliche Instrumente aus Novaesium.* Cologne: Clemens-Sels Museum.
Watermann, R. A. 1974. Von römischer medizin der Rheinlande. *Materia Medica Nordmark* 26 (11/12): 343-363.
Watermann, R. A. 1978. *Valetudinarium das römische Legionskrankenhaus.* Neuss: Clemens-Sels-Museum.
Watermann, R. A, 1980. *Mensch und Medizin Zwischen Macht und Militär der römischen Kaiserzeit.* Frankfurt am Main: Gerhard Michter Verlag.
Watson, G. R. 1969. *The Roman Soldier.* Ithaca: Cornell University Press.
Webster, G. 1981 (2nd edition). *The Roman Imperial Army.* 2nd Edition. London: Adam and Charles Black
Webster, J. 1994. The Just War: Greco-Roman Texts as Colonial Discourse. In S. Cottam, D. Dungworth, S. Scott and J. Taylor (eds.) *TRAC 94: Proceedings of the Fourth Annual Theoretical Roman Archaeology Conference, Durham 1994.* Oxford: Oxbow Books, pp. 1-10.
Webster, J. 1999. Here be Dragons! The Continuing Influence of Roman Attitudes Towards Northern Britain. In B. Bevan (ed.) *Northern Exposure: Interpretative Devolution and the Iron Ages in Britain.* Leicester Archaeology Monograph No. 4. Leicester: School of Archaeological Studies, pp. 21-32.
Wells, C. 1972. *The German Policy of Augustus.* Oxford: Clarendon Press.
Wells, P. S. 1995. Identities, material culture, and change: 'Celts' and 'Germans' in Late-Iron-Age Europe. *Journal of European Archaeology* 3 (2): 169-85.
Wells, P. S. 1999. *The Barbarians Speak: How the Conquered Peoples Shaped Roman Europe.* Princeton: Princeton University Press.
Wheeler, R. E. M. 1928. The Roman Amphitheatre at Caerleon, Monmouthshire. *Archaeologia* 78: 111-28.
Whittaker, C. R. 1994. *Frontiers of the Roman Empire: A Social and Economic Study.* Baltimore and London: The Johns Hopkins University Press.
Whittle, A., J. Pollard and C. Grigson 1999. *The Harmony of Symbols: the Windmill Hill*

Causewayed Enclosure. Oxford: Oxbow Books.
Wigg, D. G. 1999. The Development of the Monetary Economy in N. Gaul in the Late La Tène and Early Roman Periods. In J. D. Creighton and R. Wilson (eds.) *Roman Germany Studies in Cultural Interaction*. Portsmouth, Rhode Island: Journal of Roman Archaeology Supplementary Series, no. 32, pp. 99-124.
Wilmanns, J. C. 1995a. Der Arzt in der römischen Armee der frühen und hohen Kaiserzeit. In Ph. J. van der Eijk, H. F. J. Horstmannshoff and P. H. Schrijvers (eds). *Ancient Medicine in its Socio-cultural Context*. Amsterdam and Atlanta: Rodopi Press, pp. 171-88.
Wilmanns, J. C. 1995b. *Der Sanitätsdienst im römischen Reich*. Medizin der Antike (2). Hildesheim, Zürich and New York: Olms Weidmann.
Wilmott, C. T. and L. Hird 1997. *Birdoswald: Excavation of a Roman Fort on Hadrian's Wall and its Successor Settlements 1987-92*. Archaeological Report 14. London: English Heritage.
Wilmott, C. T. 1997. A New Building Type in an Auxiliary Fort: the Biroswald Basilica and its Discovery. In W. Groenman-van Waateringe, B. L. van Beek, W. J. H. Willems and S. L. Wynia (eds.) *Roman Frontier Studies 1995*. Oxbow Monograph 91. Oxford: Oxbow Books, pp. 581-86.
Wilson, D. R. 1965. Roman Britain in 1964 (Caerleon). *Journal of Roman Studies* 55: 199.
Wilson, D. R. 1971. Roman Britain in 1970, Sites Explored. *Britannia* 2: 243-88.
Wilson, D. R. 1972. Roman Britain in 1971, Sites Explored. *Britannia* 4: 298-351.
Wilson, R. 1997. Behind the Frontier: Romans and Natives in the Military Zone of Northern England. Case Study- North East Yorkshire. In W. Groenman-van Waateringe, B. L. van Beek, W. J. H. Willems and S. L. Wynia (eds.) *Roman Frontier Studies 1995*. Oxbow Monograph 91. Oxford: Oxbow Books, pp. 587-94.
Winkelmann, F. and J. Jacobs 1901. Das Kastell Pfünz. *Der Obergermanisch-Raetische Limes des Roemerreiches*. Heildelberg: Verlag von Otto Petters.
Wolff, G. 1897. Das Kastell Hofheim und die anderen Befestigungen daselbst. *Der Obergermanisch-Raetische Limes des Roemerreiches*. Heildelberg: Verlag von Otto Petters.
Woolf, G. 1902. Das Kastell Okarben. *Der Obergermanisch-Raetische Limes des Roemerreiches*. Heildelberg: Verlag von Otto Petters.
Woolf, G. and J. Jacobi 1903. Das Kastell Gross-Krotzenburg. *Der Obergermanisch-Raetische Limes des Roemerreiches*. Heildelberg: Verlag von Otto Petters.
Woolf, G. 1998. *Becoming Roman the Origins of Provincial Civilisation in Gaul*. Cambridge: Cambridge University Press.
Wright, R. P. 1969. Roman Britain in 1968. Inscriptions. *Journal of Roman Studies* 59, 198-246.
Zanier, W. 1992. Das römische Kastell Ellingen. *Limesforschungen 23*. Mainz: Verlag Philipp von Zabern.
Zienkiewicz, J. D. Forthcoming Report on Caerleon 29.
Zienkiewicz, J. D. Forthcoming Report on Caerleon 39.
Zienkiewicz, J. D. 1986. *The Legionary Fortress Baths at Caerleon II: The Finds*. Cardiff: Cadw, Welsh Historical Monuments.
Zsidi, P. 1995. *Gods, Soldiers and Citizens in Aquincum*. Budapest: Pro Aquinco Foundation.
http://www.fortlock.com
http://horshoecc.com

www.ingramcontent.com/pod-product-compliance
Ingram Content Group UK Ltd.
Pitfield, Milton Keynes, MK11 3LW, UK
UKHW061848041026
15591UKWH00015B/962

9 781841 713786